FOOD AND YOUR FUTURE

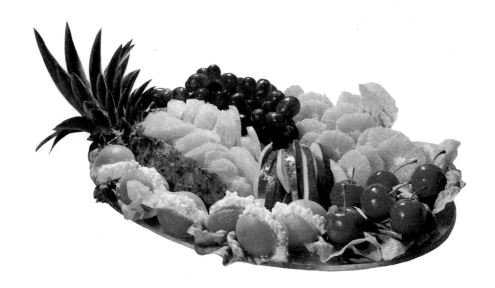

RELATED PRENTICE-HALL BOOKS

EXPLORING HOMEMAKING AND PERSONAL LIVING *Henrietta Fleck and Louise Fernandez*
PERSONAL ADJUSTMENT, MARRIAGE, AND FAMILY LIVING *Judson T. Landis and Mary G. Landis*
UNDERSTANDING AND GUIDING YOUNG CHILDREN *Katherine Read Baker and Xenia F. Fane*
YOU AND YOUR FOOD *Ruth Bennett White*

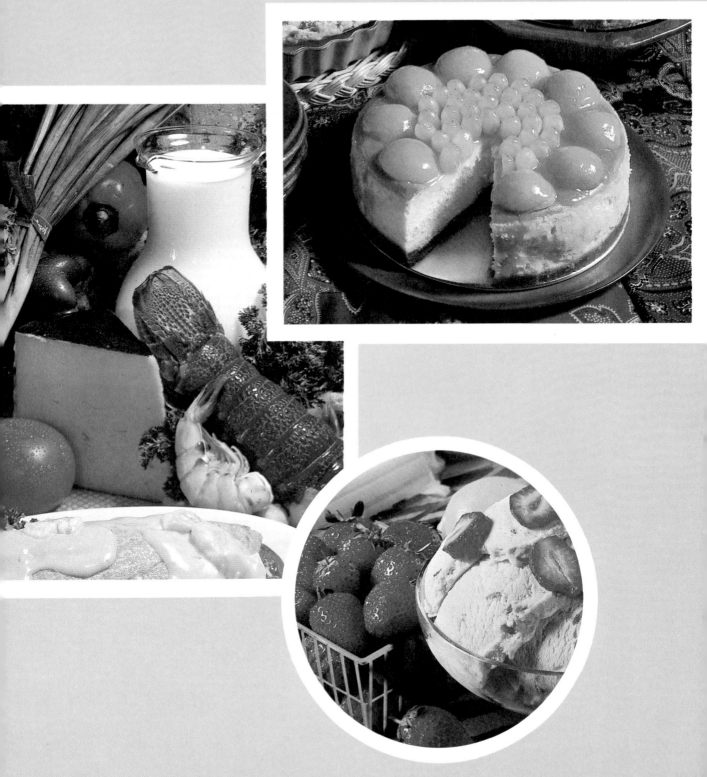

PRENTICE-HALL, INC.   ENGLEWOOD CLIFFS, NEW JERSEY

Ruth Bennett White

FOOD
and your future

Second edition

CONSULTANTS

BARBARA BRADSTREET
Gloucester High School, Gloucester, Massachusetts

JUDY HATH
Orange County Department of Education, Santa Ana, California

MATTIE JACKSON
Jefferson Township High School, Dayton, Ohio

TEDDY POPE
Houston Independent School District, Houston, Texas

BETTY H. TRUSSELL
Denver Public Schools, Denver, Colorado

FOOD AND YOUR FUTURE, Second Edition

Ruth Bennett White

Ruth Bennett White has taught courses in foods, nutrition, and general home economics at all levels of education in the United States and abroad, and has conducted research at the University of Iowa, Cornell University, and Columbia University. She is a member of local, state, and national home economics associations and of the American Association of University Women. She has contributed articles to both scientific and popular publications.

SUPPLEMENTARY MATERIALS

    Teacher's Guide
    Spirit Duplicating Masters

Library of Congress Cataloging in Publication Data

White, Ruth Bennett.
    Food and your future.

    Includes bibliographies and index.
    SUMMARY: Discusses present-day eating habits; nutritional contributions of the basic foods; the relationship of diet to weight, heart disease, aging, and pregnancy; and the feeding of children.
    1. Nutrition. 2. Food. [1. Nutrition. 2. Food. 3. Diet] I. Title
TX354.W46 1978 641.1 78-14853
ISBN 0-13-322925-4

10 9 8 7 6 5

PRENTICE-HALL INTERNATIONAL, INC., *London*
PRENTICE-HALL OF AUSTRALIA, PTY. LTD., *Sydney*
PRENTICE-HALL OF CANADA, LTD., *Toronto*
PRENTICE-HALL OF INDIA PRIVATE LTD., *New Delhi*
PRENTICE-HALL OF JAPAN, INC., *Tokyo*
PRENTICE-HALL OF SOUTHEAST ASIA PTE. LTD., *Singapore*
WHITEHALL BOOKS LIMITED, Wellington, *New Zealand*

PHOTO CREDITS

Cover: Lewis & Neale, Inc.
Page 1: Shostal Associates **2** *top:* DPI
2 *center:* American Dairy Association **2** *bottom:* United Dairy Industry Association **5, 6, 7, 8:** J. Gerard Smith **13:** J. Gerard Smith **14-15:** J. Gerard Smith **16:** Thomas J. Lipton Co. **17** *top:* Peter Vandermark, Stock/Boston **17** *bottom:* Wally McNamee, Woodfin Camp & Associates **18** *left:* Frank Siteman, Stock/Boston **18** *right:* O. Christian Irgens **19** *top:* Hal McKusick, DPI **19** *bottom:* Shostal Associates **20:** Freda Leinwand, Monkmeyer Press **21** *top left:* T. Fujihara, Monkmeyer Press **21** *top right:* Paul Fusco, Magnum **21** *bottom:* William Hubbell, Woodfin Camp & Associates **22:** Dunn, DPI **23:** DPI **24** *left:* DPI **24** *right:* Paul Conklin, Monkmeyer Press **25** *top:* Jon Sinish, DPI **25** *bottom:* Shostal Associates **26** *top:* Henry Deters, Monkmeyer Press **26** *bottom:* Oscar Mayer & Co. **27:** Erich Hartmann, Magnum Photos **28:** Los Angeles Metropolitan Water District **29** *top:* Hal McKusick, DPI **29** *bottom:* Paul Stephanos, DPI **32-33:** Culver Pictures **35:** Costa Manos, Magnum Photos **36:** Costa Manos, Magnum Photos **37:** Corlett, DPI **38** *left:* U.S. Department of Agriculture **38** *right:* Rick Winsor, Woodfin Camp & Associates **40** *top:* Rhoda Sidney, Monkmeyer Press **40** *bottom:* DPI **41** *left:* William Hubbel, Woodfin Camp & Associates **41** *right:* U.S. Department of Agriculture **44-45:** J. Gerard Smith **47** *top:* Erich Hartmann, Magnum Photos **47** *bottom:* Costa Manos, Magnum Photos **48:** John Bintliff, DPI **49** *left:* U.S. Department of Agriculture **49** *right:* National Oceanic and Atmospheric Administration **50:** U.S. Department of Agriculture **53** *top:* J. Alex Langley, DPI **53** *bottom:* Eric Wilson, DPI **54** *left:* Bruce Davidson, Magnum Photos **54** *right:* Roger Malloch, Magnum Photos **55** *top:* Tana Hoban, DPI **55** *bottom:* U.S.

Continued on page 448.

The metric system used in this text is in accordance with the standards set forth in the *Handbook of Metric Usage in Home Economics*, published by the American Home Economics Association, 2010 Massachusetts Avenue, N.W., Washington, D.C. 20036.

Contents

UNIT 1   Your food in a changing world

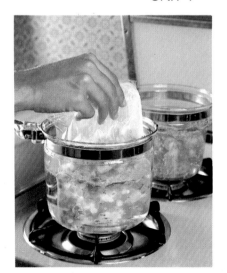

UNIT 2   Your food and your nutrition

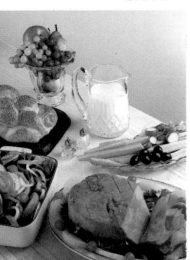

UNIT 3   Successful meal management

UNIT 4   **Nutrition and the early years**

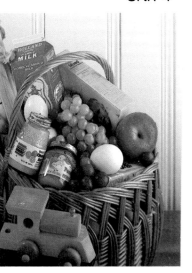

UNIT 5   **Research**

Tables

Figures

Food and Your Future, Second Edition, is designed to meet the need for integrating the continually changing scientific knowledge of nutrition with practical use of nutritional principles. In the United States, we have experienced in the last decade dramatic changes in life styles that have significantly altered our views of food and nutrition. Pollution of the land, air, and water has had detrimental effects on the safety of our food. The spiraling cost of living has driven food prices up. More women are working outside the home and spending less time preparing meals, with a consequent increase in convenience foods, fast meals, and snacks. With more single heads of households, more meals are eaten away from home. Interest in food and nutrition has increased among Americans of all ages and professions. People are investigating new ways to prepare and enjoy food, as well as new ways to control weight without sacrificing nutrition.

The past **century** has revealed more about nutrition than all previous time. Because of this new knowledge, it is possible for all people in the United States, regardless of income, to eat well, if they choose foods wisely. And yet over a million Americans eat less than a good diet. Our failure to reap the full benefits of sound nutrition is not the result of any lack of food or money but of the often confusing technical nature of scientific data and the difficulty of applying it to everyday life. The trend of increasing interest in nutrition has brought with it a vast assortment of half-truths, generalizations, and outright falsehoods about nutrition, generated by those unable to interpret the available information correctly.

Good nutrition is good preventive medicine. Food makes every cell in our bodies and is therefore the basis of sound health, physical appearance, mental development, and sense of well-being. Studies show that it also enables us to retain longer the characteristics of youth as we grow older. As a young person, you have the most to gain from good nutritional habits. The aim of this book is to provide you with a fundamental knowledge and understanding of the science of nutrition to ensure good health and longer life.

To facilitate the teaching and learning process, this edition of *Food and Your Future* is organized in five units. Unit 1 examines the practices of good nutrition in the world today. It presents current problems, such as world overpopulation and underproduction of food, fad diets, and contamination of the food supply.

Unit 2 focuses on each of the major food groups — fruits and vegetables, milk, meat, and grain foods. Each group is treated in two chapters. The first is a look at the nutritional values and forms of each; the second presents ways of using the foods in balanced meals for the greatest nutritional value.

Other chapters discuss the positive and negative values of sugar and fat, two important but often misunderstood food types.

Unit 3 details major ideas on managing meals and then applies them in nutritional programs to prevent and correct overweight and some types of heart disease. A separate new chapter deals with the relationship between aging and nutrition and meal management for the elderly. A special chapter on gourmet cooking shows how good nutrition can mean interesting meals, no matter how little time or money you have to spend.

Unit 4 is devoted to the special nutritional requirements of the expectant mother and young children. It traces the effects of diet on the expectant mother, as well as on the nourishment of the baby during gestation. It shows how good eating habits are established in the preschool years and the responsibility that parents have in raising a well-nourished child.

Unit 5 is a reference section providing a low-calorie, low-saturated-fat cookbook, a glossary, and an index, as well as metric conversion, weight-height, RDA, and nutritive values of foods tables.

All of the chapters have been updated. New in this edition are behavioral objectives at the beginning of each chapter. The end of each chapter includes a variety of activities that act as a guide and stimulus in acquiring skills in the management of time, energy, and money in planning menus, shopping for food, and planning and preparing balanced meals and snacks. Each chapter also includes brief career capsules and an annotated bibliography.

Food and Your Future, Second Edition, has been carefully controlled for readability (see the statement inside the front cover). Content, design, tables, and pictures are integrated to present the science of nutrition comprehensively to the nonscientist. In anticipation of the conversion of the United States to the metric system of measurement, quantities are given in metrics, followed by their customary equivalents in parentheses. Key vocabulary words appear in text in boldface type and color; they are listed for review at the end of each chapter and are defined in the glossary.

Among the many people who were instrumental in the preparation of the book, particular acknowledgment should be made to James McClintock, Frances Zuill, and the late Amy L. Daniels of the University of Iowa; Martha Van Rensselaer, Flora Rose, and Leonard Maynard, Cornell University; Julia Outhouse and Janice Smith, University of Illinois; Helen Judy Bond, Clara Taylor, and Charles Glen King, Columbia University; Henry Borsook, University of California, Berkeley; Velma Farrand, St. Louis, Missouri; Virginia Fowler, Audrey Hallett, Elizabeth Tillman, Barbara Morgan, and Aina Summerfelt, San Diego, California; Alice Mittermiller, La Jolla, California; Cedona Kendall, Ferguson, Missouri; Donna Newberry Creasy, Ossining, New York.

Scientific knowledge in nutrition is constantly growing. You are encouraged to seek new knowledge from reliable sources as it changes. If this book helps you to attain and maintain good eating habits, it will have fufilled its purpose.

R.B.W.

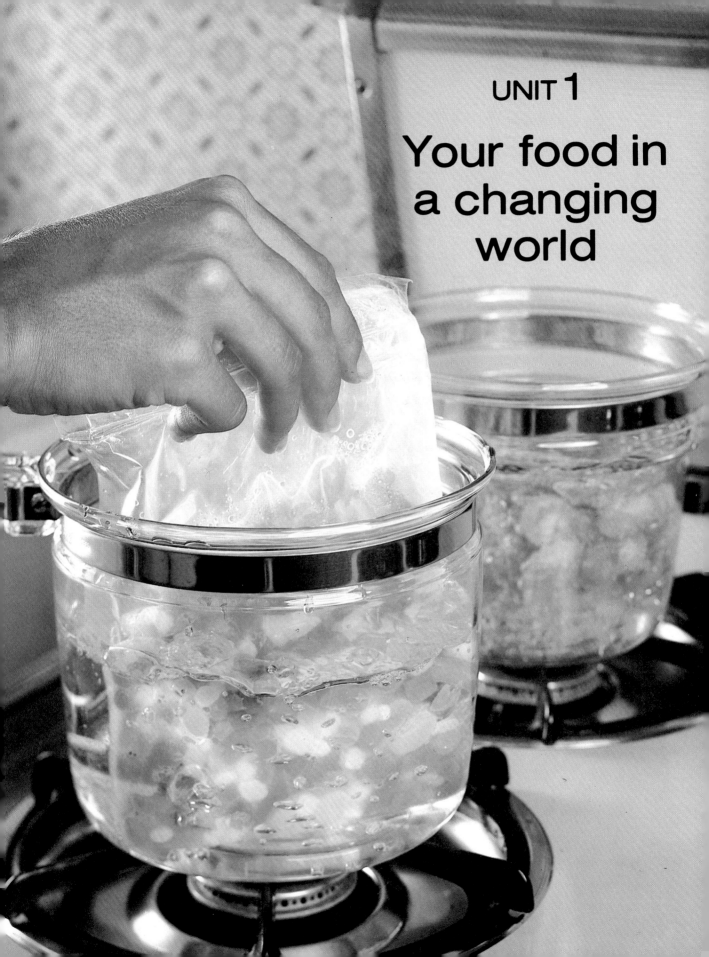

Your food in a changing world

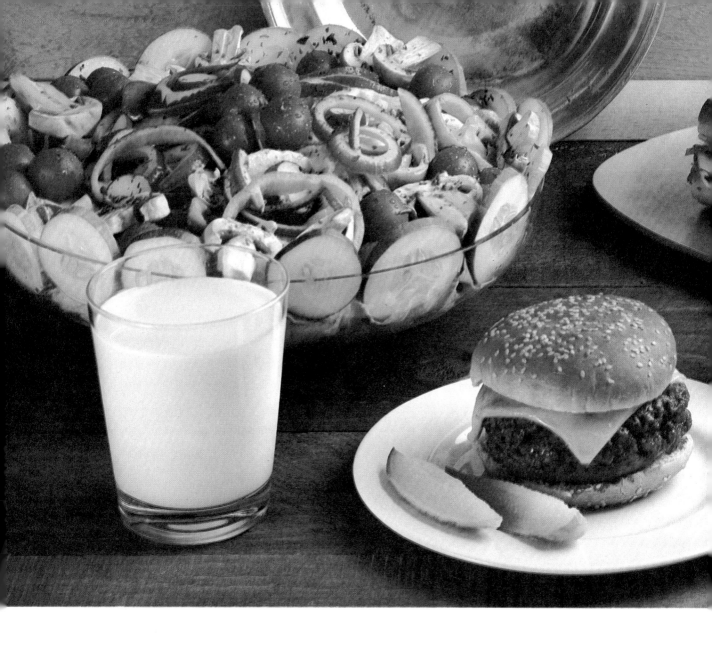

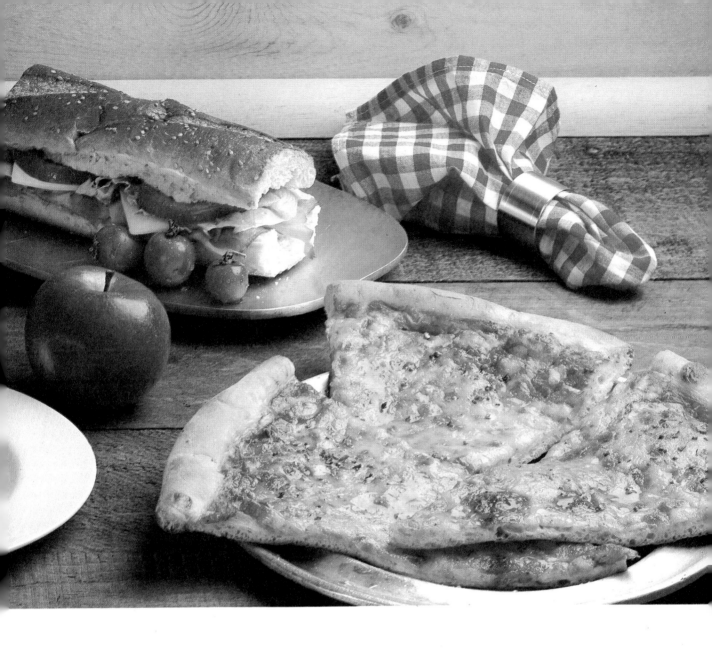

CHAPTER 1

Life styles and your food

After studying this chapter, you will be able to

- list physiological, emotional, and social reasons for eating.
- describe cultural, religious, and geographical influences on eating.
- demonstrate how today's family meal patterns have evolved.
- describe two developments in food processing that have made quick meals possible.
- predict a probable future change in land use that will affect food production.

WHY DO WE EAT?

A number of years ago, there was a popular saying: "You are what you eat." In many ways, this statement is literally true. On a physical level, each of us is a combination of nutrients—fats, proteins, sugars, starches, vitamins, and minerals—that we must continually replace and keep in balance so that we may continue to live and be healthy.

Physiological reasons for eating

The process of nutrition begins long before birth. A woman's health and nutritional state and her diet during pregnancy are among the most important factors in her baby's growth and development in the uterus and in later life. The subject is so important Unit 4 is

The hamburger—epitome of the American way of eating.

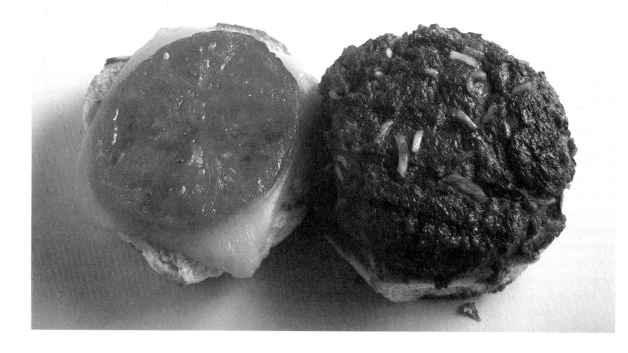

devoted to it. See pages 402–403 for needs for calories and nutrients during pregnancy and lactation.

After birth, of course, nutrition continues to be a basic need. Though now free to accept or reject a particular food that is offered, infants in general will instinctively accept enough foods to satisfy hunger.

As we leave infancy and childhood, however, we begin to become consciously aware of our nutritional needs. We also become increasingly responsible for seeing that these needs are met.

Emotional and social reasons for eating

No matter how central it is to our survival, food is even more than that. Food is a source of pleasure and satisfaction to most people. By eating, we are not just doing something that we must do to survive; we are, in addition, satisfying our desire for pleasure. We like to eat things that taste good, have an appealing texture, and are attractive to look at.

Psychologists have observed that eating is more pleasurable when it is a social act, that is, when we eat with others and share warmth and companionship along with a meal. In most societies, eating generally is a social act. Because food is so important in our lives, sharing food becomes a way of showing concern for, interest in, and enjoyment of people we care about. As a result, foods have a special place in any culture.

All life's important events are marked by celebrations in which

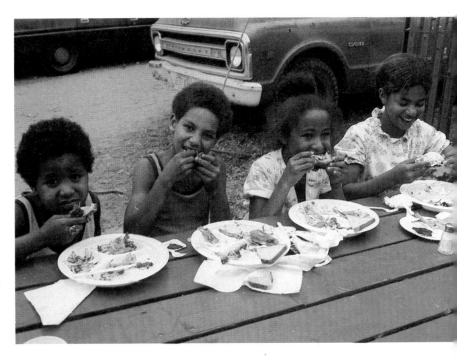

As we leave infancy and childhood, we become more responsible for meeting our own nutritional needs.

A picnic in the park is an example of eating as a social act.

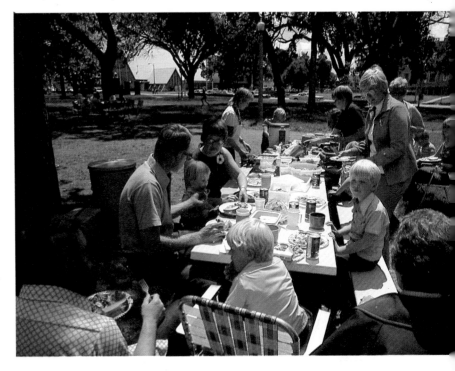

Life styles and your food **17**

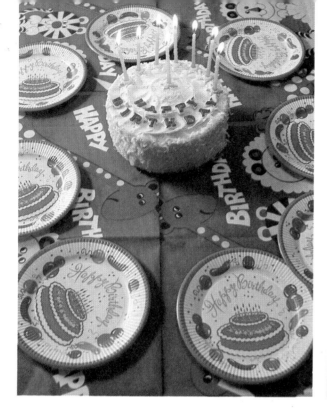
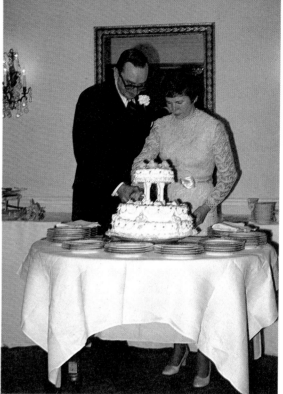

In the United States, traditionally decorated cakes are associated with birthdays and weddings.

food is shared. Who ever heard of a birthday party without cake and ice cream? Or a wedding without wedding cake? Every year, thousands of people have anniversary parties, graduation parties, or even neighborhood cookouts—all occasions when friends come together to share food and companionship or to celebrate an event.

Think for a moment of the two most important milestones of life—birth and death. When these events occur, people show their interest and concern by sharing food. Neighbors, friends, and relatives prepare food and bring it to the home so that the new parents or the grieving family do not have to prepare food when they are occupied with other concerns. More than simply being kind or providing something that the family must have, however, the

friends and relatives are showing their desire to share in the family's experience, whether it is happy or sad.

National and other holidays are associated with **traditional foods**: black-eyed peas on New Year's Day, cherry pie on Washington's Birthday, corned beef and cabbage on St. Patrick's Day, hot dogs and hamburgers on the Fourth of July. One holiday is completely devoted to foods. On the fourth Thursday in November, most Americans sit down to a traditional dinner of roast stuffed turkey, winter vegetables, pie, cranberries, and "all the trimmings." Thanksgiving is a celebration of food and a day on which we recognize its importance in our lives—not just the life of the body, but the life of society as well. Families and friends gather together to give thanks for the food on the table, for life in a free society, and for the love and friendship that have brought them together.

Influence of customs on eating

Although the turkey is almost always present on the Thanksgiving table, "all the trimmings" may vary depending on local and family custom. Whether the bird is stuffed with cornbread, oysters, chestnuts, rice, or herb-seasoned bread; whether the vegetables are potatoes, onions, corn, cauliflower, sauerkraut, or turnips; whether the pies are apple with Cheddar cheese, pumpkin, or mincemeat—all these things depend to a large extent on the area of the country in which the meal is served. The chances are, how-

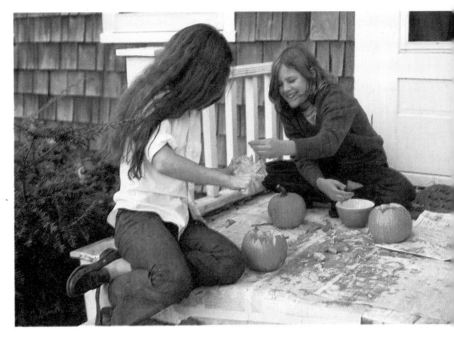

Pumpkins are as much a part of Halloween in the United States as witches and ghosts.

A turkey appears on almost every American family table on Thanksgiving Day, but the foods that accompany it are influenced by cultural, religious, and geographical customs.

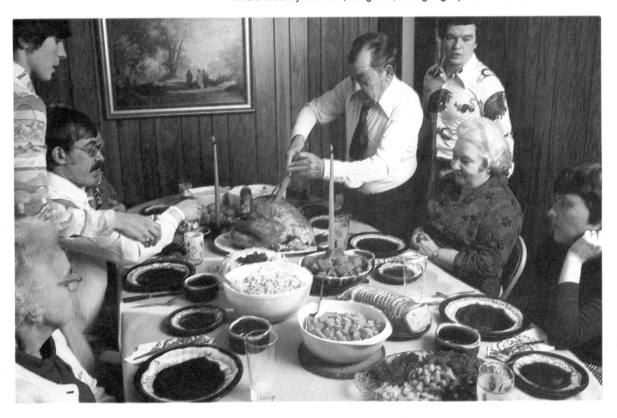

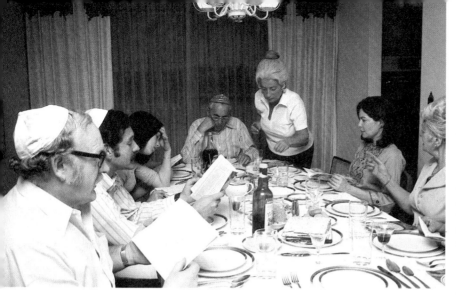

Foods served at the Passover Seder have a long tradition of religious significance.

ever, that the combination will become a tradition within that family. Year after year what *your* family eats for Thanksgiving dinner will probably be the same.

Cultural traditions. If you are living in the Chesapeake Bay area (Maryland, Delaware, Virginia, and Washington, D.C.), your turkey is likely to have oyster stuffing—partly because oysters are plentiful in the region and partly because it is a local tradition. If you come from a family with an Italian heritage, you may very well have an antipasto platter, minestrone soup, and lasagne before the turkey dinner. Many of the foods we eat are traditional, and the traditions are established by the cultures in which people have lived.

Cultural traditions in foods are so strong, in fact, that people may develop a prejudice for or against a certain food because of customs. We all learn to like the foods we are taught to eat and to like the methods of preparation we are used to. If you have never eaten raw fish, for example, chances are you will not be eager to try it. Yet in many parts of the world, it is acceptable and even

desirable to eat fish raw. It is important to remember, however, that since people learn certain tastes in foods, they can also learn to change their tastes.

Religious traditions. Besides cultural traditions, religion also helps to determine what people eat. In India, for example, the devout Hindu eats no beef because cows are sacred in the Hindu religion. Some religious groups eat no animal flesh at all, relying instead on egg, dairy, vegetable, and grain products to supply the essential fats and proteins in their diets.

Religions recognize that food is a central part of the human experience. Christian religions, for example, remember the Lord's Last Supper as a central part of their worship. The meal they are remembering is, in fact, the Seder meal for Passover in the Jewish religion. Many religious holidays and festivals have traditional foods associated with them—for example, Easter eggs, Passover matzoh , or the ten-course dinner of the Chinese New Year celebration.

Geography. As the oyster dressing of the Chesapeake Bay region suggests, availability of foods also plays a key role in determining people's eating habits. Certain foods grow well in one part of the world but poorly in another. Salt-water fish of seas and oceans differ from freshwater fish of lakes and rivers. Geographical facts also explain why the Chinese eat rice and Eskimos eat blubber. People learn to survive on foods that are near at hand, and in doing so they acquire a taste for the foods that they know.

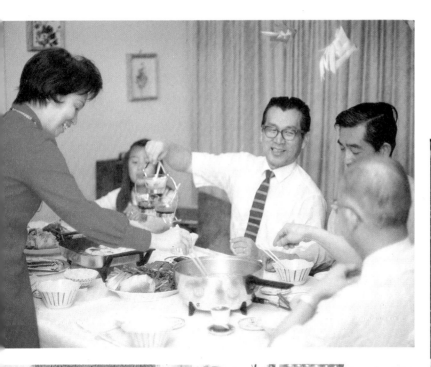

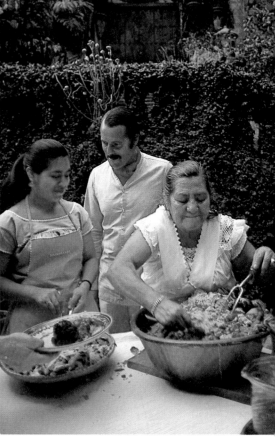

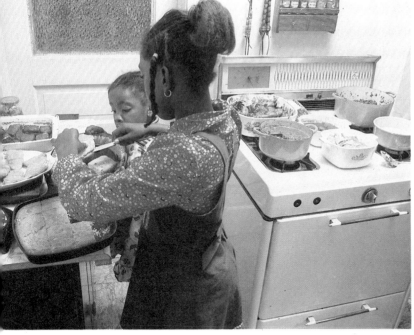

Ethnic culture and geographical heritage influence the kinds of foods we eat and the ways we prepare it. *Top left:* A family enjoys an Oriental meal. *Top right:* A Mexican family prepares to sit down to dinner. *Bottom left:* A family prepares "soul" food, developed in the South.

Throughout human history, our eating patterns—what we eat and when and how we eat it—have been influenced by culture, religion, and geography. In the modern world, a number of other things also affect our eating patterns.

Family meals on the run

In the rural and small-town societies of an earlier America, people worked and lived either at the same place or very close by. In this earlier society, mothers usually stayed at home; children came home from school promptly and did their chores and studying; fathers returned home immediately at the end of the workday. The family then settled down to a large dinner and a quiet evening in one another's company. The food was usually grown in their garden and prepared at home; the children had probably helped; the fathers had come home at a predictable hour; no one usually went out during the evening.

In today's world, there is an increasing number of one-parent families in which the parent must

An outgrowth of developing food preparation and eating habits in the United States is the backyard cookout or barbecue.

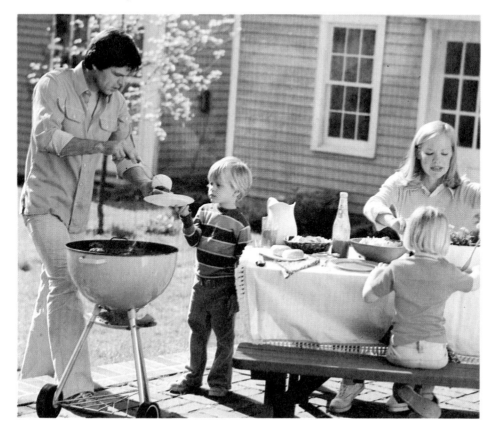

work. Even in two-parent families, economic and personal considerations bring more and more women into the working force outside the home. Working people have less time to spend in meal preparation than the at-home mothers of earlier times.

Other pressures also complicate modern family life. Every year an increasing number of people find jobs in major cities that require them to commute long distances and lengthen their working day. Both schools and jobs tend to be farther from where people actually live. Parents of both sexes are more involved in leisure-time activities or other commitments outside the home that demand an increasing amount of their time and energy. Children's lives, too, especially teen-agers' lives, are busier than they were in earlier times. The total amount of time that many families spend together is steadily decreasing.

Compare a dinner hour in the life of a modern family with that of the one examined earlier. At 4:45 in the afternoon Mother picks Jason up from rehearsal for the senior play. (She has already stopped at the supermarket on her way to the school.) The next stop is the junior high, where Jenny finishes track at 5:15. As the family walks in the door at 5:30, the phone is ringing. Dad has called to say that he is tied up with a client and will be getting home on the 7:05 train in time for his meeting at church at 8:00. Jason must be back for dress rehearsal at 7:15, Mother has a school board meeting at 7:30, and Jenny is going out to baby-sit at 8:30. The pork chops go di-

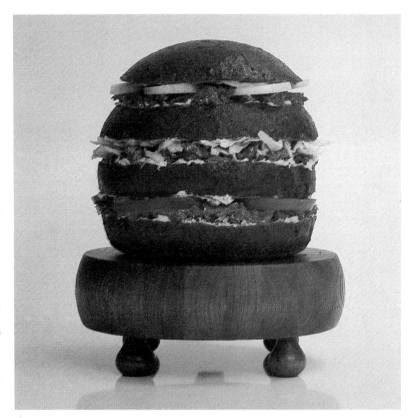

Sandwiches are one of the oldest foods for meals on the run.

rectly into the freezer right from the supermarket bag; out come four frozen meat pies, and Mother starts to clean the salad greens. She and Jason will eat now, and Jenny will wait and keep Dad company when he gets in.

Foods for meals on the run

Being too busy to sit down to a full meal is not a problem that began in contemporary America. In eighteenth-century England, John Montagu, Fourth Earl of Sandwich, refused to stop gambling even for meals. He asked his servant to bring him two pieces of bread with some meat between them so he could eat while he

continued to play cards. Napoleon Bonaparte was said to have offered a reward to anyone who came up with a method of providing fresh meat to his troops on the march. During World War I and World War II, the United States government needed to transport milk, eggs, meat, and produce to its troops overseas in such a way that the foods would not spoil during shipping.

Convenience foods. Out of the need for quick meals and the extensive availability of food has come a wide range of conven-ience foods. Milk may now be purchased in powdered, dry, canned, or condensed forms. Eggs and egg substitutes are also available in powdered or frozen forms. Main courses—stews, chicken and dumplings, spaghetti

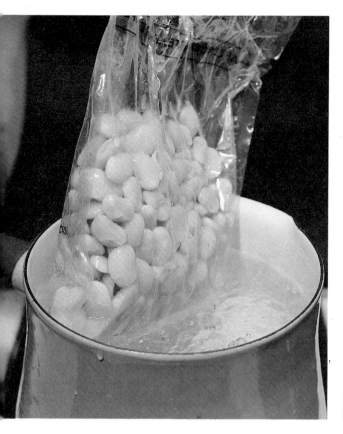
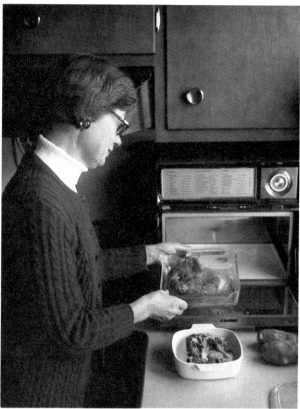

Frozen foods of all kinds and microwave ovens are two modern developments that have responded to the trend to decrease food preparation and cooking time in the home.

and meatballs—are available canned or frozen.

Fast freezing alone has revolutionized modern eating habits. Rather than being seasonal items or off-season luxuries in some areas, vegetables and fruits are now available everywhere at reasonable prices year round. Frozen vegetables and fruits retain much of the taste, texture, color, and nutritional value of their fresh counterparts.

Taking the fast-freezing process one step further, the industry developed a variety of complete meals, from frozen meat pies to TV dinners (complete with dessert) to meals in a plastic bag—stews or main courses that are heated in boiling water or a microwave oven. Such developments have made it possible for Jason and Jenny's mother to provide a main course in a matter of minutes and simply add a salad, bread and butter, beverage, and fresh fruit for dessert. Both seatings of the family's dinner will have a well-balanced meal in a minimum of preparation time.

Fast foods. In the past ten to fifteen years, a new industry has arisen to meet the needs of a society on the move. Fast-food chains try to encourage the habit of eating out. "No time to cook tonight? Bring the family out for fried chicken." "You deserve a break today." "Have it your way." The slogans are as numerous as the fast-food chains, and the prices are set low to make them attractive to everyone. Few parents would consider taking the family out once a week to a restaurant where dinner would cost $5.00 to $10.00 per person. Few parents would consider taking a toddler to an elegant restaurant or suggesting that everyone dress up tonight and go to the best place in town—at least not very often. Few teen-agers would think of having lunch or a post-game snack at a formal restaurant.

Fast-food chains have overcome all these objections to eating out. The food is inexpensive, the atmosphere is informal, and the food can even be taken out and eaten at home or in the car. Chain managements check individual restaurants continually to maintain standards of quality, freshness, portion control, cleanliness, and service.

The chains worked hard to establish their products, and the American public literally ate them up. As the demand for fast foods increased, so did the number and variety of chains. On many highways in the United States, a family looking for a half-hour break at dinner time can choose—within a mile or so—from numerous possibilities: Greek or Syrian sandwiches, pizza, hot dogs, submarine sandwiches (heroes, hoagies, grinders), tacos, roast beef, fish and chips, fried chicken, shrimp, ribs, and probably four different brands of the good old American hamburger—charcoal broiled or otherwise. The family knows that with computerized ordering and superspeed cooking, they will not have to sit and wait for twenty minutes while the baby whines for food. Their meals will be on their

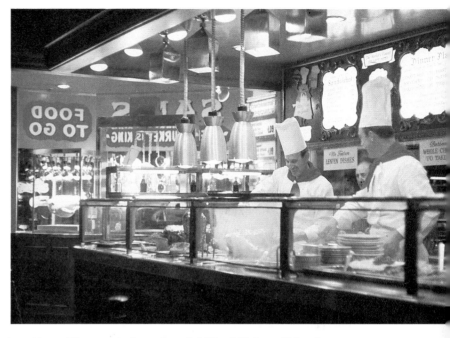

Above: The popularity and availability of "take-out" food to eat while working, studying, playing, or traveling clearly reflect modern American life styles. *Below:* Pizza is an American adaptation of Italian foods and is available frozen and in mix form to make quickly at home, as well as in fast-food chain restaurants.

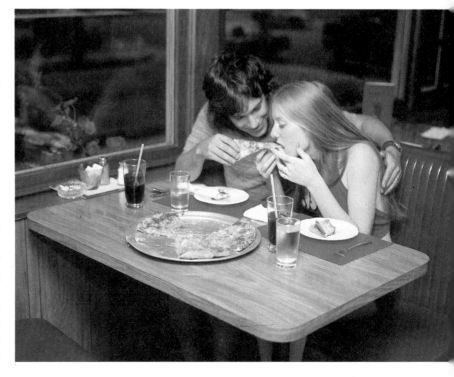

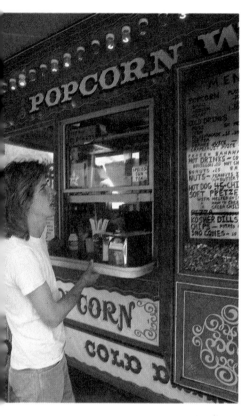

Above: Street vendors sell food throughout American cities.

Below: A sandwich with fruit and a glass of milk make a nutritious, quick meal.

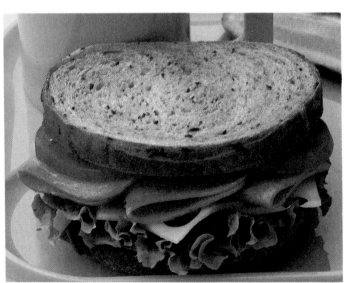

trays in minutes and will be exactly what they ordered. And if the family is traveling across the country, they know that the food they ordered will taste just like the food at the place back home. If a store of the fast-food chain of their choice is not in sight, it is surely around the next bend.

Nutritional effects of modern eating patterns

Quick meals, whether prepared at home from convenience foods or purchased ready-made at a fast-food chain, seem to be increasing in popularity almost daily. Given the basic importance of food for maintaining life, it is most important that we be sure that quick meals are also nutritious meals. The Earl of Sandwich didn't have a bad idea. A sandwich made of whole-grain bread, meat, cheese, or eggs, and raw vegetables, eaten with a glass of milk or fruit juice, meets the standards of good nutrition. The problem arises when we fail to plan our quick meals around nutritional requirements. The person who habitually has coffee for breakfast, two slices of pizza and a soft drink for lunch, and a hamburger, French fries, and a milkshake for dinner is not getting vital nutrients. Busy schedules and the unquestionable appeal of fast foods are making such a day-in day-out pattern all too common in modern life.

Taking both nutritional needs and the appeal of fast foods into account, the public high schools in Las Vegas, Nevada, began a lunch program for students that would satisfy both these requirements. A similar program in New York City schools offered a number of appealing fast-food items—tacos, hamburgers, French fries, hero sandwiches, milkshakes, and pizza—at moderate prices in the school cafeteria. In order for schools to be reimbursed by the government for student lunches, lunches must meet U.S. Department of Agriculture standards: 56 g (2 oz) protein, 180 mL (¾ c) raw vegetables, a roll or slice of bread, and 240 mL (8 oz) milk. About 45 percent of Las Vegas students actually bought lunches meeting the standard. Given a choice, many substituted French fries for a green salad.

U.S. Department of Agriculture regulations do not permit schools where it funds lunches to serve soft drinks. In the future, junk foods also may be banned from these schools. One of the ways in which the Las Vegas and New York school programs are meeting the government requirements, how-

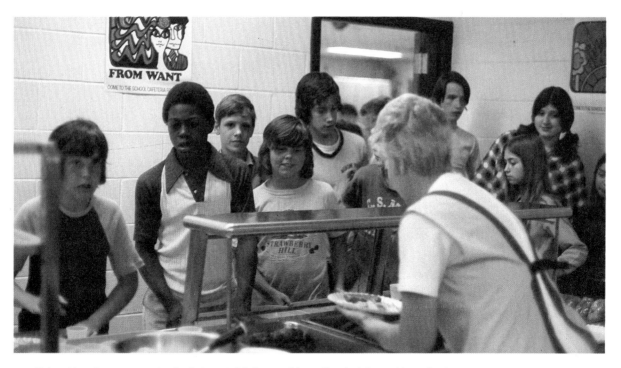

School lunch programs try both to establish sensible eating habits and to reflect modern eating patterns.

ever, goes unnoticed by the students. Without changing the flavor, the fast-food products sold in the school cafeterias are enriched to bring them up to government standards. Wheat germ is added to fortify hamburger buns and pizza dough. Extra iron and vitamin A reinforce the food value of the French fries. Clearly, then, students who eat these school lunches—even without a salad— are getting more nutrients than the students who may eat the same thing at a fast-food spot around the corner.

This fact has brought about one of the major criticisms of the fast-food lunch programs. Critics suggest that the schools are encouraging students to think that fast food is nutritious by not letting them know that nutrients have been added to their familiar burgers and pizza. The critics say that the schools are deceiving students and failing to teach them to recognize the elements of good nuturition.

An alternate to fast-food programs is in effect in the schools in Milwaukee, Wisconsin. Here the schools serve only one hot-meal choice a day—one that meets government requirements. The menus, however, are planned by the student council so that students have a voice in selecting—in advance—the meals they are served. Because preparing and serving only one hot meal allows the school to purchase ingredients in greater quantity and minimize waste, the schools can offer the meal to students for nearly half the Las Vegas price. Participation rate in Milwaukee is 70 to 75 percent of students.

A school in Oakham, Massachusetts combined a nutrition education program in the classrooms with service of family-style lunches because less than one-third of the students were eating school lunches.

Family-style lunches were then served by students assigned on a rotating basis. Servers were excused from class 10 minutes early to set tables. At lunch, servers brought food in serving dishes to their tables. Students could choose amounts of each food they wanted. Participation in the lunch program rose by half, and food waste declined by half. In addition, regular tests showed students were learning about nutrition. Other programs of family-style lunches and nutrition education have had similar results: high involvement and low waste.

We have already glanced at the importance of food in our lives and at some of the factors that influence eating patterns. The changes that are going on in our use of available food-producing resources will determine what we may eat in the future and what the next generation may eat.

When farming began, each family grew its own food. Soon people realized that not everyone needed to farm. Gradually farming was turned over to one group in the tribe or community, while others hunted, built shelters, or tended to health needs. As society became more complex, jobs became more diversified and more specialized. Food production was left in the hands of relatively few people, while all the others were the consumers of the food produced.

Future history and future eating patterns may be largely determined more by the decrease in the amount of available land than by the decrease in the number of food producers. At present, it is estimated that there is only .40 hectare (1 acre) of arable land (land on which crops may be grown) per person. Of that land, 10 percent (an amount equal to all the arable land in Europe) is used for growing what are called nonfood crops—crops such as tobacco, rubber, or non-nutritious foods such as coffee or tea. These crops produce revenue for the growers and are central to their economic survival, but they contribute no food to the world's population. The population is expected to double in the next thirty to forty years, and the arable land

per person will be reduced to less than .20 hectare or half an acre (given the need to build additional housing).

It seems unlikely that the production of these crops will be reduced significantly. The most likely change that will insure adequate food production on shrinking arable land is a decrease in the amount of livestock raised for food. Consider the space that cows, pigs, sheep, and other livestock occupy on a farm or ranch—space that could be devoted to producing other kinds of food products. Another kind of waste occurs in raising livestock for food. To produce a single .45-kg (1-lb) steak, the farmer must feed a steer 7.2 kg (16 lb) of grain protein (corn, soy, etc.) Only .45 kg (1 lb) of feed protein goes toward meat. The rest produces nonedible parts of the steer—hair, bones—or is thrown off in its waste matter. By contrast, a milk cow requires only .45 kg (1 lb) of vegetable protein to produce 240 mL (8 oz) milk—a far more economical use of animal feed.

By contrast with people in other countries, Americans often fail to think of protein sources other than meat. In China and Japan, rice, vegetables, and soy products are the basic sources of proteins, vitamins, and minerals, while meat is used only in an incidental way. If we gave meat a less important place in our diet, an astounding amount of land could be utilized for crop production. Each acre of land now used for meat production could yield 5 times as much protein in cereal

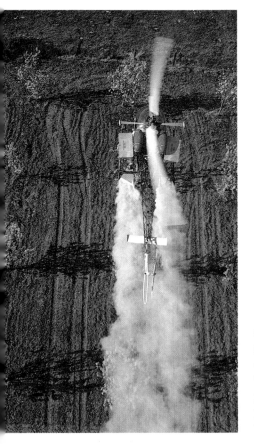

Pollination of fruit trees by helicopter instead of insects is a modern and efficient way of getting the most out of food crops.

28

crops (corn, wheat, barley), 10 times as much in legumes (peas, beans, lentils, etc.), or 15 times as much in leafy vegetables. Some foods in each group offer an even higher yield; an acre devoted to growing spinach, for example, would yield *26 times* as much protein as one used for meat production.

Millions of people in the world—including many in the United States—subsist on a poor diet or suffer starvation. Although the United States leads the world in exports of grain, much grain that could have been shared with the world's poor has been lost in the production of livestock.

As the world's population continues to expand while its arable land cannot, it is clear that we will have to discover new food sources, make greater use of foods that are underutilized at present, and develop new ways of

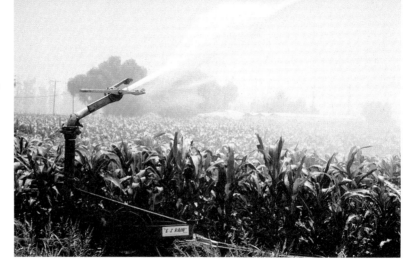

Irrigation, a method of reclaiming arable land, has been developed and improved for centuries.

processing and preparing the foods that are most economical and most nutritious. Already on the market is a **meat extender** made of soy protein and intended to be mixed with ground meat for use in hamburgers, meatloaf, and the like, in order to reduce the family food budget without compromising nutrition. It is entirely

possible that eggs, dairy products, and vegetable proteins will come to replace meat entirely in our diet—not just because they are cheaper to buy, but because our survival in a world of shrinking farmlands and expanding population may depend on it.

How technology and the needs of our "society on the go" will

The current interest in camping and survival tactics, both of which necessitate a minimum number of foods that are light in weight and small in bulk, may lead to developments in food processing and packaging that will affect our future eating patterns.

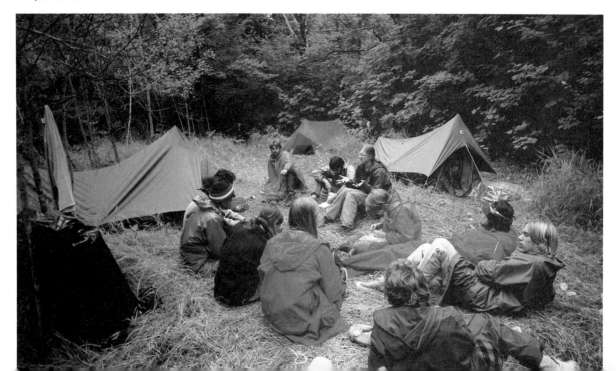

affect future food products is more difficult to predict. Science fiction shows us a society in which once a day people take a pill containing all the vital nutrients instead of eating conventional meals. History and the place that food has traditionally had in feasts and ceremonies suggest that such a dramatic change may be a long time in coming. But come it may. Only the future holds the answer.

RECAP

Why do we eat?

Physiological reasons for eating   **Emotional and social reasons for eating**   **Influence of customs on eating**   *Cultural traditions*   *Religious traditions*   *Geography*

Modern eating patterns

Family meals on the run   **Foods for meals on the run**   *Convenience foods*   *Fast foods*   **Nutritional effects of modern eating patterns**

Food in the future

THINKING AND EVALUATING

1. What is the basis of truth in the saying "We are what we eat"?

2. Compare social or holiday food traditions in your family with those of other members of the class. Does your family have birthday meal traditions? Salmon and peas on the Fourth of July, or a clambake?

3. What effect have cultural and religious customs and geographical location had on the foods served in your family and your own food likes and dislikes?

4. Does your family make a point of having dinner at home together? If so, explain the reasons why it's possible. If not, why not?

5. From this chapter you have learned that convenience foods and fast foods are not necessarily "junk" foods—they can be nutritious if used in well-balanced meals. How would you change your own consumption of convenience or fast foods in order to improve your meals "on the run," without actually changing your eating patterns?

6. Can you think of workable ways the land used for non-food crops could be turned over to food production?

APPLYING AND SHARING

1. For one week, experiment with your own nutritional instincts. Within the limits of the foods available to you at home,

---

VOCABULARY

arable land
convenience food
eating patterns
fast-food chains
meat extender
nutrients
nutritional needs
traditional food

at school, and elsewhere, eat only the things you feel like eating. Within the limits of family and school schedules, eat only at times you feel like eating. Keep a record of the kinds and quantities of foods you eat, and the total amounts for each day.

2. Choose a religion other than your own or a holiday that is not celebrated in your family and see what you can find out about the food traditions of the religion or holiday. Use reference works and periodical indexes in the library; talk with people who might have experience with the tradition; check the yellow pages for organizations (consulates, religious groups, ethnic societies) that might be able to send you materials. Report your findings to the class in a paper or a talk.

3. Conduct the same kind of research on a geographical area of the United States other than your own, or on another country.

4. Choose a fast-food chain restaurant near you and evaluate its menu. If you select menu items carefully, can you get a meal at the restaurant that includes meat or eggs, milk or a milk food, a salad, vegetable, or fruit, and bread or another grain food like rice or spaghetti? Compare your findings with those of other members of the class on other fast-food chains.

5. Watch the newspaper and check magazines for articles that describe technological developments in food production that may affect our future eating patterns. The condensed semiliquid foods in tubes created for astronauts is one past development; so was manufactured meatless bacon. Post articles in the classroom.

CAREER CAPSULES

Food technologist Usually works for a food company; develops new products. Four-year college education in mathematics and sciences required.

Food editor/writer Works for a newspaper, magazine, or book publisher, or as a free lance; plans, researches, and writes articles or books on food. Four-year college education in home economics and/or journalism usually required.

RELATED READING

Borgstrom, Georg. *Harvesting the Earth.* New York: Abelard-Schuman, 1973. Suggests a global plan in the use of the world's resources for the future survival of human beings.

Sargent, Frederic O. "Planning for a New Life Style." *People—A Good Life for More: Yearbook of Agriculture, 1971.* Washington, D.C.: USDA, 1971. Presents suggestions for environmental planning, with emphasis on people and their needs.

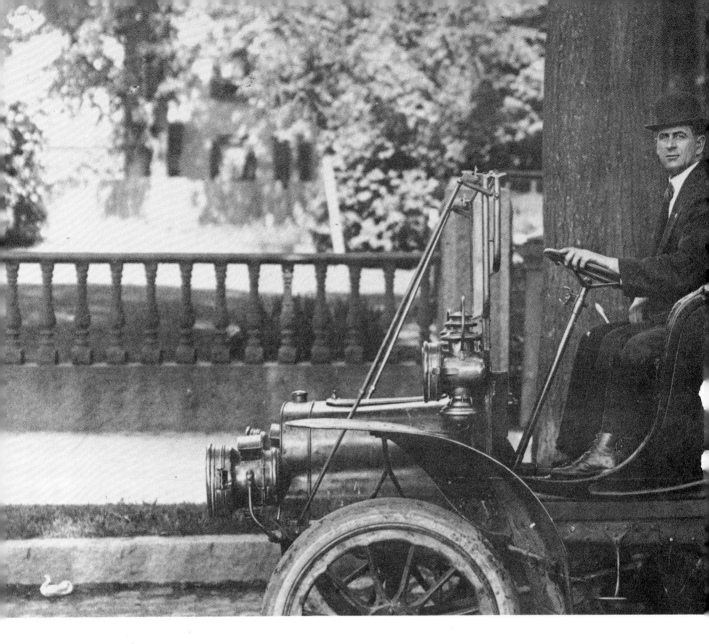

CHAPTER 2

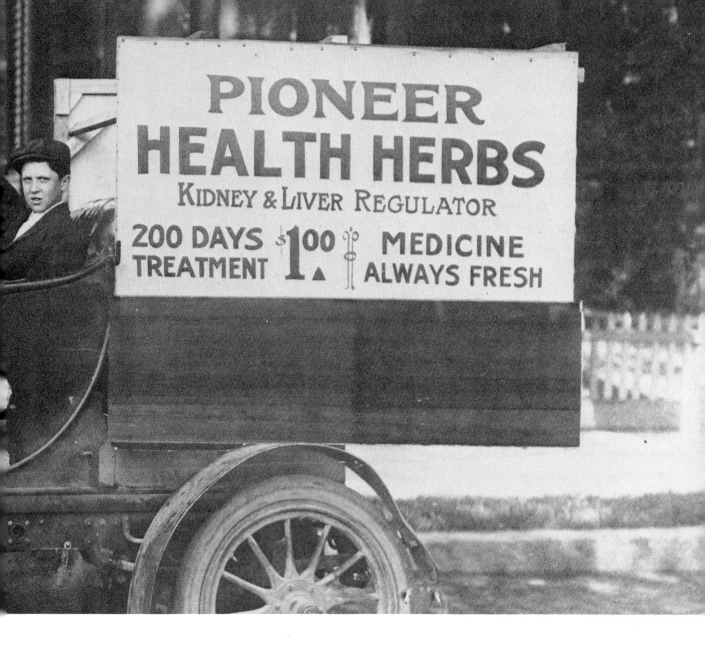

Fads, fallacies, and facts

After studying this chapter, you will be able to

- identify some food fads and food scares.
- recognize the signs of a food quack.
- identify sources of dependable information on food.
- make a personal contribution toward protecting or raising our food standards.

FOOD FADS AND FALLACIES

Every once in a while, people in the United States seem to plunge into a food craze. Friends announce that they have been eating nothing but one special food for weeks and feel like Superman or Wonder Woman. Every magazine suddenly seems to carry articles about the health-giving power of food x or vitamin y. Invalids rise from their sickbeds to testify to the benefits of a new cure-all food or food supplement. It seems that the elimination of all our ailments is just around the corner with the help of this long-overlooked food or that underrated food supplement.

In the same way, food scares also sweep the country. At various times in the past few years, we have been told that it is dangerous to eat cranberry sauce, clam chowder, maraschino cherries, milk, eggs, and a host of other foods. It sometimes seems that there is scarcely anything we can take from the grocery shelf without wondering if it is safe to eat.

Sometimes food crazes and food scares are based on facts. Sometimes they are based on a "crank" theory—a theory with little or no scientific basis. Often, they stem from a misunderstanding of facts, wrong interpretations of facts, or incomplete knowledge of facts.

When food fads sweep the country, we need to be able to distinguish between **fallacy** (error) and fact. We should question the sources of the fad. We should consider past knowledge of nutrition and the latest scientific research on food. We should greet any new discovery, whether authoritative or not, with careful thought. Even science—far less a food craze—rarely produces a fact that overturns everything we have learned about food. Solid new evidence generally adds only a little at a time to our knowledge. Hence discoveries that seem "revolutionary" should be viewed with skepticism.

Fad diets

Each year many people reactivate old health disorders or create new problems by following fad diets. A **fad diet** is an eating plan that is followed with great zeal, even though it lacks a nutritionally sound foundation. A fad diet is often based on a fad food—one

thought to have near-magical powers.

Most fad foods and diets would be harmless if used only for a few days. However, a kind of fanaticism usually grips the followers of a fad diet. They refuse to abandon the diet even when their health fails. Deaf to the warnings of friends and relatives, they can end up in a hospital, with doctors and nurses trying to rebuild their health.

One 36-year-old woman decided to follow a diet often called the "Zen diet," though many who practice Zen Buddhism disagree with it. She ate only ground oatmeal, cornmeal, and buckwheat, bread made from rice, and 12 ounces of soup or tea daily. She refused meat, eggs, milk, vegetables, and fruit. After eight months, she became bedridden with a serious case of **scurvy** caused by a lack of vitamin C. Still she refused to change her diet, believing that it would cure her "temporary" weakness. When at last she was hospitalized, it was found that in addition to scurvy she had deficiencies of other essential nutrients, including protein and folic acid. She was suffering from general **malnutrition,** or poor nourishment. A simple switch to an adequate diet saved her life.

Similarly, people attempting to lose weight sometimes follow harmful diet plans. Many overweight people seize on any diet that promises to shorten the painful period of self-restraint. Hoping for a shortcut to slenderness, they too can endanger their health. Some fad diets do not include necessary foods. If followed for any length of time, they result in malnutrition. Shortcut diets usually do not work. Once the dieter returns to previous eating habits, all the lost pounds return, also.

Quacks and quackery

Sometimes people are led into fad diets by **food quacks**—persons who claim knowledge they do not possess. Sometimes food quacks believe the claims they make. Often, however, they deliberately spread misinformation for profit. They profit from lectures, books, consultations, or from products bought at their suggestion.

One well-known example of food quackery is a book on weight reduction titled *Calories Don't Count* by Dr. Herman Taller. For a time the book was a best-seller, partly because of its misleading title. Eventually, however, the U. S. Food and Drug Administration seized the books and the safflower oil capsules that were sold with them. Dr. Taller was brought to trial and given a jail sentence.

Dr. Taller's book was financially successful despite the fact that his colleagues in the medical profession rejected his ideas. The general public continued to buy Dr. Taller's book and follow its suggestions. When people allow themselves to be taken in so easily, it is not surprising if others also try to enrich themselves through false claims.

In the Food and Drug Administration records there is a story of a "health" lecturer who invited the public to an introductory free talk. At this talk, he sold tickets to a series of lectures. He urged his audiences to buy only his brand of

The exaggerated claims of quacks for the healthful properties of certain foods can be not only misleading but also fraudulent.

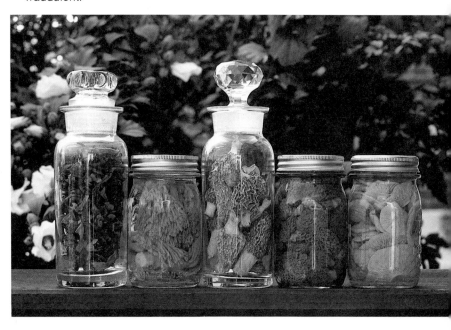

whole-wheat flour, peppermint tea, wheat germ, and honey. He claimed that these foods would prevent or cure cancer, arthritis, liver trouble, heart disease, and many other illnesses. The foods cost about 90 percent more than the cost of similar products in grocery stores.

After a nine-month trial, a jury found the lecturer guilty of fraud. While free on bail, he conducted another lecture tour. He begged his audiences for funds to keep up his struggle against "persecution" by the medical profession, the Better Business Bureau, and the Food and Drug Administration. Some people-believed his claims. After he was sentenced to a year and a day in jail, he appealed the verdict and sued the judge. However, the appeals court upheld the first verdict, despite the popular support he had gained.

Food quacks cost the public over a million dollars annually in the effort required to prove the quacks wrong and to force them to stop their practices. In addition, food quackery has other harmful effects. If sick people follow a fraudulent claim instead of seeking good medical diagnosis and treatment, their lives are doubly endangered.

The soil depletion myth

One favorite subject of food quacks is soil depletion. They would have us believe that our farmland is so worn out and deprived of nutrients that it cannot produce foods with enough vitamins, minerals, and protein. According to the picture they paint, our fruits and vegetables are like brightly colored, hollow vessels containing little but water.

Of course the picture is false. The plant is a kind of factory that manufactures nutrients. It is not just a conduit or canal for the transport of nutrients from the soil. The plant itself produces the nutrients you need through the process of photosynthesis. In photosynthesis, the green leaf of a plant uses the radiant energy of sunshine, oxygen from the air, and water to create vitamins, sugars, starches, and fats. Fertilizers support the process of photosynthesis by adding nitrogen and minerals to the soil. With the help of nitrogen from the soil, the plant also makes proteins.

"Organic" foods

Because of concern about the misuse of fertilizers, many people have recently become interested

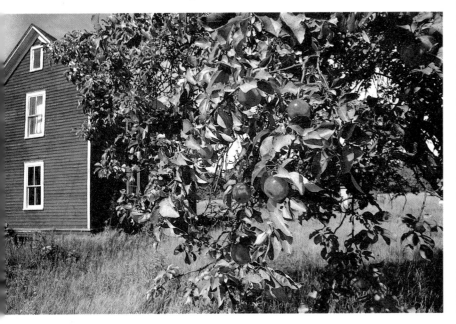

Plants draw minerals and nitrogen from the soil and manufacture other nutrients.

in "organic" and "natural" foods. Organic is a term for foods grown without the aid of any commercial fertilizer or pesticide (poison used to kill insects). Some think that organic foods, usually sold in "health" food stores, are more nutritious as well as free from the poisonous residue of insect-killing sprays.

Some buyers of organic foods seem to believe that since organic farming avoids the use of commercial fertilizers, it introduces no chemicals to the soil. Buyers approve the use of manure (fertilizer made from animal excrement) and compost (fertilizer made from decayed plants) instead of commercial fertilizers. Both compost and manure provide moisture-holding bulk or humus (decaying vegetable or animal matter) to the soil. They are both good fertilizers under the right conditions. However, compost and manure cannot be used by plants directly. These organic fertilizers must first be broken down into their inorganic chemical elements. This happens in the soil over a period of time through the action of bacteria (tiny organisms naturally present in soil). Thus, "organic" fertilizers do indeed add chemicals to soil. Moreover, manure can contribute to the spread of infectious diseases if not properly managed.

It is desirable to avoid pesticide residues, but the purchase of organic foods does not always achieve this purpose. The agriculture department of one state studied the pesticide residues on products in a health food store and in other kinds of food markets. It found that 20 percent of the foods studied in ordinary markets had pesticide residue. In the health food store, 30 percent of the same kinds of foods had pesticides on them. Furthermore, the products in the health food store were often more expensive.

"Natural" foods

While "organic" foods are found mostly in health food stores, "natural" foods are found nearly everywhere. As soon as advertisers noticed that the word "natural" attracted buyers, they used it to describe everything from lipsticks to house shingles. As a result, the meaning of "natural" is vague and unreliable, at least in food advertising.

In general, "natural" foods are those supposed to have been packaged or processed without additives by the processor. An additive might be a preservative or a coloring agent to make the food attractive. Even a cucumber can be sprayed with paraffin to look shiny or an orange can be dyed a brighter color. Many consumers feel that these changes are unnecessary and perhaps harmful.

In fact, few foods are completely "natural." Even when they are, their "naturalness" does not necessarily make them better than other foods. For instance, food faddists sometimes claim that honey, made by the bee, is superior to refined sugar, made in a factory from sugar beets or sugar cane. From a nutritional standpoint, this claim is a fallacy. Honey is itself a form of sugar. For the purposes of nutrition, honey is no better than refined sugar and no worse.

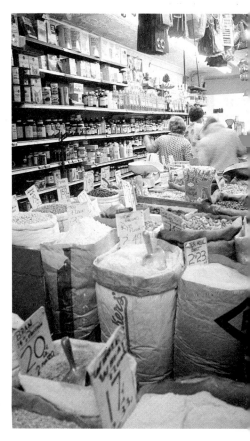

"Health" food stores often specialize in "organic" foods, said to be grown without the aid of commercial fertilizers or pesticides.

A food faddist who insists on a "natural" product may be dismayed by facts a scientist could point out. For instance, many people look for "natural" vitamins. One popular "natural" source of vitamin C is rose hips, the red balls that form on roses after the blooms fade. Rose hips are indeed a good source of vitamin C. However, roses are usually sprayed to destroy pests and plant diseases that might prevent the production of luxuriant flowers. The spraying of roses is not done under government regulations, as is the spraying of citrus trees. Therefore, a person who buys rose hips as a source of vita-

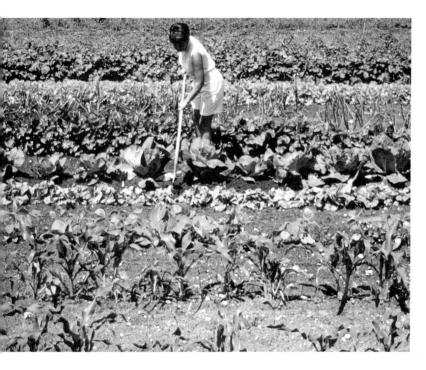
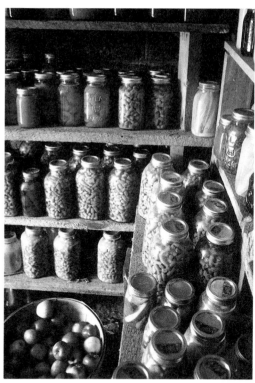

"Natural" foods grown and canned at home with no additives or artificial color are not necessarily better than other foods.

min C may get more pesticide spray residue than those who eat citrus fruits sprayed according to government regulations.

Food faddists often enthusiastically support **food supplements,** such as vitamin and mineral tablets. Again, these enthusiasms have a kernel of truth. Growing children and older people may need food supplements, particularly when food intake is low. Persons who have been ill or whose intestinal absorption is impaired may need additional nutrients.

However, we know that excessive amounts of vitamins A and D can be toxic. Too much vitamin B_6 has been found to interfere with drugs used to treat Parkinson's disease. It is not possible at present to prepare one all-purpose supplement that can be given to everyone. We do not yet know enough about food supplements to devise a formula that could suit the needs of people of different ages and health.

Vitamins and minerals are not substitutes for food. They are meant to work with food to build and rebuild our bodies. For those who wish to take supplementary vitamins, intake should not exceed the recommendations of the most reliable authorities (see the RDA table on pages 402-403). The best way to get vitamins and minerals is to eat a variety of wholesome foods every day. Food supplements cannot take the place of real food. Food fads should not replace sensible eating habits that support good health for a lifetime.

How can we learn to build sensible eating habits? Among all the claims we hear from food faddists, quacks, alarmists, and enthusiasts, how can we tell truths from half-truths or falsehoods? When the next food craze or food scare sweeps the country, will we be able to judge it calmly?

Sources of information

It is important to become well-informed about nutrition. When you hear an alarming or amazing message about food, ask questions such as the following.

Is the speaker a qualified nutritionist? Has he or she studied at reputable universities and earned an advanced degree in nutrition?

Does the person promote a product that sells for a high price? Is it available only through certain stores or by mail?

Does the person promote certain foods to the exclusion of others?

Does the person try to make you fear the consequences of not following his or her advice?

Does the person ridicule or condemn prominent authorities, such as the U. S. Food and Drug Administration or the American Medical Association?

Have you noticed any untrue or misleading information in books or articles written by this person?

A "yes" answer to any but the first question should warn you to consider the person's message with great caution. Meanwhile, you may continue to search out sources of good information. Some reliable sources of information follow.

Nutritionists who are government employees or hospital consultants

The American Medical Association's Council on Food and Nutrition

College teachers and research scientists in food and nutrition

The Federal Trade Commission, in the area of fraudulent and misleading advertising

The U. S. Food and Drug Administration for advice on labeling and safeguards against contamination of food

The Consumer and Food Economics Research Division of the U. S. Department of Agriculture

A national or state consumer representative

Books and articles written by recognized authorities and published by reliable publishers (usually those who have been in business for a number of years and are not privately subsidized)

Government protection

In judging the claims of food faddists, it is important to realize the extent to which the government protects you. Many people have been working hard for many years to protect the wholesomeness and safety of your food. A wide variety of laws provides a framework of protection that you may temporarily overlook when threatened by a food scare.

More laws protect food than any other consumer item. Two divisions of the federal government have major responsibilities as guardians of food—the Department of Health, Education and Welfare and the Department of Agriculture.

As an example of services provided by the government, the U. S. Department of Agriculture's symbol on meat and poultry indicates a high standard of wholesomeness. It means that diseased animals are rejected before slaughter. It means that food workers in plants where the meat or poultry is processed follow certain rules. They must wear hairnets and may not wear rings, earrings, or nail polish. If they leave their work stations, they must sanitize their hands in a special solution when they return. These rules are enforced by government inspectors.

The federal Food and Drug Administration enforces many of the government food regulations. Federal labeling laws apply to all foods made in one state but sold in others. Companies that violate the labeling law may be prosecuted. Their products may be seized and removed from the market.

The law makes the following requirements.

Both the picture and the written description on the label must accurately represent the contents.

The ingredients must be listed with the largest amount first and the rest in descending order. For instance, if a margarine contains more liquid safflower oil than hydrogenated oil, the safflower oil must be listed first, then the hydrogenated oil. If there is more gravy than chicken in

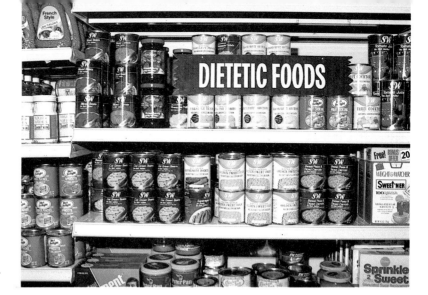

Government regulations require foods prepared for people with special food needs to be carefully labeled and their ingredients listed.

A government standard of identity controlling nationwide production of butter requires certain ingredients to be present (or not present) in butter and therefore does not require the ingredients to be listed on the packages.

a can of chicken fricassee, "gravy" must be listed first, followed by "chicken."

The contents must be stated in units of measure that are in common use, such as ounces or grams.

The package must not be larger than the contents. The product must fill the container at the time it is packaged, even though the contents may settle later.

Statements must be in English, must be easy to read in clear type, and must give the name of the product and the style of its preparation (such as thick, thin, or medium syrup in canned fruits).

The name and address of the manufacturer, packer, or distributor must be on the label.

Special foods, such as those prepared for diabetic patients, persons with heart disease, or those who are subject to allergies, have special labeling laws. Among these is the specification of the amount of ingredients for each unit of measure.

Manufacturers are not required to list all the ingredients in some 300 foods. These foods are covered by "standards of identity" that have been set up by the FDA.

A standard of identity is like a recipe that must be followed at risk of prosecution. For instance, a package of butter does not have to state that color has been added. The color is included in the standard the FDA has set as acceptable for butter. The ingredients of a bottle of catsup or a jar of mayonnaise need not be listed on the label because these foods

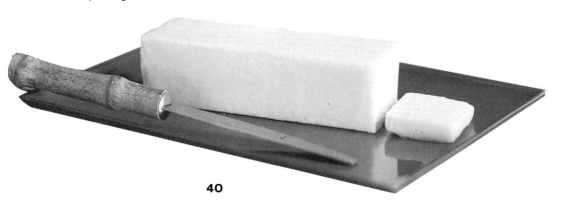

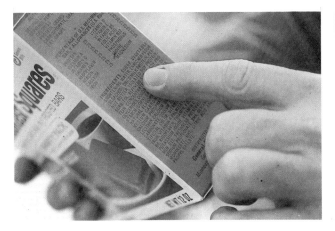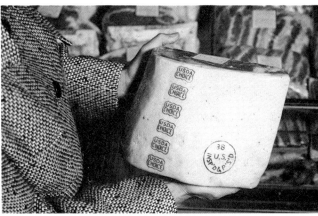

Left: Nutritional panels on food packages list, among other things, the percentages of recommended daily allowances of nutrients the foods contain per serving. *Right:* Government regulations require certain food products, such as meat, poultry, eggs, and butter, to be graded and labeled with their grades.

follow an FDA standard. Only a mixture with certain ingredients may be called "catsup" or "mayonnaise."

Nevertheless, because consumers are becoming more aware of nutrition, many manufacturers now · list ingredients even on products that follow an FDA standard. They often volunteer other information that consumers find useful. As a result, you may find the following items on labels.

A nutritional panel, which is sometimes required, sometimes voluntary. It lists the amount of protein, carbohydrates, and fat, and the calories per serving. It may also give amounts of vitamins and minerals. These are given as a percentage of the total needed daily by the average adul., according to the RDA.

A grade, not always required by law, but used on some foods. The grade indicates a standard of quality set up by the U. S. Department of Agriculture. The grade, which for a product such as butter could be "AA," "A," or "B," is shown on an official mark shaped like a shield.

A Universal Product Code—a row of little lines about 1 inch (2.4 cm) wide, used in some markets with computerized checkout stations. The computer at the checkout scans the lines, which tell the name, price, and weight of the product. This information then appears on your sales receipt.

Consumer contributions

Government agencies depend on consumers to help set standards for food. We can help improve the nutritional value of our food by expressing our needs to our government representatives. Consumer suggestions helped bring about the labeling laws. Consumers could exert pressure to have standards set for all kinds of processed foods. They could ask that complete nutritional information be listed on the 300 foods that now come under a standard of identity. When consumers want further information and express their wishes in a convincing manner, the food industry often responds voluntarily.

Another way we can enforce high standards is by reporting violations of the law. Responsible agencies cannot enforce the law without the help of concerned citizens. When you see a violation, you should write to the responsible agency, stating the facts briefly and courteously.

If you see false or misleading advertising, write the U. S. Federal Trade Commission.

If you see substandard meat and poultry products, write the U. S. Department of Agriculture.

If you see unsanitary conditions in restaurants and other public eating places, write your local city or state department of health.

For unclean or unwholesome food made and sold within your state, write your state department of health.

If you suffer food poisoning from food bought in a store or restaurant, notify your local department of health and the U. S. Food and Drug Administration.

If you observe instances of air or water pollution, write the U. S. Environmental Protection Agency.

Life styles and your food **41**

It is often a good idea to make copies of your letter and send them to others who may help. For instance, you can send copies to your state and local consumer representative, your senator or congressperson, local officials, supermarket managers, or the president of the food processing company.

You may also want to write legislators in order to argue for the passage of better laws. If so, state in your letter the condition you want to correct. Use facts to support your argument. If you refer to a particular bill under discussion, identify it by number and sponsor. Make clear how a new law could help the consumer.

In the past, concern over the quality of foods has led to higher and higher standards. When the public is aroused, scientists investigate, facts are found, and, if necessary, regulations or laws follow. If, after study, we learn how to nourish ourselves better, then even a food craze or a food scare will have served a useful purpose.

RECAP

Food fads and fallacies

Fad diets   Quacks and quackery   The soil depletion myth   "Organic" foods   "Natural" foods

Distinguishing fallacy from fact

Sources of information   Government protection Consumer contributions

THINKING AND EVALUATING

1. Describe three ways you can recognize a food quack or an untrustworthy claim.

2. Describe at least one way in which false food claims can be harmful.

3. Name three sources of trustworthy food information.

4. State four requirements of federal labeling laws.

5. Name at least two government agencies that help supply us with reliable food information. Describe the function of each.

6. Describe two ways in which we as consumers can help improve the quality of our food.

APPLYING AND SHARING

1. Bring to class a food advertisement from a magazine or newspaper, or a tape recording of a food advertisement on television or radio. For each ad, ask the following questions: What nutri-

VOCABULARY

bacteria
fad diet
fallacy
food grade
food quack
food supplement
humus
malnutrition
"natural" food
"organic" food
pesticide
photosynthesis
scurvy
soil depletion
standard of identity

tional information does the ad offer? What feelings does the ad attempt to arouse? Does the ad give you enough information to justify purchase of the food product? If not, what information do you think it should offer?

2. Some people think that food advertising on programs for small children should be severely limited. After the whole class has done research on this question, split into two groups, one group to argue for this proposition, the other group against it.

3. As a group, study the prices of products on sale in local markets and health food shops. Make a chart comparing costs of the same foods at different stores.

4. Study the labels on several different brands of the same kind of food. Which offers the best information? Which do you think is the best food in the group?

5. Look in the *Reader's Guide to Periodical Literature* for current articles on nutrition. Read six of these articles and write a synopsis of each. Does any one of these articles seem to promote a food fad? How do you know?

CAREER CAPSULES

Dietician for food service facility Works in commercial, industrial, educational, nursing, business or government operations; plans, controls, and evaluates diets. Four-year college education in dietetics and R.D. (certificate of registration in the American Dietetic Association) required.

Publicist for food company Works in publicity section of home economics department; writes news releases, conducts press conferences, supplies advertising and marketing departments with promotion materials. Required education varies; ability to write and communicate orally essential.

RELATED READING

Goldbeck, Nikki, and David Goldbeck. *The Supermarket Handbook: Access to Whole Foods.* New York: Harper & Row, 1973. Recommends foods readily available that do not contain a high percentage of additives and synthetics.

Packard, V. S. *Processed Foods and the Consumer: Additives, Labeling Standards, and Nutrition.* St. Paul: University of Minnesota Press, 1976. Discusses topics included in title and such others as "natural" and "organic" foods and toxicants that occur naturally in foods.

Whelan, Elizabeth M., and Fredrick J. Stare. *Panic in the Pantry—Food Facts, Fads, and Fallacies.* New York: Atheneum, 1976. Humorously presents facts about the "health" food movement, food additives, food processing techniques, and the safest and most effective ways of feeding the world's population.

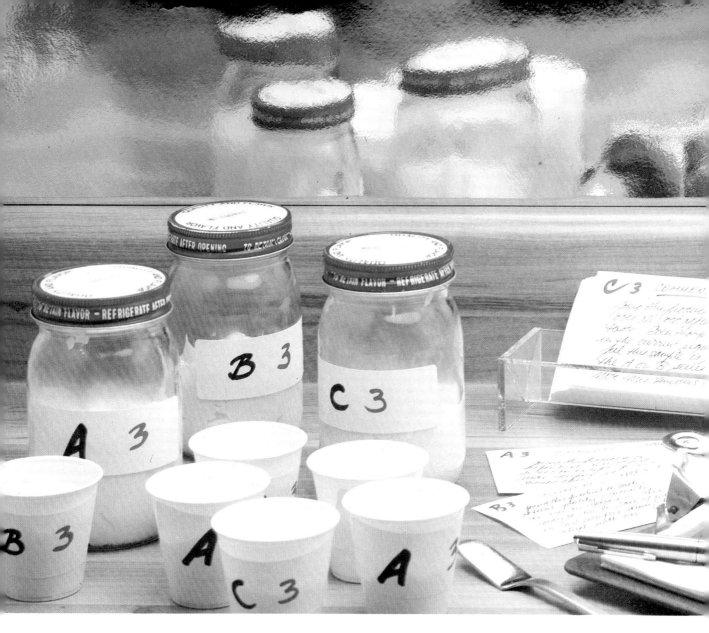

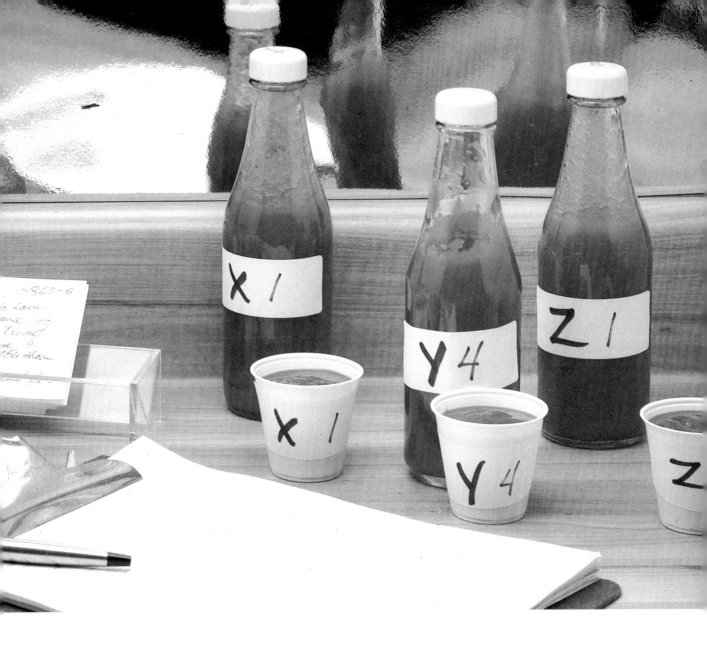

A safe food supply

After studying this chapter, you will be able to

- identify four food poisoning bacteria.
- describe ways to avoid food poisoning at home and in restaurants.
- describe several sources of food contamination.
- identify the responsibilities of scientists, the food industry, individual consumers, and government agencies in preserving the safety of our food.

Over 2 million people suffer from food poisoning every year, according to the U. S. Public Health Service. A person may be slightly ill or seriously ill with food poisoning. It may cause cramps, vomiting, diarrhea, and fever. Symptoms can occur within a few hours after eating or as long as three days later. Certain rare kinds of food poisoning can be fatal.

Food can carry other diseases as well. The U. S. Public Health Service lists 24 diseases carried by bacteria found in contaminated food or water (Table 3-1). In addition, food may contain residues from pesticides, toxins from industrial wastes, residues from antibiotics and chemicals used on ranches and farms, and excessive radioactive fallout. All are hazardous to health.

Concern with the cleanliness and safety of our food supply has a long history. In the seventeenth century, the government of Massachusetts Bay Colony required slaughterhouses to follow certain sanitary standards. With increases in population and new hazards in the twentieth century, we have become increasingly concerned about contamination of our food supply. Many dangers can be overcome by following safeguards at home and in public places. Others require intervention by public interest groups or by the government.

Bacteria that cause food poisoning

Four bacteria are the major causes of food poisoning in the United States. A bacterium called Salmonella causes a common kind of food poisoning. As a rule, it is not fatal. There are 1200

Table 3-1 **Foodborne and waterborne diseases by type of infections**

TYPE OF DISEASE	OUTBREAKS	CASES	PERCENT OF TOTAL CASES
Typhoid fever	65	603	0.6
Salmonellosis	209	10,699	11.7
Shigellosis	99	10,354	11.0
Botulism	56	116	0.1
Staphylococcal food poisoning	633	28,331	30.0
Gastroenteritis, undetermined cause	839	44,083	46.6
Total	1901	94,186	100.0

Reported in a 1952–1960 study by Aimee N. Moore, "Meals away from Home," *Protecting Our Food: Yearbook of Agriculture, 1966* (Washington, D.C.: USDA, 1966), p. 182.

known strains of Salmonella. One or more of these strains may occur in raw meat, fish, poultry, eggs, milk, and products made from these foods. Infected pets may transmit Salmonella to people who handle them.

Salmonella bacteria multiply in the stomach and intestines. However, Salmonella bacteria can easily be destroyed by heating food to 74 °C (165 °F). Thus, bringing most foods to a boil (212 °F) for several minutes kills Salmonella bacteria. Pasteurization kills Salmonella in milk.

About one-third of food-poisoning illnesses are caused by Staphylococcus. This bacterium can grow in all meats, meat products, salads, sandwiches, and particularly in cream fillings in desserts such as cream puffs and chocolate eclairs. "Staph" bacteria form a toxin that is not destroyed by boiling or baking. Proper sanitation and storage are extremely important in preventing the growth of staph bacteria in foods. Refrigerating foods up to the time of serving is the best way to avoid food poisoning caused by Staphylococcus.

The bacterium Clostridia perfringens is widespread in animal feces (excrement), soil, and sewage. Meats that are handled several times—such as chops, ground meat, or stew meat—are particularly vulnerable to Clostridia perfringens. It also occurs in precooked and frozen foods, such as poultry, meats, meat stuffings and gravies, and meat-and-vegetable mixtures.

To avoid diseases from Clostridia perfringens, cool leftovers quickly and refrigerate them at a temperature below 4 °C (40 °F). (You can check the temperature of your refrigerator by putting a thermometer in it.) Since boiling or baking kills Clostridia perfringens as well as Salmonella, reheat leftovers quickly up to at least 60 °C (140 °F) and serve at once.

The food poisoning called botulism, caused by the bacterium Clostridia botulini, is usually fatal. Fortunately, it is rare. It is the result of poor canning methods and seldom shows up in commercially canned food. Deaths from botulism can almost always be traced to home-canned food.

People who can their own foods at home should can non-acid vegetables and meats only in a pressure canner, following the instructions carefully. Botulism bacteria survive boiling temperatures. A higher temperature is necessary to destroy them.

When you are aware of the conditions that encourage the growth of harmful bacteria, you can easily devise some common-sense rules for your protection. Cleanliness of dishes, pots and pans, tabletops, sponges, and dish towels is essential. Always wash your hands before handling food. Much as you love your pets, you should not touch them while you are cooking or eating. Unwashed feeding dishes, toys, or bedding for pets should not come into contact with cooking utensils, working surfaces used in the preparation of food, or with the food itself.

Pesticides

An estimated 625,000 to 1.5 million different kinds of insects share the earth with us, and they want to eat many of the same

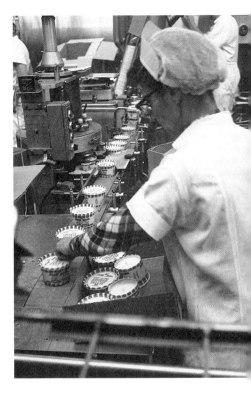

Modern practices in food processing attempt to ensure cleanliness and absence of elements that cause food poisoning.

Proper home canning methods eliminate the possibility of botulism, a form of food poisoning.

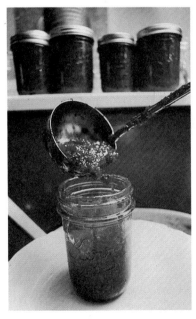

things we do. Insecticides were invented to protect our food supply. However, the methods used to get rid of insect pests have often had damaging effects. Some insecticides have contaminated our food supply, causing illness or other bad effects. For instance, inspectors found that an oil used in making chicken feed contained high residues of the pesticide dieldrin. The FDA removed the contaminated oil from the market, as well as the contaminated feed. In addition, 6.5 million chickens had to be destroyed.

Certain kinds of pesticides have been banned by the U. S. government. One of these is DDT. Scientists discovered that DDT disrupted the reproductive cycle of birds and fish. It has caused cancer and birth deformi-

ties in rats. Though no human deaths from DDT have been reported, DDT has been found in human milk.

The presence of DDT in human beings is a natural result of the way the food chain works. DDT sprayed on crops remains in the soil for many years. DDT becomes a part of plants grown in the contaminated soil. When these plants are eaten by birds and animals, DDT remains in their bodies. And when we eat these contaminated plants, birds, and animals, DDT becomes a part of us. Thus, it became necessary to ban DDT.

Because of the way the food chain works, anything used on crops may eventually be consumed by human beings. For this reason, the federal government tries to control the use of insecticides and weed killers on farms.

Insecticides sprayed or dusted on crops may eventually be consumed by people, and their ingredients and use are controlled by the federal government.

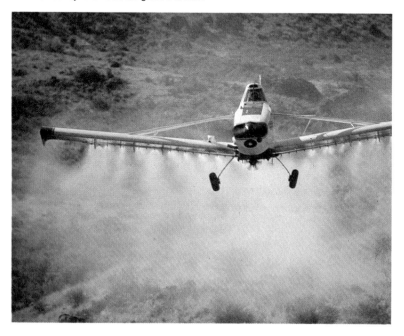

Industrial wastes

In recent years, we have become increasingly aware of the contamination of our environment from many sources. Industrial wastes have polluted the air and water. These wastes enter the food chain and ultimately are eaten by human beings.

The Senate Subcommittee on Energy, National Resources, and the Environment investigates pollution. One expert testified that 27 metals to which we are exposed are even more harmful than pesticides and weed killers. Among these metals are lead and mercury.

Gasoline fumes along heavily traveled highways have a high lead content. Lead also seeps into

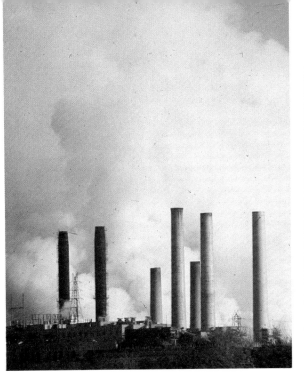
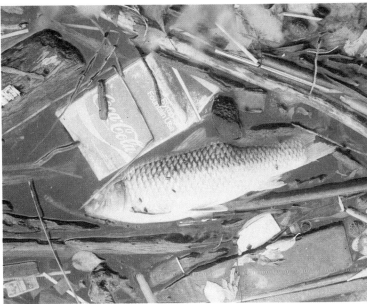

Industrial wastes that pollute the air and water may contaminate the foods we eat.

water carried by lead water pipes. In these and other ways, dangerously high levels of lead enter the food chain.

In 1970, the government officials analyzed the chemical content of certain fish and shellfish. They found that the amount of mercury in these fish was far greater than the amount thought safe for human consumption. Like insecticides, mercury moves along the food chain from water to fish, plants, birds, animals, and human beings.

In Japan, between 1953 and 1960, 43 persons died from mercury poisoning. Many more were severely damaged and handicapped as a result. The mercury came from fish and shellfish caught in Minimata Bay. The mercury was discovered to have originally come from a plastics factory that discharged its wastes into the waters of the bay.

Mercury pollution also comes from the wastes from paper and paint manufacturing, smoke from incinerators and factories, automobile fumes, and sewage. Mercury originates in cinnabar ore. It is estimated that this ore, eroding naturally, causes about 5000 tons of mercury to move through our environment each year.

Scientists continue to be on the lookout for excessive amounts of mercury. For instance, when toxic levels of mercury were found in the livers of Alaskan fur seals, the FDA examined products made from seal livers. It was found that iron supplement pills made from seal livers contained mercury up to 60 times the safe level. These pills were withdrawn from the market.

Currently, researchers are looking for ways to halt mercury pollution. Research is sponsored by the Food and Drug Adminis-

tration, the National Oceanic and Atmosphere Agency, and the fish canning industry.

Additives in animal feeds

Another possible source of contamination is the antibiotics used in animal and poultry feed. Scientists find that antibiotics control diseases and speed up growth. However, long-term feeding of antibiotics to animals could cause them to build up intestinal bacteria that are resistant to antibiotics. If this happens, a new hazard would exist for human beings who eat the animals. We would be exposed to bacteria that our antibiotics cannot fight.

In 1970–1972, a team of scientists appointed by the FDA studied this possibility. As a result

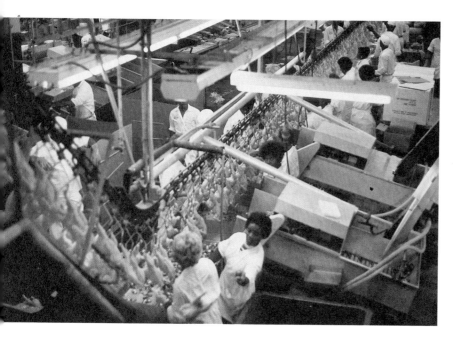

Additives to animal feeds and processing chemicals must not leave a residue in animal food products that will harm people.

animals. They must show that the proposed rate of use will not leave any harmful residue in milk, meat, or eggs. The feed label must show specific directions for use. Farmers and ranchers must follow the directions.

Additives in human foods

Another possible source of contamination that worries many people is the chemical additives used by the food industry (Table 3-2). Most additives make food more attractive and tasty or preserve it longer. Some chemicals become part of the food by accident. Chemicals from wrappings, for instance, sometimes get into the food itself.

Nitrates and nitrites used to process meats, poultry, and fish are currently under study. Nitrates and nitrites preserve foods and prevent botulism. They help retain the red color of meats. They also improve the flavor and texture of some foods.

Researchers have found that nitrites and amines (a natural product of digestion) can combine in the human digestive tract to form chemicals called nitrosamines. According to the U. S. Department of Health, Education, and Welfare, nitrosamines can cause cancer in animals. There is no substitute for nitrites but vitamin C helps reduce the amount needed to process meat products. Meanwhile, nitrates or nitrites added to processed meats such as frankfurters or smoked meats must be listed on the label. Consumers can thus avoid them if they wish.

of their research, almost a thousand drugs were banned from use in animal feed. Certain antibiotics that are important in human medicine were taken out of animal feeds. Others may be given only on a veterinarian's prescription.

Another result of the study was that the animal feed industry was ordered to find substitute drugs that could increase growth rate in animals. The industry was also asked to do further research on the use of antibiotics in animal feed. There is no firm evidence that the meat supply is in danger. It may be that early alertness has forestalled future problems.

Every chemical added to the food of livestock must be approved by the FDA. Manufacturers of animal feed must show that a proposed additive meets certain standards. Manufacturers must conduct tests by feeding their product to at least two species of

Table 3-2 Selected examples of chemical additives in foods[1]

ADDITIVE	PURPOSE OF ADDITIVE	FOOD USING ADDITIVE
Natural herbs, spices, extracts, carvone, benzaldehyde, amyl acetate	To enhance flavor, making many foods more enjoyable to the taste	Cakes, confections, gelatins, beverages, toppings, desserts, meats
Carotene, cochineal, chlorophyll, annatto	To enhance color, making foods more appealing in appearance	Butter, margarine, cheese, pastries, beverages, confections, ice creams, jams
Mono- and diglycerides, lecithin, agar-agar, starch, pectin, gum arabic, gelatin, methylcellulose, sorbitol	To stabilize, emulsify, thicken, or make a smooth texture	Frozen desserts, salad dressings, chocolate milk, ice cream, cake mixes
Sodium and calcium propionate, BHT (butylated hydroxytoluene), BHA (butylated hydroxyanisole), vitamin E (antioxidant)	To prevent oxidation and spoilage; to delay spoilage by molds, yeasts, bacteria, and to retard rancidity in fats	Breads, cereals, baked grain foods, fats, oils, fatty foods, cheese, fruit juices, syrups, frozen and dried fruit, cake mixes, pie fillings
Sodium bicarbonate, potassium tartrate, tartaric acid, lactic acid, citric acid	To alter acidity or alkalinity; to act as a leavening agent in baking; and to add flavor	Cake, cookies, other baked foods, cheese spread, processed cheese, chocolates, confections, beverages
Chlorine, chlorinedioxide, potassium bromate, and iodate potassium	To bleach or mature; to make cream-colored flour white	White flour, some cheeses
Sorbitol	To retain moisture; to act as an anticaking agent; and to improve flavor	Mixes, salad dressings, bread, cakes
Riboflavin, thiamin, niacin, vitamin B6, vitamin B12, vitamins A, D, C (ascorbic acid), potassium iodide, iron	To increase nutritive value	Flour, cereals, cornmeal, pastas, baby foods, margarine, nonfat milk, iodized salt, beverages, other foods

[1] Other chemicals are added to foods to retain moisture; to prevent caking, drying, sticking, hardening, or foaming; to act as noncaloric sweeteners; to whip foods; and to propel food from cans under pressure.

All chemicals added to food must undergo rigorous tests, according to a 1958 Food Additives Amendment to the Food, Drug, and Cosmetic Act. A food processor who wants to use a chemical must test it on at least two species of animals and then present proof of its safety to FDA scientists. The FDA approves, rejects, or returns the chemical for further research. Any additive that is found to induce cancer in either animals or humans must be removed from the market.

Radiation

The effects of radioactivity in our food are a source of concern. The sun constantly gives off radioactivity. We have added to the amount of radiation in our environment by testing nuclear bombs. Some appliances, such as microwave ovens and color television sets, also add to radiation levels in the atmosphere. We know that there is a definite relationship between radiation and cancer.

Table 3-3 shows the kinds of fallout from nuclear tests that are most harmful to us. Fruits and vegetables above the earth catch

Table 3-3 Important fallout isotopes in food and water

ELEMENT	HALF-LIFE[1]	CHARACTERISTICS
IODINE 133	22 hours	Chemically similar to iodine, which is an essential nutrient.
IODINE 131	8 days	Accumulates in the thyroid gland.
CESIUM 137	29.7 years	Chemically similar to potassium, which is an essential nutrient. Locates in muscles and can cause cell damage, including genetic. Not contained in the body long, as it enters and leaves the body continually, like potassium.
STRONTIUM 89	50.5 days	Both behave chemically like calcium in plants and animals.
STRONTIUM 90	27.7 years	Laid down in the bones, as explained in Chapter 7. Can cause serious illness, such as bone cancer. Children more affected than adults, because of influence on growth.

A. B. Park, "Fallout and Food," *Protecting Our Food: Yearbook of Agriculture, 1966* (Washington, D.C.: USDA, 1966), pp. 340–341.
[1] When the reading of radioactive fallout is measured, the term "half-life" is used to measure the rate of radioactive decay. It is the time lapse during which a radioactive mass loses one-half its radioactivity.

and hold fallout. Moved by wind and rain, fallout penetrates the soil and surface water all over the world. Eventually the fallout in the soil is absorbed by plants. Soil that receives heavy rainfall shows more fallout than drier soil.

We are not certain at present that normal levels of radiation in the atmosphere were or are a danger. Certainly the banning of nuclear tests should help prevent further increases in radiation. For those who are still concerned about radiation, washing and peeling most foods usually gets rid of most of their radioactive contamination.

CONTROL OF CONTAMINATION

With so many different kinds of food contamination, the task of guaranteeing a safe food supply is enormous. To succeed, we must all contribute to the effort. First of all, scientists can help by doing extensive research. Second, the food industry must be responsible for its products. Third, consumers must learn to be alert to dangers and to make intelligent choices. Fourth, the government may be required to take action.

Food-production research

Scientists continue to search for safe and effective ways to destroy insects harmful to food without contaminating the food. One method is attractants, poisons placed not on growing foods but near them. In an experiment on a Pacific island, male fruit flies were attracted to a bait which destroyed them. In less than six months, fruit flies disappeared from the island. This safe and inexpensive technique might be adapted for use with other insect pests. Other methods include sterilization of insects by radiation, and the introduction of predators (the insects' natural enemies).

By careful breeding, we have developed plants and animals better able to resist disease. Strong, healthy plants grown in nourishing soil and animals fed a well-balanced diet are more resistant to disease and insects.

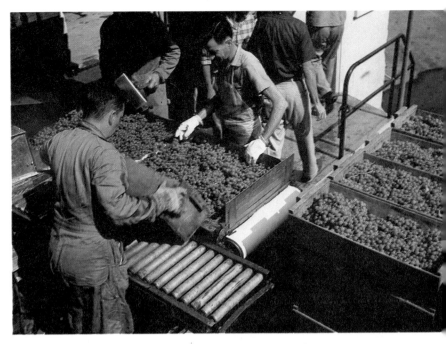

Industry self-regulation

Food industries and restaurants have practical reasons for ensuring a safe and nutritious food product. A good reputation means profit. Food processors whose food has been removed from the market lose money and also lose their reputation. If the FDA is forced to remove a food from grocery shelves, the resulting publicity can hurt a company's sales for years afterwards. It can even drive a firm out of business.

Similarly, restaurants and other public or institutional eating places do not want to be responsible for food poisoning. Most train their employees to observe high standards of cleanliness. In addition, state and federal government health codes regulate food institutions. Eating places

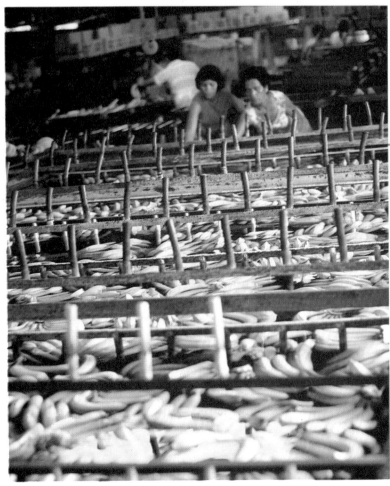

New ways of growing and processing foods more safely are continually being developed in scientific research.

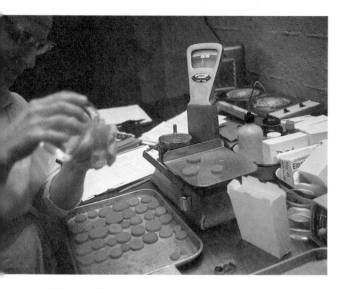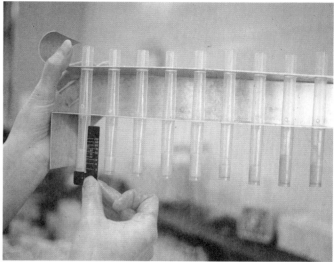

The food industries, including vegetable and milk processors, voluntarily strive to improve their standards for food safety in order to protect their reputations.

are inspected regularly. If they do not observe the law, they can be closed down.

Consumer awareness and action

The individual person must learn to avoid illness from unclean food and water in the home. In addition, consumers should report any violations of the law to the government.

When eating out, choose a clean place. If you have a choice between a restaurant where you see dishes and silverware being washed by hand and a restaurant that has an electric dishwasher, the eating place with an automatic dishwasher is generally safer. Refuse to eat from an unclean or cracked serving dish. Reject a food that smells or tastes spoiled. If you observe a food worker doing anything that might con-

taminate food, report the incident to the manager.

At home, always wash your hands before handling food. Do not sneeze or cough on food. If you have a cut or sore, keep it thoroughly bandaged while working with food or eating.

Scrub chopping blocks and counter tops with a strong detergent. Wash dishcloths with strong detergent and chlorine bleach. Use only clean utensils.

Most molds are not harmful. However, except for cheeses, throw away moldy food.

Foods that stand at room temperature for four hours can develop toxins. Be sure to heat all leftover, precooked, and frozen foods thoroughly. Bacteria that cause food poisoning can be destroyed by boiling food on top of the stove or by heating it in the oven to an internal temperature of 74 °C or 165 °F. You can use a meat thermometer (a ther-

54

mometer that pierces meat to reach the center) to be sure of internal temperature.

Keep foods that contain a thick mixture of eggs—such as cream puffs, eclairs, cream pies, and mayonnaise—in the refrigerator. Take them out of the refrigerator only at the time of serving.

Before traveling in foreign countries, find out from the U. S. Public Health Service if the water in the countries you will be visiting is considered safe to drink. If it is not, drink only boiled or bottled water. Unless you are very sure of high standards of cleanliness in a foreign country, avoid raw salads and cold cooked foods. Peel any fresh fruit that you eat. Never eat unwashed fresh fruit anywhere.

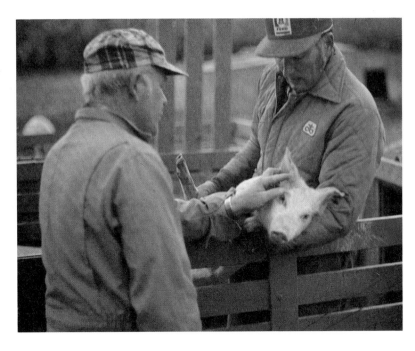

Government legislation and enforcement

Federal, state, and local laws govern all aspects of food production and marketing. As voters, we can see that these laws are updated as needed. Some of the most important federal laws follow.

The Food, Drug, and Cosmetic Act, first passed in 1906, has been revised and amended many times. The Food Additive Amendment, which regulates the addition of chemicals to foods, was one of these additions. Another amendment in 1960 gave the FDA authority to control how much and what kind of artificial colorings may be added to foods. As a result, some food dyes have been banned.

The Fair Labeling and Packaging Act of 1966 states that the accurate weight or volume must appear on a food product label. This law is enforced by the FDA.

The Wholesome Meat Act of 1967 and the Wholesome Poultry Act of 1968 set standards for meat and poultry. The U. S. Department of Agriculture enforces these laws.

The Insecticide, Fungicide, and Rodenticide Act was passed in 1947. Amended in 1972, it became the Environmental Pesticide Control Act. The U. S. Environmental Protection Agency is entrusted with the law's enforcement.

The Radiation Control for Health and Safety Act of 1968 sets standards for safety of electronic products such as microwave ovens. The FDA enforces this law.

The Public Health Service Act of 1944 helps to ensure the safety of pasteurized milk and shellfish. It regulates sanitation of food, water, and food services, as well as sanitary facilities on trains, planes, and buses.

Government legislation sets standards for meat and poultry, and the USDA controls inspection

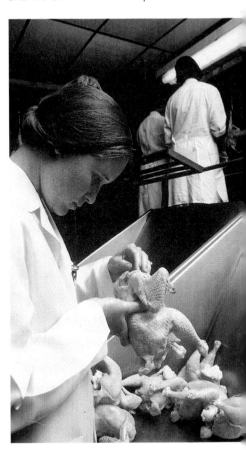

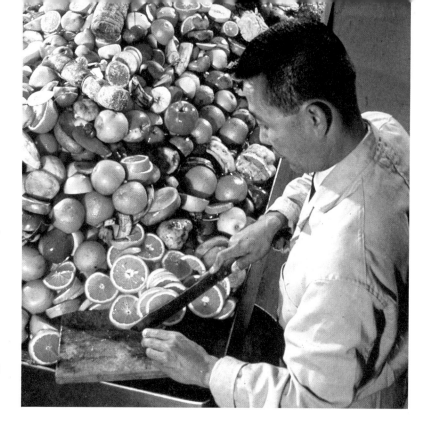

Foods imported from other countries must meet standards set by the U.S. government.

The Model Ordinance and Code for Food Service Sanitation aims to identify and exclude from public food service any person with a communicable disease. With its revisions, it excludes persons "affected with boils, infected wounds, sores, or an acute infection." It also tries to promote good habits of personal cleanliness among food workers.

The Nutritional Labeling Act of 1973 aims to provide consumers with nutritional information to help them buy wisely. Nutritional labeling is required on foods for which the processor makes a nutritional claim and on foods to which nutrients have been added.

In addition to these laws, which cover domestic production of food, the federal government also inspects imported food. Officials do not permit food that does not meet set standards to enter the country. For instance, government inspectors once rejected a shipment of cheese from a foreign country because tests showed that the cheese contained too much of a poisonous spray. The officials in the foreign country then did much the same kind of detective work we do to find the source of the poisonous spray. They finally discovered that a spray used on the timbers of a barn to kill insects had dripped onto stored hay. The hay was fed to cows that produced the milk from which the cheese had been made.

Occurrences such as this show that all of us—scientists, workers in the food industry, consumers, and government officials—must remain alert to find and eliminate threats to our food supply.

Dangers to our food supply

Bacteria that cause food poisoning   Pesticides
Industrial wastes   Additives in animal feeds   Additives in human foods

Control of contamination

Food production research   Industry self-regulation
Consumer awareness and action   Government legislation and enforcement

THINKING AND EVALUATING

1. Name four bacteria that commonly cause food poisoning. Describe some symptoms of food poisoning.

2. Describe three ways in which food poisoning can be avoided in the home kitchen.

3. Name five sources of food contamination other than bacteria. Describe how each contaminant enters our food supply.

4. Describe the responsibilities to protect the safety of food of (a) scientists, (b) food industry workers, and (c) consumers.

5. Describe three ways in which you can avoid food poisoning in restaurants and public eating places.

6. Name at least five federal laws that protect our food supply. Describe the purpose of each.

APPLYING AND SHARING

1. What do you think should be done in the future to improve the safety of our food supply? Write an essay supporting your suggestions with facts. Identify the source of your facts (the person or publication).

2. You may have observed a violation of food laws in your own community. Write the agency concerned stating the facts. Read your letter in class and send copies of your letter to others who can help.

3. Ask a government representative to speak to your class on food safety. Some agencies you might contact with this request are the U. S. Public Health Service, the U. S. Department of Agriculture Extension Office, a local office of the Environmental Protection Agency, a local office of the Food and Drug Administration.

4. As a group, visit food markets and restaurants in your neighborhood, rating them for food safety. Discuss the results of this survey in class. Your school newspaper may be willing to publish the results of your study.

VOCABULARY

antibiotics
botulism
Clostridia botulini
Clostridia perfringens
DDT
food chain
insecticides
predators
Salmonella
Staphylococcus

5. Divide the class into two groups. One group may devise a menu for a holiday dinner at home. The group should describe safety precautions for purchasing and cooking the foods for the dinner. The second group may decide how to use leftovers remaining from each dish offered on the menu. Describe how each leftover should be stored and how it should be later prepared for eating.

CAREER CAPSULES

Environmental scientist Works in laboratory, experimental farm, and "in the field"; researches soil and water conservation, relationship to plants and animals of insects, fertilizers, air and water pollution. Four-year college education in science required; higher degree required for some specialities.

Food production manager Manages plant, sales district, or personnel; oversees operations, purchasing, quality control, distribution. Two- or four-year college education and/or extensive on-the-job training required.

RELATED READING

Leverton, Ruth M. "Consumer Responsibility." *Protecting Our Food: Yearbook of Agriculture, 1966.* Washington, D.C.: USDA, 1966. Discusses the dangers in discrediting our food supply by demanding our rights, instead of recognizing our own responsibilities in keeping our food supply safe.

Moore, Aime N. "Meals Away from Home." *Protecting Our Food: Yearbook of Agriculture, 1966.* Washington, D.C.: USDA, 1966. Focuses on the safety of foods served in public eating places and discusses protection from foodborne and waterborne disease, food poisoning, foreign matters in food, planning and selecting of menus.

Mrack, Emil M. "New Sciences Spring Up to Create Food Miracles." *That We May Eat: Yearbook of Agriculture, 1975.* Washington, D.C.: USDA, 1975. Shows the contributions of scientists to the more sanitary, flavorful, nutritious, safe, and easy-to-prepare diet that has helped improve the quality of life in this century.

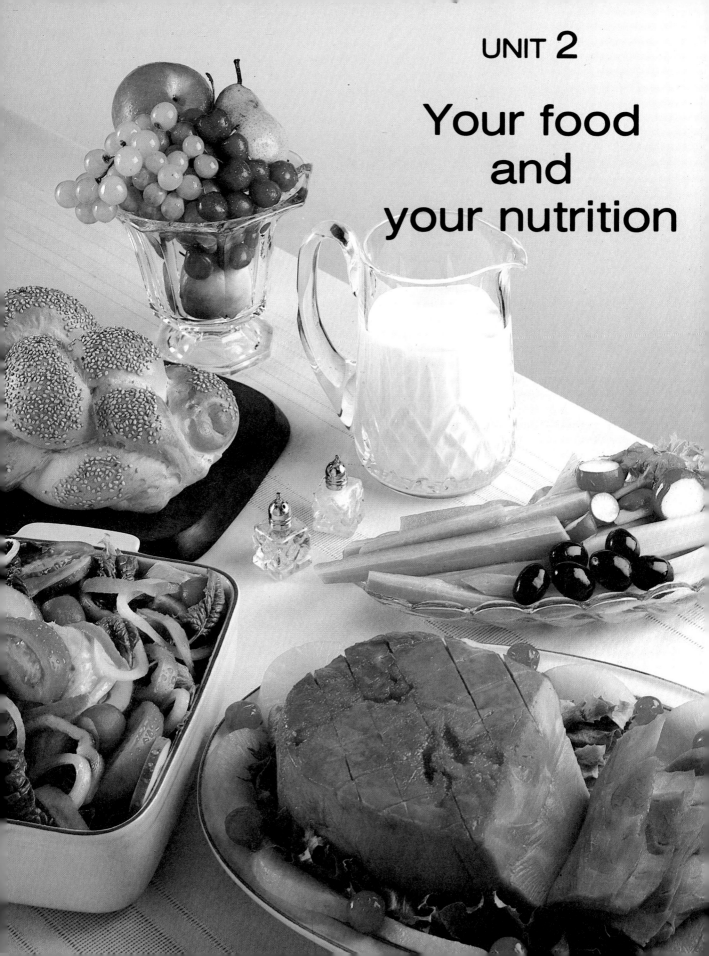

UNIT 2

Your food and your nutrition

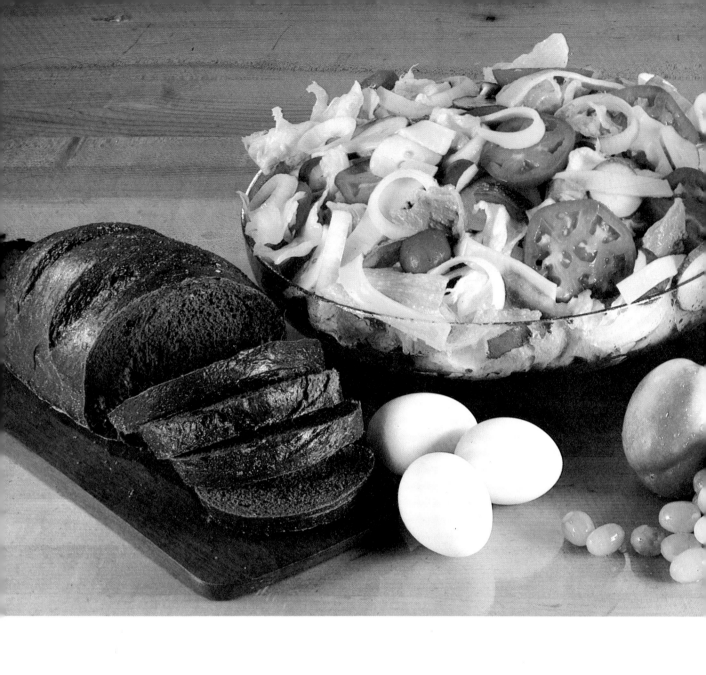

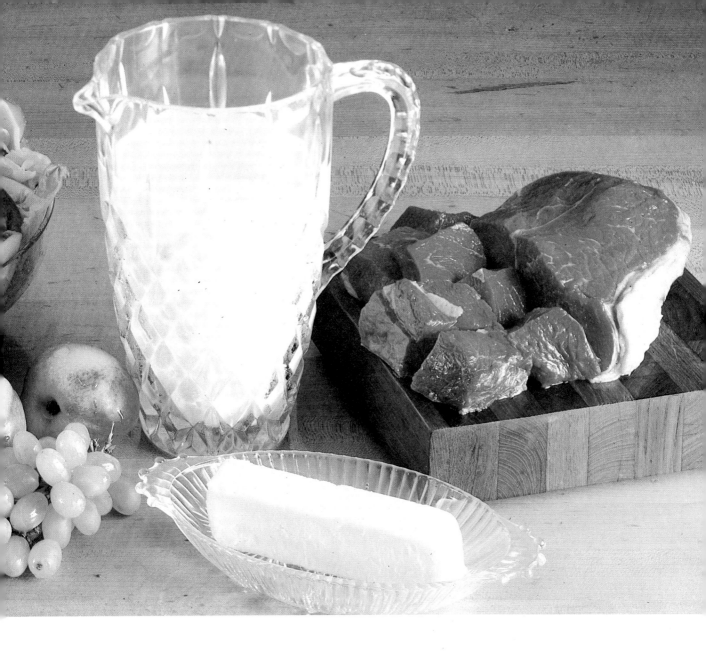

Balancing your diet

HOW DOES THE BODY USE FOOD?

Nutrition is the study of how the body uses food. It has also been defined as the chemistry of life, or the study of how health, appearance, mental alertness, and physical vitality depend upon diet.

What happens when you lift a piece of toast to your mouth and crunch down on it? Automatically your jaws and tongue start working. The crunchy piece of toast turns into mush. Casually you swallow it and probably never think about it again.

And yet there is a lot more to the business of eating than biting, chewing, and swallowing. The most important part of eating, in fact, happens after you lose all awareness of the food passing through your system. After all, food has no value to you until it is transformed chemically and becomes part of your body. How does this amazing transformation take place?

Food is changed by the body in three processes. It is changed by (1) digestion, (2) absorption, and (3) metabolism.

Digestion

Digestion refers to the way food is broken down, both mechanically and chemically, so that the body can absorb it and distribute it (Table 4-1 and Figure 4-1). Digestion begins in the mouth, continues in the stomach, and is completed in the small intestine.

The chewing of food starts the digestive process. Chewing grinds food into small particles, moistens it with saliva, and releases nutrients. In the saliva, an enzyme

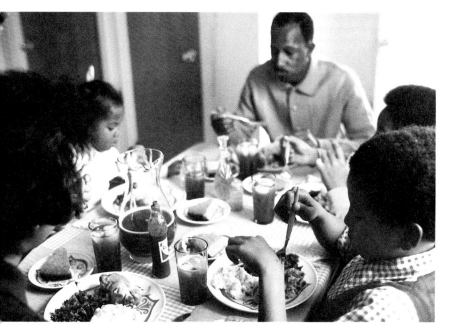

A good diet results from knowing how to plan each meal of the day.

Table 4-1 **Process of digestion**

NUTRIENT	FOOD	SPLIT BY DIGESTIVE JUICES DURING DIGESTION	FUNCTIONS IN BODY
PROTEINS	Meat, poultry, fish, organs, milk, cheese, eggs, legumes, nuts, cereal grains, others	Amino acids absorbed into bloodstream	Build tissues in all parts of body for growth and repair. Help to build hormones, enzymes, antibodies, and some vitamins. Help regulate body functioning. Used as energy, if needed.
FATS	Oils; hard, soft, and semi-soft fats; fats in foods, visible and invisible	Fatty acids and glycerols absorbed by blood and lymph after being finely emulsified in small intestines	Concentrated energy-heat. Provide essential fatty acids. Help in absorption and use of fat-soluble vitamins. Give flavor and satiety to diet. Perform other functions.
CARBOHYDRATES	Starch and sugars	Glucose—absorbed by blood Fructose Galactose	Simple sugar gives only energy-heat, flavor. "Complex" starch carries many other nutrients.

Figure 4-1   Food must be processed in the digestive tract in order to be used by the body.

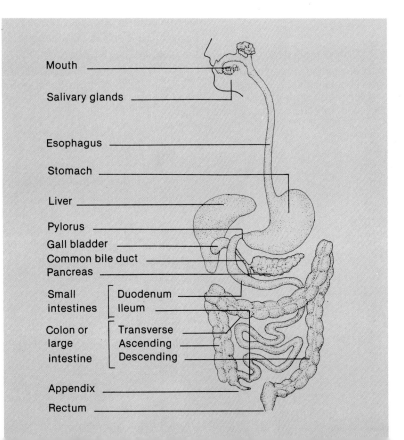

Mouth
Salivary glands
Esophagus
Stomach
Liver
Pylorus
Gall bladder
Common bile duct
Pancreas
Small intestines   Duodenum   Ileum
Colon or large intestine   Transverse   Ascending   Descending
Appendix
Rectum

called **ptyalin** begins to digest starches and sugars. Ptyalin splits up simple sugars and breaks starch into smaller molecules. It thereby prepares these foods for absorption.

Food now moves from the mouth into the stomach. Here begins an amazing process that the body performs automatically without aid from our conscious brain. The food pulp in the stomach is churned about by strong muscular contractions called

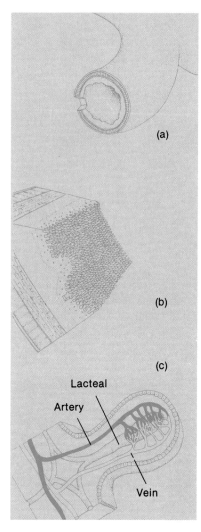

Lacteal

Artery

Vein

Figure 4-2 Food is absorbed into the body by the small intestine. (a) Wall of small intestine. (b) Lining of intestinal wall, showing villi. (c) Structure of villus.

peristaltic waves. Swallowed saliva mixes with the food pulp. In the upper part of the stomach, the digestion of carbohydrates continues. Gastric juice flows in and protein and fat now begin to be digested. At the same time, the acid in the gastric juice stops the action of the ptyalin. This in turn stops the digestion of starch and sugar.

Now the food is slowly pushed out of the stomach into the small intestine (Figure 4-2). Though narrow in width, the small intestine is approximately 720 cm (24 ft) long. It carries out the major part of the digestive process. A number of enzymes are secreted by different organs of the body to aid the final stage of digestion. For example, the liver produces bile, and the gall bladder, which stores bile, gradually releases it. The bile mixes with fat and produces a fine emulsion of fats. Enzymes can now split the complex fat molecules into smaller and separate parts. The pancreas also adds its enzymes to those in the intestinal juice. Finally the work of the small intestine—digesting protein, carbohydrate, and fat—is complete.

Absorption

The next step is for the digested food in the small intestine to become absorbed into the blood stream. The process depends upon tiny folds of fingerlike tissue, called villi, which line the intestine wall (Figure 4-2). There are more than five million of these villi. If they could be stretched out, they would represent a total surface area of about 4 m² (45 sq ft) or more. As food moves down the intestine, indigestible material from fruits, vegetables, and whole grains form bulk. Peristaltic waves push the bulk against the sides of the small intestine and the millions of villi. The villi close around the nutrients pressed against them and absorb almost all the nutrients into the bloodstream.

Metabolism

Metabolism refers to all the chemical changes that take place in the tissues of the body. There are really two processes in metabolism. The first is called anabolism. It is the process of building up new cells. The second is called catabolism. It is the process of breaking down old cells. Through anabolism, food is changed by chemical means into body tissue (Figure 4-3). Healthy cells are maintained; deteriorated cells are repaired. At the same time the process of catabolism is at work destroying old, useless tissues. Waste products are broken down into simple substances—oxygen, hydrogen, carbon, and nitrogen products. These are then eliminated in excretions.

Through the process of metabolism, the foods we eat are chemically taken apart and built into new tissues. Food is also immediately used as energy. The surplus is stored as fat.

Physicians often talk about something they call your basal metabolism. Do not confuse this with the concept of metabolism. Basal metabolism is something that can be measured. Physicians define it as the very least amount

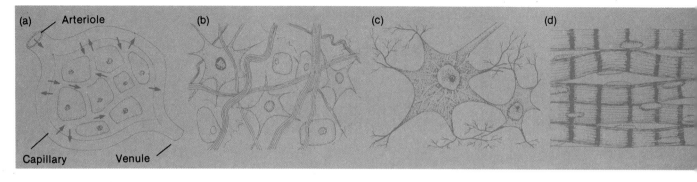

(a) Arteriole

Capillary   Venule

(b)

(c)

(d)

Figure 4-3   Different kinds of cells make different kinds of tissues from the nutrients supplied by the blood. (a) Cell. The arrows indicate the constant movement through tiny porous capillaries of nutrients to cells and waste from cells. (b) Connective tissue. (c) Nerve tissue. (d) Muscle tissue.

of energy required to keep the internal life processes going. It is the least energy needed to keep the heart beating, the blood circulating, the lungs breathing, and the temperature controlled. In fact it is the energy needed for all the body's involuntary or automatic systems.

WHAT IS A BALANCED DIET?

A balanced diet is the variety of foods in the correct proportions needed to provide all the necessary nutrients for growth, energy, and health. The aim of a balanced diet is to keep the supply of food eaten for energy in balance with your needs for good nutrition.

Food, when digested and absorbed, helps your body develop according to your hereditary pattern. **Nutrients** are the different parts of a food that are supplied to the body for the purpose of nourishment. They include proteins, carbohydrates, fats, vitamins, and minerals. Protein, car-

A variety of foods in the correct proportions is needed to provide the nutrients for maintaining good health.

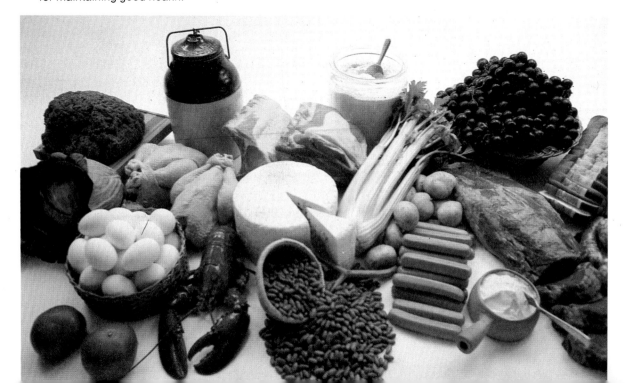

Table 4-2 How the body uses energy-heat nutrients

NUTRIENT (1 g)	CALORIE YIELD	MAIN FUNCTION IN THE BODY	HOW EXCESS AMOUNTS ARE USED
CARBOHYDRATE	4	Burned to yield energy-heat. Spares the use of protein. Helps use fat.	Stored as glycogen in small amounts. Changed to fat and stored as body fat.
FAT	9	Burned to yield energy-heat. Forms tissue fat. Has other necessary functions.	Stored as body fat. Burned for energy as needed.
PROTEIN	4	Builds and repairs body tissues. Essential for life and growth. Part of team to form hormones, enzymes, antibodies, and cells. Small amount burned to yield energy (after eliminating nitrogen), if needed.	Burned for energy or stored as fat.

bohydrates, and fats provide energy heat in the form of calories (Table 4-2). Vitamins and minerals are necessary to tissue building and to body functions.

Chemists tell us that the body needs some 50 nutrients. A well-nourished body is capable of manufacturing 25 of these nutrients. Aided by enzymes and hormones, different tissues select different combinations of nutrients to build and repair the body.

Recommended Dietary Allowances (RDA)

How can we determine how much food provides an adequate supply of the necessary nutrients? The United States government has been studying the question of dietary goals since 1936. During that depression year, a nationwide survey of eating habits revealed that about one-third of the American people had poor diets. Then, in 1940, the Food and Nutrition Board of the National Academy of Sciences' National Research Council was developed to guide the government in its nutrition program. The Food and Nutrition Board published the government's first guidelines for improving Americans' eating habits. The Food and Nutrition Board's guidelines were titled Recommended Dietary Allowances. They are listed in detail on pages 402-403.

The Food and Nutrition Board meets at least once every five years to review and refine its recommendations based on current research and current need. Members of the board, appointed by the National Research Council, are selected for their ability to interpret nutrition research and for their sound judgment.

In 1968, the board added seven new nutrients to those formerly recommended. They were three B vitamins (B_6, B_{12}, and folacin [folic acid]); one fat-soluble vitamin (E); and three minerals (phosphorous, iodine, and magnesium). In 1973, the board added another mineral, zinc, to its recommended list and lowered its calorie recommendations.

A summary of the foundation foods and recommended daily requirements is shown in Table 4-3. Each group provides many different nutrients, but not in the same proportions. The milk group is particularly rich in calcium, for example. The meat group is an excellent source of protein. Vegetables and fruits are high in vitamins C and A. The grains provide carbohydrates, and some proteins, and vitamins.

Calorie requirements

A calorie is a measure of energy or heat released from food. Whenever fat, carbohydrate, or protein is oxidized (burned) in body tissue, heat is given off.

Because of modern conveniences people today burn up less energy than in the past. In pioneer America, children often walked 3 to 8 km (2 to 5 mi) a day to school. Their parents burned up energy in rugged activity. Today machines do the heavy work on the job. We have labor-saving appliances and foods in the home, we do little outdoor work, and we rarely walk when we can ride in cars, buses, and planes. As a result of advanced technology, people tend to be less physically active.

Therefore, in 1974 the Food and Nutrition Board recommended that people reduce their calorie intake. It recommended that males age 15 or older consume only 2400 to 3000 calories a day (in 1948, 4500 calories were recommended), depending on age and body size and structure. For females age 15 or older, the board recommended between 1800 to 2100 calories a day (in 1948, 3000 calories were recommended for women). For more details, see the RDA tables on pages 402-403.

Of course, the purpose of reducing caloric intake is to keep from becoming overweight. At the same time, medical experts advise us to use up body energy in physical exercise. It is important to burn up the calories we eat. If we eat as the physically active do and yet are physically inactive, we are certain to add excess weight.

Table 4-3 **Foundation foods: Daily recommendations for all ages**

FOOD GROUP	DAILY RECOMMENDATION
MILK	3 or more servings (a serving equals 240 mL [8 oz] milk or yogurt, or a calcium equivalent such as 42 g [1½ oz] Cheddar cheese, 240 mL [8 oz] pudding, 420 g [14 oz] ice cream, or 480 mL [16 oz] cottage cheese)
MEATS	2 or more servings (a serving equals 56 g [2 oz] cooked lean meat, fish or poultry, or a protein equivalent such as 2 eggs, 56 g [2 oz] Cheddar cheese, 240 mL [1 c] dried beans, or 60 mL [4 T] peanut butter)
VEGETABLES AND FRUIT	4 or more servings (a serving cooked is 120 mL [½ c] or a portion commonly served such as a whole potato, a medium apple, orange, or banana). A dark green or deep yellow vegetable at least every other day. A citrus fruit, tomato, raw cabbage or other vitamin C-rich foods. A potato or equivalent. Other vegetables and fruits.
GRAINS	4 or more servings of a fortified, enriched or whole grain (a serving equals 1 slice of bread, 160 mL [½ c] cooked cereal, or 240 mL [1 c] ready-to-eat cereal)
FATS	Some in the form of vegetable oil high in linoleic acid to season food
SWEETS	In proportion to individual need to make the diet more palatable and satisfying

Figure 4-4   Different foods contain different amounts of water.

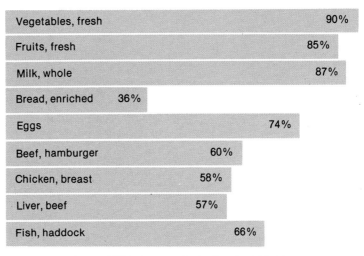

Nutritive Value of Foods, USDA Home and Garden Bulletin 72 (Washington, D.C.: Government Printing Office, 1963).

Water in the diet

As a substance water is an important part of every cell in the body. Water constitutes 55 to 70 percent of the body weight. It is needed for every body function, including the use of all the nutrients and the removal of waste products. Water helps regulate body temperature. It even helps in moving the joints and in other mechanical functions the body performs.

When the food we eat daily is oxidized or burned, about 360 mL (1½ c) of water is formed in the end products. Study Figure 4-4 to see the amount of water present in different foods.

IMPORTANCE OF BALANCED MEALS

We've seen how food is transformed through digestion and absorption. We've also learned what a balanced diet is. Now we can put the two ideas together and see how a balanced diet assists the process of digesting and absorbing food.

Whether our meals are balanced or unbalanced, the body takes full control over the way the food is digested and absorbed. Determining what we eat is the only way to control digestion and absorption. Therefore, our food choices are important to the growth and maintenance of our bodies.

Planning balanced meals

A good diet results from knowing how to plan each meal and snack of the day. Table 4-4 shows how the foundation foods may be chosen for individual meals to provide a balanced diet. Follow-

**Table 4-4 Translating the pattern for a balanced diet
into balanced daily meals and snacks**

PATTERN	BREAKFAST MENU	MENU ALTERNATES
FRUIT OR JUICE (rich in vitamin C)	Whole orange	½ grapefruit, citrus juices, tomato juice, ½ cantaloupe, berries, other fruits in season
MAIN DISH (protein)	Scrambled egg with cottage cheese	Whole-grain or enriched cereal cooked with nonfat dry milk; ready-to-eat cereal and milk; French toast; pancakes, waffles, spoon bread; lean ham, broiled chops, liver, kidneys, or fish; cheese, peanut butter, cottage cheese
MILK (fortified with vitamin D)	240 mL (8 oz), whole or skim	Cheese, yogurt (nonfat, low-fat, or whole), hot chocolate, milk shake
BREAD (whole-grain or enriched)	1 slice or more	Toast, plain; hot quick breads; sweet breads (if calories permit)
SOFT MARGARINE, BUTTER, OR VEGETABLE OIL	5–10 mL (1–2 t)	More or less, according to need
SWEET	5–15 mL (1 t–1 T) jam	More or less, according to need
HOT BEVERAGE	Coffee, tea, or others	Sugar, milk, or lemon added, according to taste and need

PATTERN	LUNCH OR SUPPER MENU	MENU ALTERNATES
MAIN DISH (protein)	Tuna fish salad	Other fish salads, chicken or turkey salad, bean or fruit salad; chef's salad, egg salad; cottage cheese; hot casserole dish using cheese, baked beans, meat, fish, or poultry with any combination of vegetables and/or rice, noodles, bulgur, or macaroni products; omelet; soups, such as bean, meat-vegetable, fish or poultry chowder, pea, lentil, or minestrone; sandwiches, such as meat, fish, poultry, cheese, eggs, peanut butter, baked beans, hamburgers, frankfurters, or liverwurst; enchiladas with cheese filling; tacos with beans, meat, or cheese filling
BREAD (whole-grain or enriched)	Hot corn muffin	Other hot muffins, popovers (plain), toasted English muffins, crackers, fresh yeast bread, any quick bread
MILK	240 mL (8 oz)	Cottage cheese; other foods as suggested for breakfast
SOFT MARGARINE, BUTTER, OR VEGETABLE OIL	5 mL (1 t)	More or less, according to need
DESSERT	1 banana	Fresh fruit in season, canned, or frozen; ice cream, ice milk, pudding; cookie, gingerbread, deep-dish fruit pie

Table 4-4 cont. on next page.

Table 4-4 (cont.)

PATTERN	SNACK MENU	MENU ALTERNATES
FRUIT	1 apple	See Table 4-5 for alternates

PATTERN	DINNER OR SUPPER MENU	MENU ALTERNATES
MEAT, FISH, POULTRY, ORGAN MEAT, EGG OR ALTERNATE	Baked fresh ham	Lean pork (fresh or cured), lean beef, lamb, chicken, turkey; fish, shellfish; liver; beans, peas, lentils (dried); cheese, eggs
STARCHY VEGETABLE	1 med. baked potato	White or sweet potatoes, parsnips; hot breads; rice, macaroni products, bulgur; dumplings
GREEN OR YELLOW VEGETABLE	120 mL (½ c) cooked collards	Turnip greens, spinach, dandelion greens, kale, broccoli, Swiss chard, lettuce; yellow squash, corn, carrots; others
RAW VEGETABLE SALAD OR FRESH FRUIT	½ cantaloupe	Other fresh, canned, or frozen, fruit; raw finger vegetables or salad with lettuce or cabbage
BREAD (whole-grain or enriched)	1 slice or more	Toast, hot quick breads, sweet breads (if calories permit)
SOFT MARGARINE, BUTTER, OR VEGETABLE OIL	5–10 mL (1–2 t)	More or less, according to need
BEVERAGE	Milk, coffee, or tea	Sugar, milk, or lemon added, according to taste

PATTERN	SNACK MENU	MENU ALTERNATES
MILK AND COOKIE	Milk and cookie	Fresh fruit, before bed, if desired and needed

ing are basic principles to use for planning balanced meals.

1. Include in each meal approximately a third of the protein needed during the day. Some of this should come from animal foods, such as milk, cheese, red meat, poultry, fish, organ meats, and eggs.
2. Include in each meal a variety of foods to provide essential minerals and vitamins. Well-selected food from each food group will do this.
3. A vitamin C-rich food is desirable in one meal and helpful in each. Use at least one raw fruit or vegetable a day.
4. Use liver and seafood at least once during the week.
5. Combine foods to provide variety in nutrients so that they will nutritionally complement each

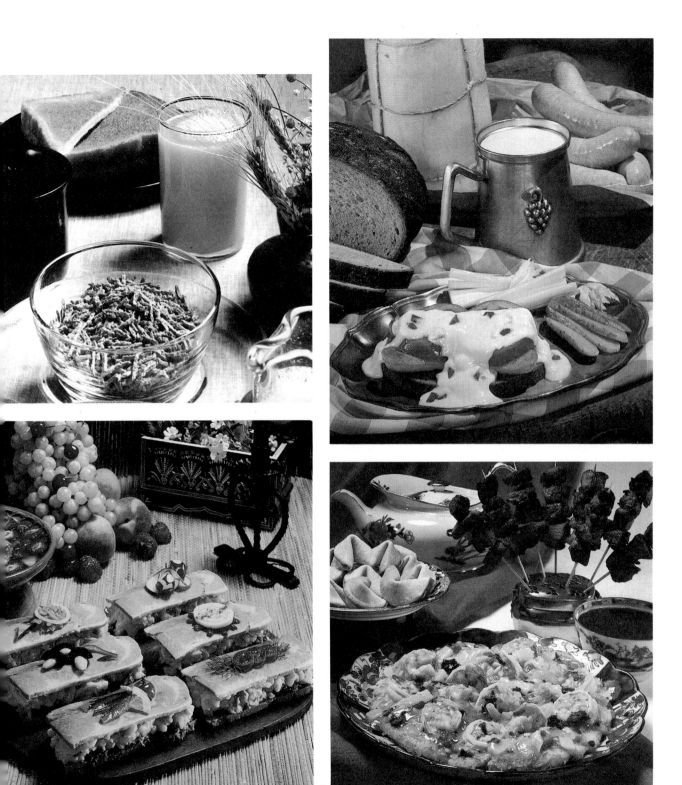

Include in each meal about one-third of your daily needs for nutrients and calories. What foods would you add to these examples to provide balanced meals? *Top left:* Breakfast. *Top right:* Lunch. *Bottom left:* Lunch or dinner. *Bottom right:* Dinner.

Table 4-5 **Nutritious low-calorie snacks for any age**

FOOD GROUP	SNACK
MILK AND MILK PRODUCTS	Plain milk, nonfat milk shake, nonfat malted milk, spiced milk, ice milk; low-fat cheese; pizza made with cheese; low-fat yogurt
FRUITS	Fruit juices; fresh raw fruit; dried fruit; canned or frozen fruit
VEGETABLES	Finger vegetables—raw celery, lettuce, cucumbers, tomatoes, radishes, carrots, green or red peppers, broccoli, cauliflower, peas, etc.
MEATS	Lean meat, poultry, fish, or other protein foods, such as eggs, peanut butter, or baked beans, in sandwiches with whole-grain or enriched bread
OTHERS	Home-popped corn with 15 mL (1 T) vegetable oil per 80 mL (⅓ c) corn added; dry-roasted peanuts (without added fat); angel food cake, sponge cake

other. Also combine a variety of foods that will complement each other in flavor (bland with sharp), texture (crisp with soft), and color (contrast for eye appeal).

6. Divide the day's food so that each meal provides a third to a quarter of the day's calories.

7. If you or any member of the family is overweight, plan meals low in fats and sweets, moderate in carbohydrates, and high in bulk.

8. Select snacks to be nutritionally beneficial and to fit into the total food need for the day (Table 4-5). Otherwise you may gain weight and deny yourself good nutrition.

As we proceed in our study, you will learn how to control weight by careful selection of each food in the diet. Consider the nutrients in each meal and think of each day as a unit. Such an understanding will protect you from fad diets.

Evaluating your diet

Until you diagnose your present eating habits, you cannot improve them. One way to do this is by a dietary study of yourself. Keep a record of the kinds of food and how much of each you eat for one week. Then analyze it and compare the results to the RDA tables on pages 402-403. Have a separate notebook for this purpose and keep it for future reference. Follow these steps for keeping a dietary record.

1. List the date, day of the week, meals, and snacks.
2. Write down everything you consume at each meal or between meals. Include every food and beverage.
3. Show the amount of what you eat. For example:

3/28/78   Tues.
Dinner
120 mL (½ c) carrots
1 baked potato
180 mL (¾) c tossed green salad
240 mL (8 oz) milk
112 g (4 oz) roast beef
1 small roll
1 pat butter
3.8 cm² (1½ sq in) gingerbread
30 mL (2 T) applesauce
1 cup black coffee

4. Estimate the amount of fat and sugar used in seasoning foods. Include it in your listing.
5. Keep your first record for seven consecutive days, if possible. Repeat this procedure at each season of the year.
6. Take one typical day's diet at each season and calculate the amount of each nutrient it contains. Use the RDA table on pages 402-403.

To calculate the calories derived from each nutrient in the food, follow a simple formula. Let us use milk as an example. In 240 mL (8 oz) of whole milk, there are 9 grams of protein, 9 grams of fat, and 12 grams of carbohydrate. Each gram of fat yields 9 calories. Each gram of protein or carbohydrate yields 4. Multiply the number of grams by the number of calories that each of the nutrients yields. This will give you the number of calories from that nutrient.

RECAP

How does the body use food?
Digestion   Absorption   Metabolism

What is a balanced diet?
Recommended Dietary Allowances   Calorie requirements   Water in the diet

Importance of balanced meals
Planning balanced meals   Evaluating your diet

THINKING AND EVALUATING

1. Explain how food is changed from the time it is eaten until it is finally used by the body.

2. What does the RDA table on pages 402-403 mean to you now? Do you think more knowledge of different foods could give it even deeper meaning? How might this help your life now? Later?

3. Explain the meaning of a balanced diet. Does eating three meals each day assure a balanced diet? Explain.

4. Explain the principles for planning a day's balanced diet, including meals and snacks. Why should snacks be considered as part of the daily food plan?

5. Using a seven-day record of the food you ate, Table 4-2, and the RDA and nutritive value of foods tables on pages 402-403, calculate the total calories you had in your diet from carbohydrates, from protein, and from fat. Save this seven-day record for future reference.

6. On the basis of your seven-day record, how would you rate your own diet? What are its weaknesses? Its strengths? Can you improve it? How?

APPLYING AND SHARING

1. Using Table 4-4 and also the principles for planning balanced meals on pages 68-72 , plan low-cost menus that you would enjoy eating and preparing. Plan menus for a guest dinner eaten at the table; on the patio; at a picnic; for a special family occasion.

2. Of the meals you planned, prepare at home three for one day. Serve, eat, and analyze them. How can you improve on your food selections or methods of preparation?

3. Using the sample outline on pages 73, record the food and beverages you consumed yesterday. For nutritional values refer to the table on pages 404-430. Analyze each meal and each snack separately. Then add up the calories, protein, fat, calcium, iron, and vitamins listed. Look up the recommended allowances for your age group in the RDA table on pages 402-403, and compare the totals for the day under each heading. How do you rate? Is this day's diet typical?

4. Try to communicate to your family what you have learned in this chapter and how it can help you. Discuss why we need balanced meals and how to plan them.

CAREER CAPSULES

Consulting nutritionist Works as advisor to nursing homes, small hospitals, doctors' offices, clinics. Advanced degree in nutrition and R.D. certification required.

Food service manager Works in restaurant, school or business cafeteria, hospital feeding program; oversees operations, personnel, purchasing, menu planning. Required education varies; knowledge of business administration and home economics essential.

RELATED READING

Hill, Mary M. "Creating Good Food Habits—Start Young, Never Quit." *Food for Us All: Yearbook of Agriculture, 1969.* Washington, D.C.: USDA, 1969. Emphasizes acceptance of a variety of foods and methods of food preparation, as well as weight maintenance.

Huenemann, R. L., et al. *Teenage Nutrition and Physique.* Springfield, Ill.: Charles C. Lawrence, 1974. Discusses three problems faced by teenagers—obesity, physical fitness, and eating habits.

White, P. L., and Nancy Sekvey, Eds. *Let's Talk About Food: Answers to Your Questions About Foods and Nutrition.* Acton, Mass.: Publishing Sciences Group. 1974. Chapter 1 concentrates on recommended daily dietary allowances, RDA and nutrition labeling, usefulness of calorie tables, nutrient density.

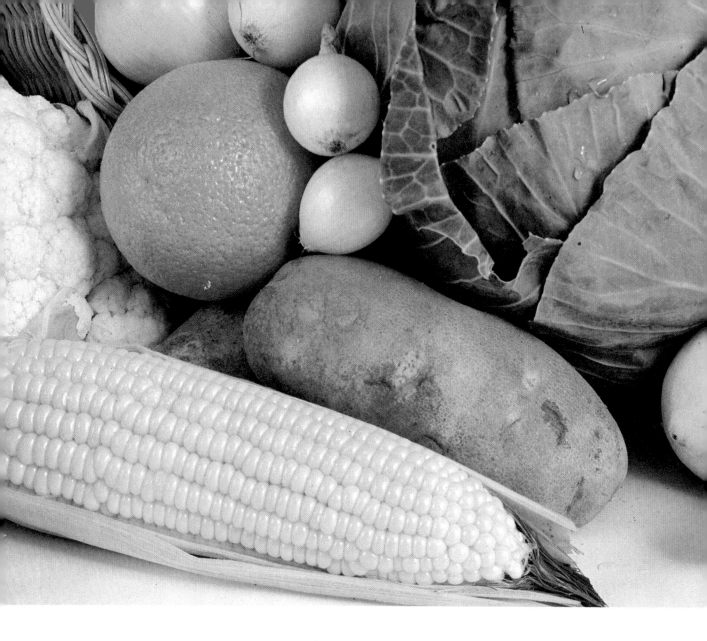

CHAPTER 5

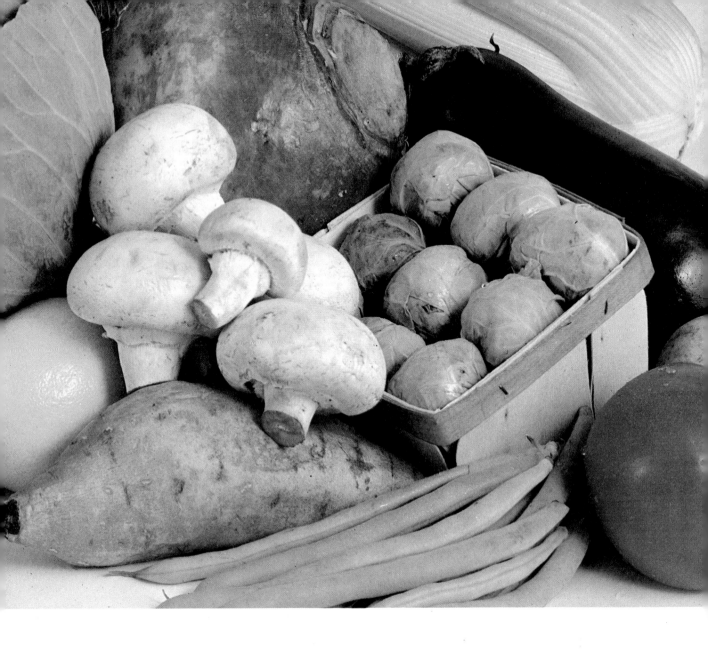

Fruits and vegetables

After studying this chapter, you will be able to

- list the fruits and vegetables that can help you maintain desirable weight and resist diseases and infections.
- explain the contributions made by fruits and vegetables to good health and attractive appearance.
- name the fruits and vegetables that are good sources of important nutrients.
- discuss the strengths and weaknesses of the vegetarian diet.

VALUE OF FRUITS AND VEGETABLES

"It is a disgrace to grow old through sheer carelessness." So said Socrates, the Greek philosopher, more than 2,000 years ago. He urged people to develop their "bodily strength and beauty to their highest limits." In this chapter, you will see how fruits and vegetables in your diet can help you to follow Socrates' advice.

Some diets include too few fruits and vegetables. But this is not due to a lack of available varieties. At certain times of the year,

Fruits and vegetables are high in nutrients and low in calories.

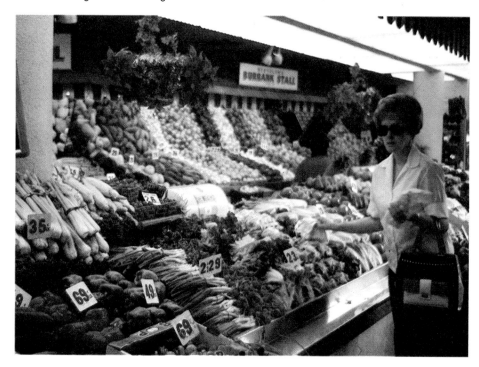

more than 70 varieties of fresh fruits and more than 200 varieties of fresh vegetables may be seen on supermarket shelves. In addition, there are hundreds of processed fruits and vegetables in convenience forms. As a group, fruits and vegetables are valuable because of the nutrients they provide.

Fruits and vegetables as sources of nutrients

Fruits and vegetables provide a variety of vitamins and minerals. You depend on them for about 90 percent of the vitamin C and two-thirds of the vitamin A in your diet. They also help keep the chemistry of your body normal. They provide the soft bulk that makes possible the natural elimination of waste from the alimentary canal. They also help you achieve and maintain desirable weight, since they are the food group lowest in calories. With the exception of olives, avocados, and coconuts, they contain no saturated fat. (Saturated fat is explained in Chapter 14.) For these reasons they may help prevent and control diseases of the heart and the circulatory system.

Healthful bacteria in vegetables and fruits help the intestinal tract to make other vitamins. These vitamins include K, folic acid, biotin, choline, and B_6. Bacteria produced from eating meat, fish, poultry, and eggs are the **putrefactive** (decay-causing) type. Fruits and vegetables are needed to counterbalance putrefaction.

Legumes are plants that take nitrogen from both the air and

soil to form protein. The protein is concentrated in the seeds. Examples of legumes are dried beans, peas, lentils, and peanuts. Other nuts are not legumes but are sources of protein too. Legumes have been called the poor person's meat. Cereal grains and legumes provide the primary source of protein for two-thirds of the people in the world. Fresh peas and beans have 4 to 6 percent protein. Dried ones have about 7 to 8 percent. Soybean flour has 10 to 15 percent protein of good quality. Recently, soybean meal has been produced with 44 percent protein.[1] Vegetables other than legumes have 1 to 4 percent protein. Fruits contain very little protein (0.05 to 2 percent).

Soybeans and peanuts almost approach meat in quality of protein. Scientists have developed a process that removes 50 to 60 percent of the fat from peanuts. Peanut butter with 26 percent protein content can now be produced. This is a major improvement. It means that peanut butter can contain less oil and fewer calories with more protein per gram. Low-fat (dry-roasted) peanuts are on the market. Ask for them. Read labels to find them in peanut products.

Soybean products can be substituted for meat (Table 5-1). If meat should become scarce, soybean products can be produced on a large scale. As discussed in Chapter 1, an acre of ground in the United States can produce 203 kg (450 lb) of protein from soybeans. Contrast this with 19 kg

[1]USDA *Agricultural Handbook*, No. 477, April 1975.

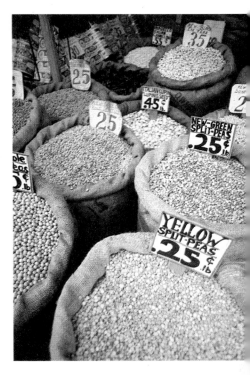

Legumes such as beans, peas, and lentils contain substantial amounts of less complete protein.

(43 lb) of protein produced per acre from the meat of animals on pasture.

Fruits and vegetables as controllers of weight

Overweight is one of the major health problems in the United States. The cause and the cure, in most cases, relate directly to food and drink. One of the benefits of fruits and vegetables is that they can help you attain and maintain a trim, slender figure.

It is important to know which fruits and vegetables are most valuable in balancing meals and to form the habit of eating them every day. The dark-green, leafy

Table 5-1 Soy-protein foods as substitutes for meat

SOY-PROTEIN FOOD	PROTEIN CONTENT (percent)	ESTIMATED 1970 U.S. PRODUCTION (million pounds)	USES
FLOUR AND GRITS	40–55	325–500	In baked foods, pet foods and sausages
CONCENTRATES	60–70	25–30	In processed meats, soy milk, baby and health foods
ISOLATES	90–95	20–25	Analogs (imitation meats), and as partial substitute for meat in meat loaves, frankfurters, etc.
TEXTURED, EXTRUDED, OR SPUN PRODUCTS	50–55 90+	25	Manufacturing analogs such as bacon strips and bits, pork, beef, chicken, fish, and other foods

Adapted from W. S. Hoofnagle and W. W. Gallimore, "Manufactured Foods, Fibers," USDA *Yearbook of Agriculture,* 1971, p. 336.

The nutrients in vegetables and fruits help to control weight and ensure fitness.

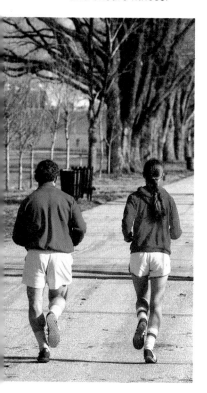
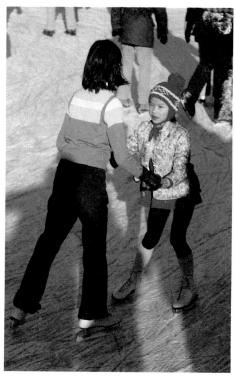

vegetables are especially good choices. They provide many vitamins and minerals, and they are low in calories.

It is a common mistake to think that potatoes are fattening. In fact, an average-sized potato contains only 90 calories. Potatoes are recommended for people in all age groups including those on weight-control diets. That is because white and sweet potatoes contain a wide variety of nutrients. (See the table of nutritive values of foods on page 428.)

A baked potato of about 140 g (5 oz) contains 22 milligrams of vitamin C. This is almost half the amount recommended daily for a child until age 12. Next to citrus fruits and tomatoes, potatoes can provide more vitamin C for the money than any other food. Potatoes provide the second largest amount of the mineral iron, rating next to dried beans and peas.

They yield more thiamin for the dollar than any other food. And all this for only 90 calories. In a day's diet, include a potato with only a small amount of fat. Or learn to eat it without fat.

Do you wish to keep your figure slender? Then you should eat generous amounts of vegetables, cooked and raw, at lunch and dinner. Having fruit or fruit juice at breakfast is helpful too. Use fruit, preferably raw, as your dessert. When you are hungry between meals, fill up on raw vegetables, such as celery, carrot sticks, and green lettuce. Drink fruit juice instead of artificial beverages. The habit of using fruits and vegetables in meals and snacks can help you keep slender and fit. (For more on ways to prevent overweight problems, see Chapter 16.)

Table 5-2 Typical low- and high-fiber foods

LOW-FIBER FOODS	HIGH-FIBER FOODS
Sugar	Vegetables
Fats	Fruits
White bread	Nuts
Nonwhole-grain cereals	Whole wheat bread
Meat, fish, poultry	Whole-grain cereals (oatmeal, dark
Peeled potatoes	farina, others)

Fruits and vegetables as guardians of fitness

Fruits, vegetables, and whole grains are natural laxatives that help keep us fit. They aid waste elimination in two ways. First, the undigested **cellulose,** or **fiber,** serves as a soft mechanical bulk (Table 5-2). It pushes the nutrients against the villi in the intestinal tract where they are absorbed into the bloodstream. The food waste is pushed on to the large intestine, which eliminates it. Second, fruits and vegetables aid by providing nutrients to build and help maintain a healthy mucous membrane lining of the intestinal tract. Good elimination requires the powerful peristaltic waves of a healthy intestinal tract. Fruits and vegetables also help prevent intestinal tract diseases.

VITAMIN C

An American researcher, Dr. Charles Glen King, made an important discovery in 1931. He isolated a material in lemon juice that cured scurvy in guinea pigs and called it **ascorbic acid.** Its more common name is vitamin C. **Scurvy** is a disease resulting from a deficiency of vitamin C in the body. Victims of the disease become weak and anemic. Gums become spongy and mucous membranes bleed. Scurvy is not common now. When it does occur, it can be reversed in three to four days by the use of vitamin C or foods rich in it.

Most animals can manufacture vitamin C from other nutrients. But human beings, monkeys, and guinea pigs must get it from their daily food. The story is told of a pet monkey that lined up with the sailors on a British ship to get his share of citrus fruit or juice. The sailors were highly amused by his behavior. But it was no joke. The monkey needed the vitamin C just as the sailors did.

About 90 percent of the vitamin C in our daily diet must come from fruits and vegetables. Unfortunately, there is no vitamin C at all in meat (except liver), eggs, dried legumes, nuts, fats, and sugars. There is only a small amount in milk.

Citrus fruits—oranges, grapefruit, lemons, limes—are our best sources of vitamin C. Tomatoes in any form are also excellent. Like citrus fruits, they protect the vitamin C with their acid content. Other good sources are collards, raw cabbage, strawberries, kale, turnip greens, mustard greens, Savoy cabbage, Brussels sprouts, cantaloupe, papayas, potatoes, broccoli, and peppers.

Functions of vitamin C

What role does vitamin C play in nutrition? How does it work for us? The broad role of vitamin C is to help form a gluelike substance called **collagen.** Collagen holds all types of body cells together. Vitamin C teams up with other nutrients, enzymes, hormones, and oxygen to build and maintain body tissues.

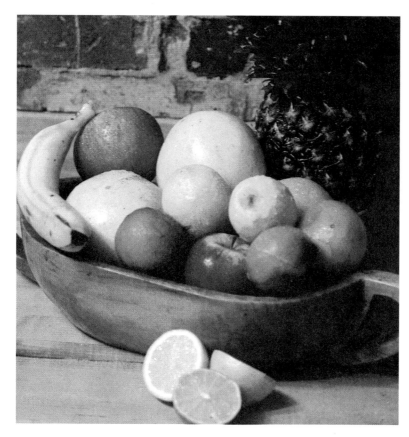

Citrus fruits are the best sources of vitamin C.

Figure 5-1   Too little vitamin C leads to badly formed bones like this porous jawbone.

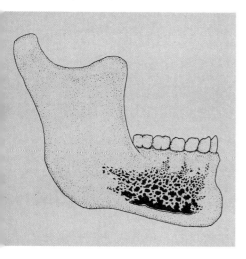

Blood vessels. A prolonged deficiency of vitamin C causes the heart to enlarge. Giving elasticity to blood vessels is a major contribution of vitamin C. One effect of the lack of this vitamin in blood vessels is blue-yellow patches, like bruises, beneath the skin. The patches show where tiny capillaries have hemorrhaged. Other bleeding may occur deeper in the body tissues or in organs such as the spleen, bladder, and kidneys, in adrenal and other glands, in muscle tissue, bone marrow, and the alimentary canal. This hemorrhaging occurs when cells "fall apart" because of insufficient vitamin C.

Red blood cells. Vitamin C works with a team of nutrients—iron, copper, protein, folic acid, and others—in forming red blood cells in the bone marrow. This team also aids the absorption of iron. Hence it helps to prevent anemia, fatigue, and loss of energy.

Resistance to infections and diseases. Vitamin C helps to prevent and heal respiratory illnesses, infections, wounds, and diseases. Earlier generations hit upon the use of hot lemonade in treating colds and other respiratory disorders. The old lemonade cure helped for two reasons. Fluids alone can help. And fluids with the high vitamin C content of lemons can help even more.

When the diet has too little vitamin C, muscle tissue becomes soft and flabby. This is because the "intercellular cement" is too watery. Vitamin C affects growth and well-being throughout life. It promotes the functioning of the sex glands and organs. It also aids in the development of firm, flexible muscles.

Bony structures. Too little vitamin C in the diet produces a loss in calcium. Too little calcium results in thin, porous, "honeycomb" bones which can break easily (Figure 5-1).

Teeth and gums. Without enough vitamin C, teeth grow in an irregular way. Also, gums bleed easily when brushed or when pressure is exerted.

Daily requirement of vitamin C

The RDA table on pages 402–403 shows that the need for vitamin C depends on many factors. Among these are age, sex, size, height, and weight. Also, the more active you are the more vitamin C you need. If you live in a hot, humid climate, you need more vitamin C. If you have a fever, you need more vitamin C. Your health and nutrition are additional factors.

The reserves of vitamin C stored in the body are quite small. The greatest concentration is in the tissues of the adrenal glands which secrete adrenalin, and in the retina of the eye. The pituitary gland and organs such as the brain, liver, and kidneys, and the bone marrow hold some vitamin C. Some vitamin C is concentrated in the hemoglobin of red corpuscles.

Vitamin C is absorbed from the small intestines and circulates to the tissues. This means each cell can use it to make the collagen that helps hold cells firmly together. When the body tissues and reserve depots are saturated, the excess is at once excreted in the urine as water and through the lungs as carbon dioxide. One cannot get too much vitamin C from food. The excess you eat at breakfast is disposed of before lunch.

Clearly you need to have a source of vitamin C daily. The best plan is to distribute the foods that contain this nutrient among all three meals in the day.

Retaining vitamin C in food preparation

Vitamin C is fragile and easily lost. It is soluble in water. Therefore, it is lost when foods soak in water. Vitamin C is also lost when the cooking water or liquid in canned vegetables and fruits is discarded. To prevent these losses, vegetables and fruits should be cooked in a minimum of water. The liquid left over from cooking or from canned fruits and vegetables should be used in soups or other cooking.

Vitamin C is easily destroyed by oxygen. The more surface exposed to the air, the greater the loss. The more bruised, wilted, or old the vegetable, the greater the loss of vitamin C by oxidation. Foods that are frozen and allowed to thaw before cooking lose a great deal of their vitamin C content. Therefore, keep vitamin C-rich foods out of the sunshine or warm places. Store fresh ones in the refrigerator, frozen ones in the freezer, and canned ones in a dry, cool place. Cook vegetables whole when possible, or cut them with a sharp knife to prevent bruising. Research shows that there is less loss by cutting in cubes than in slices. Avoid buying wilted or old vegetables and fruits. Use those that you buy before they become wilted or old.

Heat also destroys vitamin C. Studies show that vegetables lose less vitamin C if cooked in water that has been boiled one to two minutes. This causes the oxygen

Folklore and Superstition

Have you heard that
. . . raw, unsalted cucumbers are poisonous?
. . . vegetable and fruit juices are more healthful than the food from which they are made?
. . . it doesn't matter which ones you select, so long as you eat four servings of fruits and vegetables daily?
. . . rhubarb or spinach should not be eaten in a meal with milk?
. . . an apple a day keeps the doctor away?
. . . onions will cure a cold?
. . . artificial beverages with added vitamin C are as healthful as orange juice?
. . . tomato juice and citrus juices are too acid for good health?
. . . orange juice or grapefruit and milk in the same meal cause gas?
. . . strawberries purify the blood?
. . . garlic prevents high blood pressure and ulcers?
. . . onions cure insomnia?
. . . potatoes are fattening?
. . . celery is a brain food?

Don't you believe it!

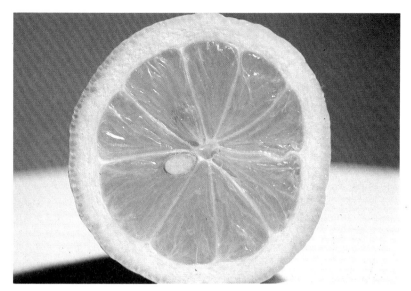

Vitamin C is easily lost from foods when foods are exposed to air.

serving them at once also helps to retain vitamin C. Leftovers should be stored at once in the freezer. Reheating should be done quickly just to the boiling point and no more.

Alkali destroys vitamin C. Therefore, don't add soda to green vegetables to retain the color, as is often done in public eating places. Contact with copper cooking utensils also destroys vitamin C.

Overripening destroys vitamin C. Buy fruits and vegetables at the peak of ripeness. Either refrigerate or store them properly to prevent overripening. Melons and fruits with thick skins lose less vitamin C than succulent, exposed fruits and vegetables such as berries, beans, or shelled green peas.

Deep-yellow vegetables are good sources of vitamin A.

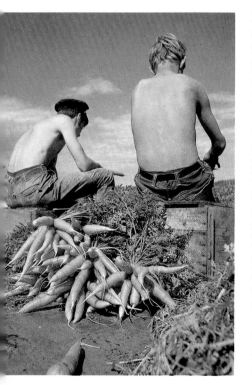

in the water to be expelled. Vegetables cooked in a pressure cooker also lose less vitamin C. Cooking vegetables quickly and

VITAMIN A

In 1912, E. V. McCollum and his associates discovered vitamin A in butterfat. This started a search that resulted in the isolation of vitamin A in crystalline form in 1936.

McCollum made his great discovery after observing two groups of cows. One group of cows ate yellow corn and green corn leaves. They grew normally and produced healthy calves. Another group ate only the stalks and seeds of wheat. They matured late and had calves that were born dead or died soon after birth. McCollum concluded that it was an unknown nutrient in the corn that made the difference.

To study the problem, he began a series of experiments with a white rat colony. These animals complete their life span

in one-thirtieth the time that human beings do. They also eat the same diet. Therefore, experimenting with them could help McCollum find the answer to this riddle.

He divided his animals into groups. He gave them identical diets with identical calories. However, one group had butter, another lard, and another olive oil. In 70 to 120 days—about 6 to 8 years in the life of a human being—the animals that were fed the lard and olive oil stopped growing. Their physical appearance also changed. They developed rough, coarse hair, sore eyes, and poor posture. They soon died.

By contrast, the animals that were fed butter had beautiful, smooth coats, bright, clear eyes, good posture, excellent growth, and a lively manner. This group had healthy, strong offspring. McCollum had proved that butter contained a nutrient that was not in the other fats. The nutrient McCollum had discovered was named vitamin A.

Later, H. Steenboch, at the University of Wisconsin, isolated a crystalline substance from carrots and called it carotene. When fed to animals, it gave the identical results as butterfat, cod-liver oil, or egg yolk had given in tests by other scientists in our country and abroad. In 1929, T. Moore found that carotene was a provitamin A and could be changed to vitamin A by the animal and human body.

Unlike vitamin C, about four months' supply of vitamin A may be stored in the body. About 95 percent is stored in the liver. That is one reason that liver is so valuable in the diet. Small amounts are stored in the lungs, kidneys, and fatty tissue. Vitamin A accumulates gradually to a peak of reserve in adulthood. Young animals and children have little or no reserve. A reserve is a great advantage when there is a shortage in the diet or when illness occurs.

Vitamins A, D, E, and K are measured in terms of International Units, referred to as IU. There are 4.5 million IU in each gram of pure vitamin A.

We should get about one-third of our vitamin A in pure form from animal fat, and two-thirds from the carotenes in fruits and vegetables. How can you tell which fruits and vegetables contain vitamin A? Color is the chief clue. Vitamin A is made from the provitamin or the yellow carotenes. The carotenes also occur in the red and deep green foods, but the stronger colors hide them. The best foods for vitamin A are the deep-green, leafy vegetables, the deep-yellow vegetables and fruits, and liver.

Look at the table of nutritive values of foods on page 425. Look for information about spinach, turnip greens, mustard greens, collards, and kale. Notice that any one of these cooked green, leafy vegetables contains from 4060 to 7290 IU of vitamin A. A serving of 120 mL (½ c) of carrots, winter squash, pumpkin, sweet potato, or half a cantaloupe has from over 4000 to over 8000 IU of vitamin A.

Functions of vitamin A

H. C. Sherman discovered in his studies of more than 80 generations of animals that vitamin A may directly affect the length of life. Let us consider its major contributions to health.

Vision. Vitamin A is essential for good vision. The connection between vision and diet was known to the Egyptians as early as 1900 B.C.

Vitamin A helps to prevent xerophthalmia, also known as "dry eye." Eyes become dry because the lachrymal gland, which normally secretes fluid to keep the eyes moist, does not function. Other problems also develop. The lids stick together, becoming scabby and swollen. In advanced cases, blindness results. Styes may be a minor effect of a deficiency of this nutrient.

Vitamin A also helps prevent night blindness. It keeps drivers from being blinded by the headlights of oncoming cars. Vitamin A combines with protein, cholesterol, and other nutrients to form visual purple. This pigment is essential for the retina. When you look at the headlights of a car, or

Too little vitamin A may lead to night blindness. *Left:* Normal night vision. *Right:* Poor night vision.

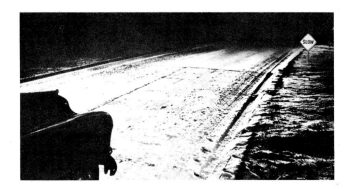
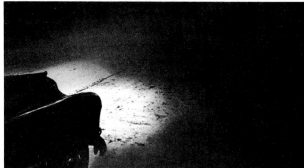

sunlight reflected on water, snow, or chrome, or when you go from a dark room to a bright one, the visual purple changes first to yellow, then to white. In the change, vitamin A is used up. The brighter the light, the faster it is used. To make visual purple, the body must draw on stored vitamin A.

Growth. Vitamin A is essential for normal growth. It was the early researchers' efforts to determine why some animals failed to grow that led to the discovery of vitamin A.

Sherman confirmed the effect of vitamin A on growth in his study of more than 80 generations of white rats. Rats fed a diet high in vitamin A grew to full adulthood. They produced normal young. But rats fed a diet with only a little vitamin A grew to almost adult size, then stopped growing. They could not reproduce young.

Skin and hair. Vitamin A is beneficial for the skin and hair. One of the first symptoms of a deficiency of this vitamin is rough, dry skin, possibly with pimples. Ancel Keys and his coworkers at the University of Minnesota examined 31 persons on a low vitamin A diet (1810 IU daily). After 23 weeks, 24 of the 31 persons showed skin eruptions, dry and scaly skin, and dull hair. Thus vitamin A plays an essential role in promoting appearance.

Defense against infection. Vitamin A guards the body against bacterial infections and diseases. A healthy, unbroken skin protects us from invasion of some bacteria. The outer layer of skin is called the epidermis. It is composed of millions of tiny epithelial cells. These cells also line the soft tissues of the mucous membrane of the respiratory tract. They are found in the mouth and alimentary tract, the urinary and genital tracts, the tear glands, and all other glands and organs in the body.

When the body is deficient in vitamin A, the cells that line the respiratory tract dry out. The mucous membrane becomes rough. The normal secretions disappear. Naturally, this lowers your ability to resist respiratory infections.

What happens when the mucous membrane of the digestive tract becomes clogged with dry, hard epithelial cells? It then becomes difficult for nutrients from digested food to be absorbed in the bloodstream. Animals having this condition get diarrhea and other digestive troubles. Furthermore, bacteria migrate in larger numbers through the alimentary canal to other parts of the body. In one experiment, typhoid-producing bacteria were inserted by a tube into the stomachs of two groups of white rats. In the group deficient in vitamin A, 93 percent of the animals soon had typhoid bacteria in the liver, lungs, kidneys, and spleen. The bacteria were found in only 38 percent of the animals who had sufficient vitamin A.

Teeth. Vitamin A helps form teeth. Poor diet and illness of the mother during pregnancy affect the development of the baby's teeth. Poor diet may affect the baby teeth that are formed before birth. The epithelial cells fold inward in the gums. They form a cap over the bud of the tooth. Vitamin A may also affect the permanent teeth, which form in the bud behind the baby teeth. The final laying down of enamel occurs during the first ten months

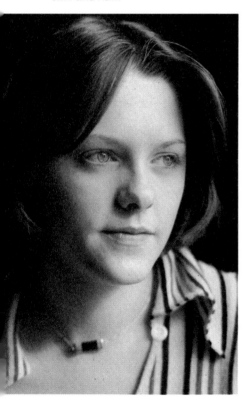

Vitamin A contributes to healthy skin and hair.

after the birth of the baby. When there is enough of vitamin A and other nutrients, the enamel is laid down in closely packed, six-sided hard prisms. This makes a smooth, attractive surface. When it is deficient, the prisms do not fit tightly together. Pits form. Food lodges in these pits and ferments. The teeth may then erode, leading to decay. About two-thirds of the pitting that occurs in poor enamel takes place during the first ten months.

Kidneys. Vitamin A helps to prevent the formation of kidney stones. Kidney stones were once so common among the poor that one doctor called them "the poor man's disease." The doctor was Dr. R. McCarrison, a medical nutritionist in India. McCarrison's patients in India ate mostly cereal, especially wheat. McCarrison fed this cereal diet to white rats. Three months after weaning, the rats developed kidney stones. McCarrison fed a second group of rats the same diet with butter, whole milk, and cod-liver oil added. All of these foods are rich in vitamin A. The second group of rats did not get kidney stones.

Daily requirement of vitamin A

The RDA table on page 402 shows the amounts of vitamin A recommended for different age groups. Your ability to absorb this vitamin depends on your state of health and the balance of your total diet.

The amount of carotene changed into vitamin A varies with the food. Cooking carrots, for instance, makes more vitamin A available. Carotene may pass directly into the bloodstream or it may be changed into vitamin A in the mucous membranes of the intestines or liver. Some ailments, such as diarrhea or liver disease, interfere with its absorption.

Vitamin A is involved in several different functions and in several major and minor ills. For this reason, Sherman suggests that 6000 to 12,000 IU of vitamin A daily would be more logical than the recommended 4000 to 5000 IU. This would allow for individual differences and would promote better health and longer life.

Can you get too much vitamin A? Food does not provide too much, but supplementary vitamin pills can mean an excess of vitamin A. Some pills are quite concentrated in vitamin A. Well-meaning mothers may give their children 40 to 50 times the recommended amount daily. If this dosage is prolonged, **hypervitaminosis** meaning an excess of vitamins, can result. Hypervitaminosis causes loss of appetite and changes in skin pigmentation. The skin becomes itchy and dry. There is loss of hair and bones are fragile and painful. Here is a strong reason for depending on foods, not pills, for vitamins.

Retaining vitamin A in food preparation

The carotenes from which vitamin A is made are deep yellow. The vitamin itself is a colorless, odorless, needlelike crystal. It resists heat, but it may be destroyed by oxygen during long, slow cooking at low temperatures. Little is destroyed when it is cooked in the absence of oxygen, as in a pressure cooker. Vitamin E protects vitamin A from oxidation, an example of teamwork in nutrients. Vitamin A retains its values better in vegetables and fruits that are kept cool and moist.

Vitamin A is not soluble in water. It needs some fat in the meal to enable it to be absorbed from the digestive tract and the bloodstream into tissues. Unfortunately, vitamin A and the other fat-soluble vitamins—D, E, and K—are absorbed by mineral oil. These vitamins, along with the mineral oil, are eliminated in evacuation of wastes. For this reason, mineral oil is not a desirable laxative.

FOLACIN

Folacin, a B vitamin, has been included in the RDA table since 1968. It is also called **folic acid.** Folic acid was discovered in the spinach leaf in 1943 and 1944 by two laboratories working independently. Research shows that folic acid performs vital functions for life. It is essential for human growth, reproduction, lactation, and the normal formation of red blood cells.

The richest sources of folacin are liver, yeast, and green, leafy vegetables (Table 5-3). Other good sources are dried beans, peas, nuts, and whole-wheat foods. Brewer's yeast is the richest source of all.

Folic acid is easily destroyed by heat. Therefore some green veg-

Table 5-3 **Sources of folacin**

FOOD	AMOUNT (micrograms)[1]
Brewer's yeast, 15 mL (1 T)	2022
Cow peas, cooked, 120 mL (½ c)	439
Rice germ (in brown rice), 28 g (1 oz)	430
Wheat germ (in whole wheat), 28 g (1 oz)	305
Liver, 56 g (2 oz)	294
Wheat bran (in whole wheat), 28 g (1 oz)	195
Rice bran (in brown rice), 28 g (1 oz)	146
Asparagus, 98 g (3½ oz)	109
Walnuts, 8–15	77
Greens, cooked, 98 g (3½ oz)	42–77
Whole wheat, cooked, 120 mL (½ c)	49
Oatmeal, cooked, 120 mL (½ c)	33
Brown rice, cooked, 120 mL (½ c)	20
Oysters, 98 g (3½ oz)	11.3
Beef, lean round, 84 g (3 oz)	10.5

[1] A microgram is 1/1000 of a milligram.

etables should be eaten raw in salads. Also remember that folacin is lost in the refining of flour. For this reason, whole-wheat and yeast breads are more valuable than breads made from refined flour.

Functions of folacin

Like other B vitamins, folacin acts as a coenzyme. As a coenzyme, folic acid is needed for the breakdown and use of some amino acids.

Folacin works with a team of nutrients, including amino acids, to make the nuclei (centers) of all cells. Cells divide for growth and each new cell needs a new nucleus. For this reason, pregnant women need more folic acid than other adults. Infants, too, have a special need for it.

Without enough folacin, a special kind of anemia develops in pregnant women and infants. The name for it is macrocytic or megablastic anemia. A person in this condition has too few red cells, and the cells contain too little hemoglobin. If folacin is taken by mouth or by injection, normal blood cells are made immediately. The person is cured, so long as the required amount of folacin is supplied. Folacin works with vitamin B_{12} in helping prevent and cure another type of anemia called pernicious anemia, discussed in Chapter 9. No doubt future research will show other uses of this vitamin.

Daily requirement of folacin

The daily need for folic acid is quite small. It ranges from 0.1 mg at age one to 0.4 mg at age ten and beyond. During pregnancy, the need is 0.8 mg. The amount is small; but seldom does so little do so much.

Retaining folacin in food preparation

Like vitamin B_6, folacin exists in several forms in food. And like B_6 and some other vitamins, it is fragile. It is soluble in water and quickly destroyed by heat in an acid solution. As much as 65 percent of the folacin in food may be lost when food is cooked at medium cooking temperature for ten minutes. When fresh, leafy greens are stored for three days at room temperature, 70 percent of the folacin is lost. Unlike most other vitamins, it is more stable in a neutral or alkaline solution.

Animals, poultry, and fish get minerals from the plant foods they eat. They use some of these minerals for their own needs, but they pass some on to us. The calcium in milk, the iron in liver and lean meats, and the iodine in seafoods are examples of plant nutrients passed on to us in animal foods.

Many minerals come to us directly from plants. Among them are iron, calcium, copper, magnesium, potassium, and small amounts of other minerals.

Calcium

Next to milk, fruits and vegetables are the best sources of calcium. A serving of 120 mL (½ c) of cooked collard greens provides 236 mg of calcium. In nations where little milk is available, people can get their calcium by eating larger amounts of fruits and vegetables. In northern Italy, for example, adults often eat a portion of a cooked, green, leafy vegetable, dried beans, a large green salad, and some cheese. Such a meal provides about half of the adult daily need for calcium.

Some leafy vegetables contain oxalic acid. These include spinach, Swiss chard, beet tops, most wild greens, and rhubarb. Oxalic acid combines with some calcium and is eliminated as waste. To preserve the calcium, place a clean whole egg in the pot with the cooking vegetables. The calcium from the egg shell "ties up" the oxalic acid and releases the calcium in the vegetables. The cooked egg may be served with the vegetables as a garnish.

Acid-alkaline balance

The normal chemistry of the body is slightly on the alkaline (base) side. You have a built-in buffer system to keep it that way. When food is oxidized by the body, the ash that remains is minerals. Some of these minerals—especially phosphorous, chlorine, and sulfur—form acids. You will find such minerals in meat, fish, poultry, and eggs. They are also pres-

Vegetables and fruits are important in maintaining the body's acid-alkaline balance.

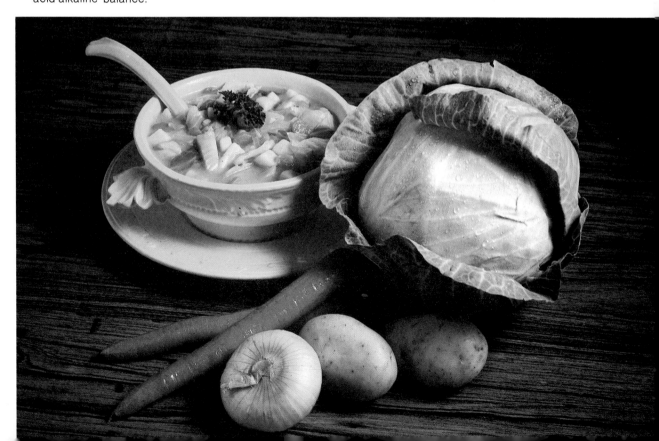

Table 5-4 **Acid-base reaction of foods**

BASE OR ALKALINE ASH	ACID OR ACID ASH	NEUTRAL
Vegetables (all except corn and lentils)	Meats, poultry, fish, shellfish	Butter
Fruits (all except cranberries, plums, and prunes)	Breads and cereals of all types	Margarine
	Macaroni products	Cooking fats and oils
Nuts: almonds, coconut, chestnuts	Cakes, cookies	Sugar
Milk, all kinds	Eggs	Syrups
Molasses	Cheese, all types[1]	Starches
Honey, jams, jellies	Cranberries, prunes, plums	
	Corn, lentils	
	Nuts: walnuts, peanuts, Brazil nuts, filberts	

[1] Much of the calcium mineral found in whole milk is lost with the whey in making cheese, leaving predominately acid-forming elements.

ent in cereals and flour and foods made from them.

When the blood is too acid, the body releases alkaline minerals to "buff down" the excess. Vegetables and fruits contain minerals that form alkaline. They tend to offset the acid-forming minerals in other foods.

You may hear a person say, "I can't eat tomatoes or citrus fruits because they are too acid." But this is contrary to scientific fact. (Some people, however, do have genuine allergies to these foods and must avoid them. This is an entirely different matter.) The citric acid in tomatoes and citrus fruits is quite mild. By contrast, the gastric juice in the body is a highly concentrated hydrochloric acid. When you take as much as 40 g (½ oz) of pure citric acid, less than 5 percent appears in the urine. Most of the citric acid has been changed by the body into carbon dioxide and water.

Eating vegetables, fruits, and milk will provide the natural alkaline needed. It is a waste of money to get alkaline in other ways. If you need more than a balanced diet gives, your physician should prescribe it. Actual harm can be done to the body by overuse of "remedies" supposed to "counteract acid."

Table 5-4 gives the foods that are potentially alkaline, potentially acid, and neutral. By a proper choice of foods, you can maintain a balance between acids and alkalis.

THE VEGETARIAN DIET

The **vegetarian** diet is as old as human beings. There are benefits to this diet. Plant foods can be grown more quickly, more easily, and more economically than animal foods. Two-thirds of the world's people today survive chiefly on plant foods. They do so mainly for economic, cultural, and religious reasons. Many of them would be glad to eat meat, fish, poultry, milk, cheese, and eggs if only they were available.

In the United States, the vegetarian diet is not a fad diet, but it can take a faddish turn. It may be a harmful diet if not properly balanced.

Dangers of the vegetarian diet

There are several weaknesses in the vegetarian diet. The chief one is that it does not provide sufficient vitamin B_{12}. This essential vitamin is found in milk, eggs, and meats. A long-term deficiency in B_{12} is detrimental to health. What happens to people who eat an all-plant diet? Studies show that nerve fibers in their spinal cords are destroyed. By the time the B_{12} deficiency shows up, it is too late. The loss of nerve function cannot be repaired.[2] (Also see pages 154–155.) Some recommend that strict vegetarians take this vitamin as a supplement. A strict vegetarian diet also may be too low in complete proteins. Complete proteins contain all the essential amino acids in the amounts needed for life and health. Neither dried beans and peas nor whole grains alone have complete protein. But eaten at the same meal, together they provide good quantities of all the essential amino acids. (See pages 148–149.) The best legumes for protein are soybeans, peanuts, and chick peas. Whole wheat lacks only one essential amino acid.

A strict vegetarian diet does not provide enough usable calcium, zinc, iron, vitamin D, and other nutrients. Women who are pregnant and lactating need more of these nutrients, and their lack will stunt children's growth. Too little iron

[2] *Family Health,* February 1974, pp. 32–48.

A diet that completely excludes milk, eggs, and fish, meat or poultry may lack necessary nutrients. What beverage and dessert could you add to make this a balanced meal?

can lead to anemia in both sexes, but especially in women during the menstrual cycle.

Balancing the vegetarian diet

Like everyone else, vegetarians should eat a balanced diet. Vegetarian meals need to be supplemented by animal proteins. If vegetarians do not wish to eat animal flesh, they may adopt a lacto-ovo (milk-egg) vegetarian diet. Milk, milk products, and eggs provide the amino acids plant foods lack and enable the body to use the plant proteins. A glass of milk in each meal supplies 9 g of complete protein. It contains calcium, vitamin D, sufficient riboflavin, and some B_{12}. These and other vitamins and minerals present in milk balance the deficiencies in a diet restricted to plant foods. Eggs also yield a wide variety of nutrients, including protein.

RECAP

Value of fruits and vegetables

Fruits and vegetables as sources of nutrients   Fruits and vegetables as weight controllers   Fruits and vegetables as guardians of fitness

Vitamin C

Functions of vitamin C   *Bony structures   Teeth and gums   Blood vessels   Red blood cells   Resistance to infections and diseases*   Daily requirement of vitamin C   Retaining vitamin C in food preparation

Vitamin A

Functions of vitamin A   *Vision   Growth   Skin and hair   Defense against infection   Teeth   Kidneys*   Daily requirement of vitamin A   Retaining vitamin A in food preparation

Folacin

Functions of folacin   Daily requirement of folacin   Retaining folacin in food preparation

Minerals

Calcium   Acid-alkaline balance

The vegetarian diet

Dangers of the vegetarian diet   Balancing the vegetarian diet

THINKING AND EVALUATING

1. List the vegetables and fruits you like best and those you like least. With the aid of the table of nutritive value of foods on pages 404-430, evaluate them for nutrient content. Are your preferences nutritionally beneficial?

2. Why is it important to know the nutritive value of various fruits and vegetables?

3. Which vitamin C-rich foods would you purchase on a low food budget? Which vitamin A-rich foods?

4. Why are fruits and vegetables important to weight control?

5. List the contributions of vitamins C and A to the body. Describe how these vitamins are absorbed, distributed, and stored in the body.

6. How may vitamins C and A be preserved in food preparation?

APPLYING AND SHARING

1. Write a report on why fruits and vegetables are important to the diet. Be prepared to discuss your ideas in class.

2. Compile a table of the richest sources of vitamins C and A for your own use by using this chapter and the table on nutritive value of foods on pages 404-430.

3. Using your list of best food sources for vitamins C and A as a reference, visit your local supermarket.

VOCABULARY

adrenal glands
alkaline
ascorbic acid
carotene
cellulose
collagen
epidermis
epithelial cells
fiber
folic acid
hypervitaminosis
legume
macrocytic anemia
oxalic acid
putrefactive
retina
scurvy
vegetarian
xerophthalmia

a. List the food sources for these vitamins in whatever forms they are sold (fresh, dry, canned, frozen), and calculate the cost per serving. Now check the nutritive labels for the amount of vitamin C and/or A per serving. Which source of these vitamins is the most economical?

b. Make a list of foods fortified with vitamins C and A, and calculate the cost per serving. Compare the results of these two exercises. Discuss your conclusions in class.

4. Keep a record of the total food you eat and drink for three days. Are you getting the recommended amount of vitamin C and vitamin A daily? In which meals or snacks? From what sources? How could you improve your diet?

5. Plan balanced menus for three days. Include a good source of vitamin C in each meal and one source of vitamin A in each day's diet, choosing foods you enjoy and can afford. Save all these menus and calculations. Total the calories for each meal and snack, and for the whole day. Does the total fit your need for weight control? How would you alter it to fit your needs more specifically, yet retain adequate balance in each meal?

6. Research the topic of vegetarian diets. How many vegetarian diets did you find? Describe three and evaluate them for nutritional adequacy.

CAREER CAPSULES

Plant scientist   Works in laboratory, on experimental farm, and "in the field"; depending on specialty, researches plant ecology, genetics, crop production, diseases. Four-year college education required; higher degree required for some specialties.

Cannery worker   Works in production department as maintenance worker, equipment operator, peeler, trimmer, packer, checker. High school education usually required; on-the-job training essential.

RELATED READING

Chrispeels, M. J., and D. Sadava. *Plants, Food, and People.* San Francisco: W. H. Freeman, 1977. Surveys the role of plants in providing food for the people of the world.

White, P. L., and Nancy Sekvey, Eds. *Let's Talk About Food: Answers to Your Questions About Foods and Nutrition.* Acton, Mass.: Publishing Sciences Group, 1974. Pages 39–40 present questions and answers on Vegan and other vegetarian diets.

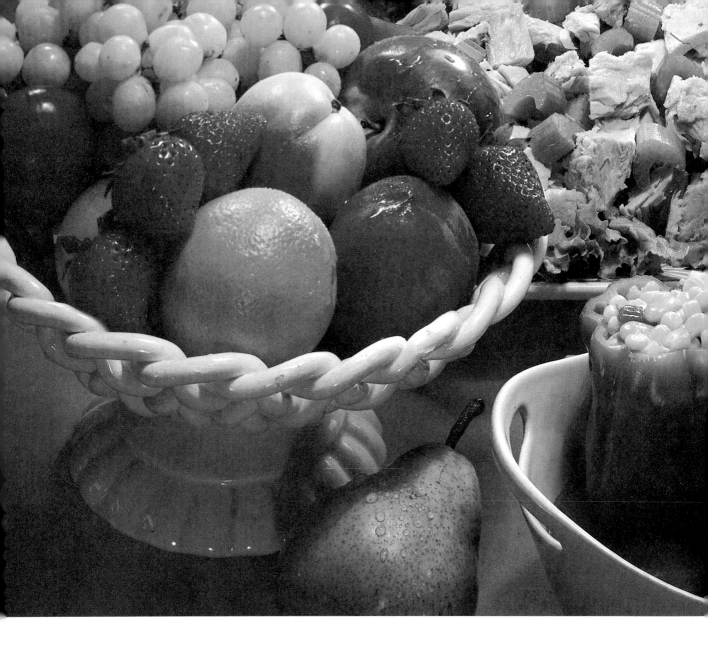

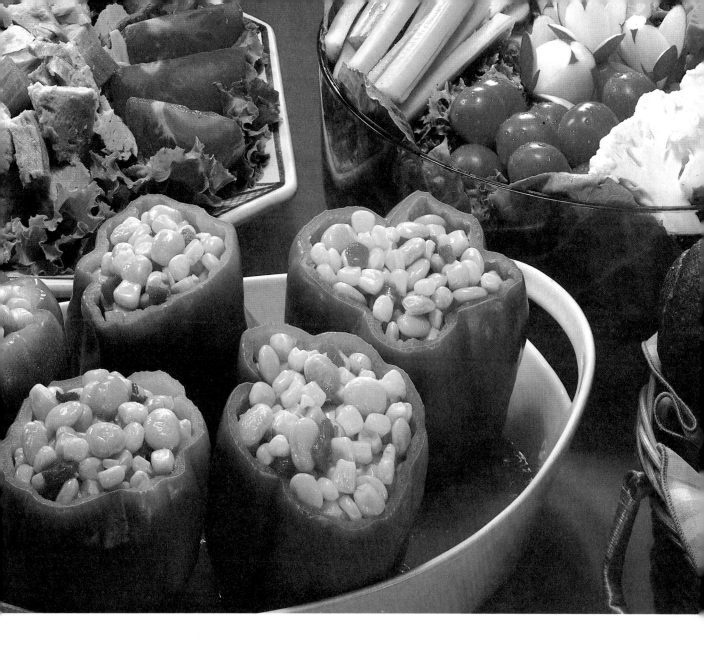

CHAPTER 6

Fruits and vegetables in meals

After studying this chapter you will be able to

- select fresh fruits and vegetables for quality.
- explain how and when processed fruits and vegetables are beneficial.
- list the principles for shopping for fruits and vegetables.
- describe how to store fresh and processed fruits and vegetables.
- cook specific fruits and vegetables to attain peak of flavor, texture, color, and food value.

ECONOMY OF FRUITS AND VEGETABLES

People are often praised for their skill and artistry in preparing meats and desserts. But fruits and vegetables are often neglected in menus in our homes and in public eating places. When they are included, they are often cooked in such a way that they are neither enjoyable nor nutritious. This is most unfortunate. You know how important these foods are in the daily diet.

As a food group, fruits and vegetables are well worth your dollar. They are relatively inexpensive, and they are rich in nutrients. Legumes rank first of all foods in the amount of protein, iron, and niacin they contain. They are third in thiamin content. Potatoes rank first in thiamin, second in vitamin C and iron, and third in calories. Citrus fruits and tomatoes are first in vitamin C, third in vitamin A, and fourth in thiamin. Dark-green and deep-yellow vegetables rank first in vitamin A, second in calcium, and fourth in iron.

In this chapter you will learn how to shop for, store, and properly prepare a wide variety of fruits and vegetables. You will learn how to retain the most

Properly cooked fruits and vegetables are economical as well as nutritious.

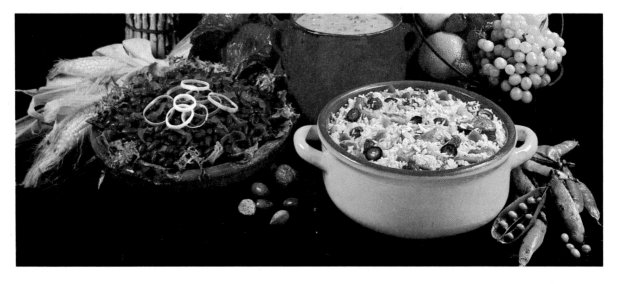

flavor and nutrients and the best appearance.

The many forms of fruits and vegetables are often bewildering to the consumer. They may be canned, frozen, dried, freeze-dried, pickled, spiced, and smoked. One may well ask, "Which is best, fresh or processed?" The answer is that both fresh and processed foods can be nourishing. But you need to know how to pick out the best of the fresh and processed fruits and vegetables.

QUALITY IN FRESH FRUITS AND VEGETABLES

First, let us consider how to judge the quality of fresh fruits and vegetables. The things to watch for are freshness, natural color, maturity, size, and weight in relation to size. Some of these characteristics affect the flavor, nutrients, and cost. Others affect the cost but not the nutrients.

Leafy vegetables should be crisp, firm, tender, and clean. They should also be untrimmed because the outside leaves protect the food against loss of vitamins. Outside leaves also protect freshness and provide vital nutrients. All fruits and vegetables should be free from soft spots. Leaves should show no brown, black, yellow, or dark spots. Finally, no withering should be apparent.

Choose green vegetables and root vegetables that are slightly undermature. Older vegetables become tough and woody and have less flavor and nutrients. Fruits are a different matter. Pick out only mature fruits, since they will probably have the best flavor. Mature but green tomatoes or hard fruit should be ripened at room temperature, out of the sun. Avoid old and withered fruits and vegetables. They have less flavor and nutrients.

In general, medium size is a good choice. Overlarge carrots, turnips, and beets may be woody. Overlarge white potatoes may have hollow centers, wireworms, or black streaks. Smaller oranges may have more juice, less thick skin, and more nutrients than large ones. A small, hard, firm head of cabbage is better than a large, loose head The former is likely to have fewer worms, less residue from spray, and less loss of vitamin C. Of course, you should also consider pricing when selecting the size of a vegetable.

Weight is a better indicator of quality than size. Heavy weight in proportion to size indicates high quality.

The color of a fruit or vegetable should be characteristic of its kind. For example, green vegetables should be deep green. The green color should be uniform and free of dark-colored spots. Yellow vegetables should be deep yellow. Cauliflower should be a clean white. A green underskin on a potato means that a toxic chemical, solanine, is present. Such potatoes are not a bargain,

Fresh fruits and vegetables should be chosen for color, size, and weight, as well as freshness.

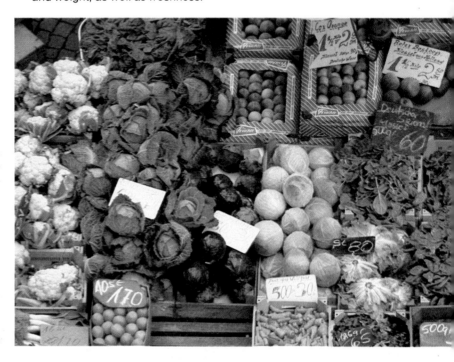

even at a low price. When fresh produce is packaged, it is protected from dirt, germs, and withering. There is less bruising from handling by customers. But pre-packaged food can cost more. Sometimes food is packaged so as to hide blemishes or spoilage. The dripping of juice in a fruit package indicates poor quality.

PROCESSED FRUITS AND VEGETABLES

Many years ago, people would often get sick early in the spring. A major reason for this was that they had not had enough fruits and vegetables to eat during the winter. As a result, they did not get enough vitamins, especially A and C. The body reserves of these vitamins were lowered. Naturally, with weaker cell tissues, people were more likely to have sickness and infections.

Fortunately, we no longer have to worry about living through long lean winters. Fruits and vegetables and their juices are now canned, frozen, and dried. They can be eaten all year long.

Processing methods

Processed fruits and vegetables usually reach the consumer in one of three forms.

Canning. New methods of canning far surpass the old "boil-and-can" method. The latest methods include pressure canning and flash canning.

Pressure canning is used for nonacid vegetables and meat products. It uses 2.7 kg (6 lb) of pressure for vegetables to reach a temperature of 110 °C (230 °F). It destroys all harmful bacteria.

A new method of flash canning is called HTST (high temperature–short time). The food is heated to a temperature of 140 °C (285 °F), which is held only seconds or a few minutes at most. Then, in an aseptic (germ-free) chamber, it is canned, sealed, and quickly cooled. Juices, baby foods, peas, corn, and all small-unit foods are canned by this method.

Other methods under study or in use include the following:

1. High-frequency electronic heating
2. The addition of antibiotics, such as nisin and subtilin
3. The addition of chemicals, such as propylene oxide and hydrogen peroxide
4. The mechanical shaking of the containers to circulate heat and decrease cooking time

Freezing. Fresh vegetables and fruits are quickly frozen and held at −18 °C (0 °F) until they are used. When frozen food thaws, it should be used at once, before harmful bacteria start to form. Refreezing causes rapid deterioration of color, texture, flavor, and nutrients. Refreezing can also allow harmful microorganisms to develop.

Drying. Drying fruits and vegetables is the oldest method of preserving them. The foods preserved by this process are concentrated sources of nutrients and energy. (See the table of nutritive

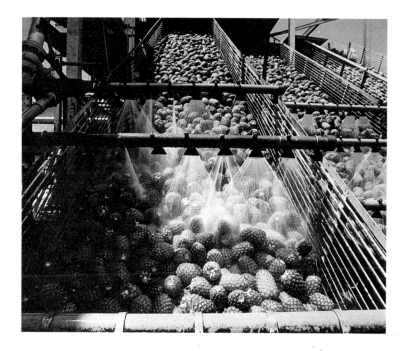

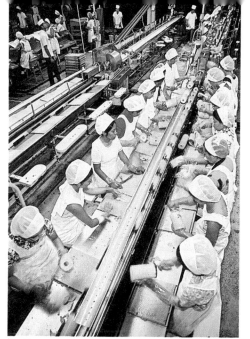

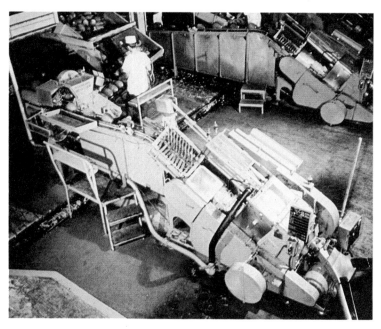

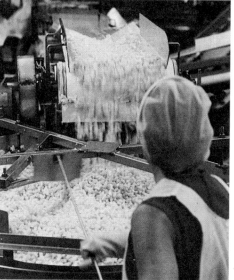

Pineapple goes through many steps before cans appear on your supermarket shelves. The fruit is washed (*top left*), peeled and cored (*bottom left*), and trimmed (*top right*). Then it is sliced or diced (*center right*). Slices are graded and packed (*bottom right*).

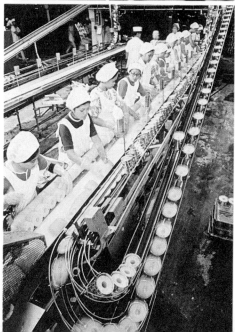

values of foods on pages 404–430.) Fruits intended for drying are harvested later than those picked for canning and freezing or for the fresh-food market. They keep well for long periods when stored in a cool, dry place. The moisture is reduced to 18 to 24 percent. The removal of moisture prevents microorganisms from growing and thus prevents decay and spoilage.

Dried foods usually cost less per serving than fresh, canned, or frozen foods. Because of their reduced weight and bulk, they cost less to package, transport, and store. For example, it takes 2.7 to 3.6 kg (6 to 8 lb) of fresh apricots to make .45 kg (1 lb) of dried ones.

Advantages of processed fruits and vegetables

Processed foods help make a good diet always available. Processed foods are also convenient, clean, and ready to be prepared quickly. In addition, dried and canned foods are easily stored and transported.

Commercial processors take care to preserve foods as soon as they are harvested. Processing plants are located in the heart of the district in which food is grown. The food is whisked from harvest to processing plant, often in a flume of water on a conveyor belt. Then, within minutes after harvest, it is prepared and then canned or frozen. Few home-makers can act so promptly unless they have their own gardens. This means a lot, especially for the juicy and leafy fruits and vegetables that spoil quickly.

Dried foods are available all year round. They keep so well, in fact, that vegetables and fruits thousands of years old have been found in the ancient tombs of Egypt. Another advantage of dried fruits and vegetables is their high mineral content. A serving of 240 mL (1 c) of dried raisins contains over four times as much iron as a serving of fresh grapes. A 240-mL (1-c) serving of uncooked dried apricots has almost seven times as much iron and four times as much vitamin A as the same amount of canned apricots.

The carbohydrates and proteins in dried fruits also make significant contributions to the diet. Dried fruit is therefore a more wholesome sweet than candy or rich cookies. The calories in dried fruits carry more than their weight in meeting the day's total nutrient needs.

Modern science is finding new ways to dry other foods. In freeze-drying, research is combining some of the best features of freezing with the drying process. Fresh frozen food is dried in a vacuum. Weight and bulk are reduced in some foods by half or more. Other freeze-dried foods keep their original size but weigh much less. A freeze-dried strawberry has only one-sixteenth the weight of a fresh one. Texture and nutrients in such foods are retained. Unfortunately, the flavor and aroma of fresh fruit are lost. Research is under way to solve this problem.

Fruits used for "fresh fruit" pies are frozen in large quantities by the freeze-drying process. The cost for such pies, however, is high for family use.

100

Drawbacks of processed fruits and vegetables

Higher cost of some canned and frozen foods can be a problem for the consumer. This is an important point to remember for anyone. It would be foolish to buy either canned or frozen potatoes or carrots if the fresh ones cost less. On the other hand, canned or frozen peas might be lower in cost than fresh ones. Thus, you must determine how much you can afford to pay. Shop for the foods that cost less per serving in your markets at different seasons of the year.

Volatile acids cannot escape from canned foods. The acids change the color of green vegetables, making them either olive or a pale green. The drab appearance of canned vegetables makes them less appealing to us. However, the volatile acids and the changed color do not affect the nutritive value or taste of the food. Canned nonacid vegetables lose vitamins if they are held too long in storage or at temperatures above 18 °C (65 °F). Loss of vitamins can be avoided by using what you buy in order of purchase within four to six months and by not overbuying. However, canned citrus and acid fruits may be kept in the home for up to a year without loss of vitamins.

Processed fruits and vegetables lose nutrients in another way. Some vitamins and minerals are lost as the freshly picked food is moved in a flume of water from farm to processing plant. More nutrients are lost when the food goes through a process called blanching. This is the process of dipping the food in boiling water or exposing it to steam and then dipping it in cold water. Blanching is needed to stop enzyme action within the food and prevent deterioration. Research is underway to improve the process to keep loss of nutrients to a minimum.

When you buy dried fruits, beware of sulfuring, a process that helps retain the color of light-colored fruits. Sulfuring also protects vitamin C—but at the expense of thiamin. One study showed that sulfuring destroys about three-fourths of the thiamin in light-colored fruits. Unsulfured fruits, such as prunes, usually lose only about 20 percent of thiamin.

The quality of processed fruits and vegetables depends on the difference between well-equipped and poorly equipped processing plants. Well-equipped plants that apply the latest knowledge lose as little as 5 to 10 percent of the water-soluble nutrients in fruits and vegetables. Plants less well equipped and less efficient lose 40 to 50 percent! Thus, when you buy canned vegetables and fruits, it is wise to note the name of the processor. Well-established firms have good modern equipment. They usually take pride in the highest-quality product.

SHOPPING FOR FRUITS AND VEGETABLES

You now have the information you need to make good choices among fruits and vegetables. The following principles will guide you in buying fresh and processed produce.

Fresh fruits and vegetables

1. Buy fresh fruits and vegetables at a market that has a rapid turnover and good refrigeration. If you can, buy at a genuine farm market where foods are harvested just before marketing.

2. Avoid stores that display fresh produce in the sun. Also avoid those that overwater fresh vegetables to give them an appearance of freshness. Too much sun and watering cause deterioration and loss of water-soluble vitamins and other nutrients.

3. Shop for fresh produce on the days when it is freshest, but at a time when you do your other food shopping.

4. Observe good shopping manners. When you examine fresh fruits and vegetables for quality, do not squeeze them. This causes bruises and rot and increases spoilage. You may be sure the loss on such produce is included in the price. In the end, consumers pay for poor shopping manners.

5. Purchase fruits and vegetables yourself for best choices and lowest cost; don't trust the judgment of others.

6. Whenever possible, buy fresh vegetables and fruits in bulk, not in packages. By buying in bulk, you can select each piece of produce to assure high quality and uniform size. Also, bulk produce usually costs less than packaged produce.

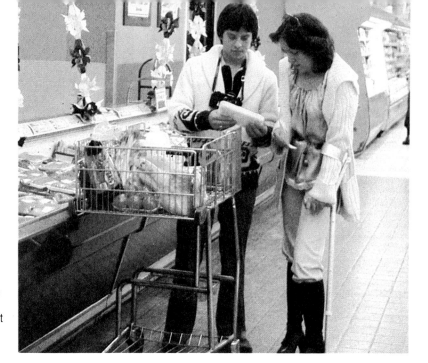

One advantage of packaged produce is that you can buy pieces of large items that would be too much to use economically if bought whole.

Processed fruits and vegetables

1. To insure quality when purchasing processed fruits and vegetables, make sure that bottles and jars are tightly sealed. Make sure there is no seepage at the seal. Do not buy canned products with rusted or bulging lids. There should be no seepage at the seams. When canned goods are opened, there should be no fermentation, off-color, or off-odor.

2. Whenever possible, buy the larger cans of food instead of the smaller cans. The larger cans usually cost less per serving than the smaller ones. Even single people will find a large can of tomatoes, juice, or fruit economical because the opened unused portion may be stored in the refrigerator.

3. Do not buy frozen fruits and vegetables that have thawed and been refrozen. You can tell thawing and refreezing has happened if the juices have run out and discolored the package or if a bag of small-unit items like beans or berries is a frozen, solid mass.

4. Compare prices on large and small packages of frozen foods. Usually large packages cost less per serving than the smaller ones. But weight and cost must be checked and compared.

5. Compare the cost per serving of processed foods with fresh foods. Dried beans and other legumes cost about one-fifth to one-tenth as much per serving as canned cooked beans. Yet you may need some canned beans as a reserve. Canned tomatoes are often less expensive per serving than fresh ones. So are processed citrus fruits when the fresh ones are out of season.

6. When sales are on, buy canned or frozen food in quantity to save money. Sales usually occur at harvest time, when the new crop is ready for canning or freezing.

7. Read the descriptive label on processed foods. On it is the list of ingredients as well as certain nutrients the food contains.

The following guidelines will help you to use fruits and vegetables economically.

Fresh fruits and vegetables

Most produce has been exposed to insecticides, sprays, sand, dirt, insects, and microorganisms. For this reason, you should be careful about washing, storing, and using fresh fruits and vegetables.

1. Sort all fruits and vegetables.
2. Wash fruits and vegetables thoroughly and dry them before storing. Fill the sink two-thirds full of water. Change water as often as necessary so that all the foods are washed in clean water. Scrub root vegetables—celery, asparagus, and the like—with a brush. Wash green leaves a few at a time. Drain them in a colander or wire basket made for the purpose. Shake off the surplus moisture.
3. Wrap fresh produce in old, clean towels or paper towels. Store it in the crisper drawer of the refrigerator. For best storage, the crisper drawer should be only two-thirds full. Fresh produce that is packaged in plastic may be stored on the refrigerator shelves.
4. Store foods with a strong odor, such as onions, cantaloupes, or pineapple, in tightly closed plastic bags so that the odor will not affect other foods. Moisture, flavor, and freshness are retained better if each kind is separately packaged or wrapped.
5. Use the ripest, most perishable fruits and vegetables first. Store them in the front part of the refrigerator. Fresh green leaves are more likely to spoil than carrots. Corn will spoil sooner than potatoes. Green onions are likely to spoil sooner than yellow ones. Late-crop potatoes keep better than new and early ones.

Canned and dried foods

1. Plan to have a variety of dried and canned fruits and vegetables on hand. A reserve helps you prepare a meal quickly and inexpensively for family or guests.
2. Store canned and dried foods in cool, dry, dark areas below 20 °C (65 °F) and above freezing. Be aware that dried fruits may spoil in hot humid weather if moisture is allowed to get through to them. Canned foods are not subject to this problem. However, over a period of time, canned foods will gradually lose their vitamin content. Cool temperatures delay this loss. Higher temperatures accelerate it.
3. Canned foods are sterilized, cooked, and ready to eat. But you may wish to add a little seasoning to some vegetables. Just before serving, heat them to below the boiling point. Don't cook them more than this or they will lose texture and vitamins.
4. Cans have been exposed to contamination in the air. Therefore, before a can is opened, it should be washed, then dried with a paper towel. Cans and the unused food in them can then be safely stored in the refrigerator.

Wash fresh fruits and vegetables before storing them in the refrigerator.

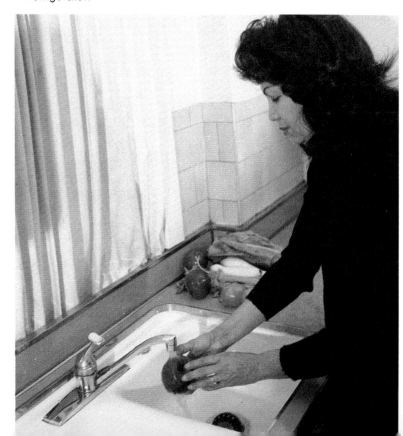

(Citrus and acid foods are an important exception. They do not keep well in opened cans.)

In spite of loss of some nutrients during processing, canned foods may offer good value. Thus, per cup, canned orange juice contains 100 milligrams of vitamin C; frozen juice, 120; and fresh juice, 124 milligrams. The relative cost is important to those with low incomes.

You should eat some vegetables and fruits raw. They give you nutrients that are destroyed by heating or cooking. At the same time, some vegetables and fruits benefit by cooking.

Some vegetables and fruits are more nutritious when eaten raw; others are more beneficial cooked.

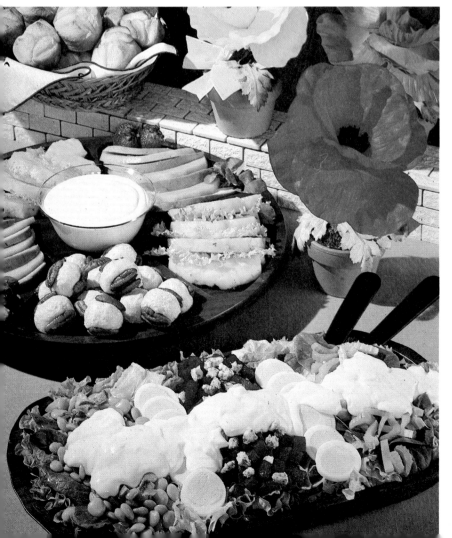

Reasons for cooking

Following are several reasons for cooking vegetables and fruits.

1. Human beings digest and absorb cooked vegetables more easily than raw ones.
2. Cooking reduces the bulk, especially of the green, leafy vegetables, enabling us to consume larger amounts.
3. It is easier for us to absorb the nutrients in cooked fruits. Cooking softens a fruit's cellulose and protopectins. **Protopectins** in fruits tend to cement the structure of fruit cells. They can interfere with the complete absorption of the nutrients in fruit. Cooking changes protopectins into **pectin** and makes absorption easier.
4. The pectins from cooked fruits combine with cholesterol and eliminate it.
5. Cooking destroys molds, yeasts, and most bacteria. In places where sanitary conditions are poor, it is safer to eat hot, cooked food or raw food that can be peeled.
6. Cooked fruits and vegetables are easier to digest for people who have trouble digesting or absorbing the nutrients in uncooked fruits and vegetables. Children, elderly people, and people with certain diseases often need cooked rather than raw produce.

7. Proper cooking improves the flavor of many vegetables and adds variety to meals.

Goals for cooking

Keep the following goals in mind when cooking fruits and vegetables.

1. Tender, yet firm, crisp texture that is neither soft and soggy nor tough and hard
2. Retention of maximum nutrients at lowest cost
3. Retention of color
4. Peak flavor

Techniques for cooking vegetables

Vegetables may be simmered, boiled, steamed, sauteed, pan fried, stir fried, baked; cooked in waterless or pressure saucepans, or in microwave ovens. The cooking time varies with each method. For example, it usually takes less time to stir fry, or use a pressure cooker or microwave oven than to cook using a variety of other methods. The following principles will serve as a guide for cooking vegetables successfully.

1. Cook in as short a time as possible to assure maximum flavor, crisp texture, and retention of color and nutrients. Table 6-1 gives the approximate cooking time for 33 vegetables. The time required depends on the size of the pot and on the size and maturity of the food. For example, small pieces or young, tender vegetables require less time than large pieces or old, tough vegetables. Timing also depends on

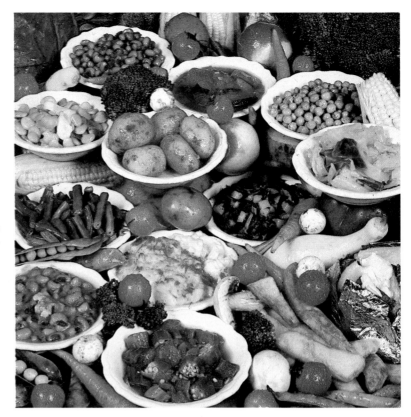

Cooked vegetables should retain texture, shape, color, nutrients, and flavor.

whether the food is fresh, frozen, or dried. Frozen foods take less time than fresh. Fresh foods take less time than dried. Overcooking produces soft, unattractive, less tasty, and less nourishing foods.
2. Cook in a thick, flat-bottomed pan with a tight-fitting lid to prevent oxidation. (Pressure cookers are based on this principle. They save time and nutrients.) Use a size of pan that fits the heat source and the amount of food to be cooked.
3. Use as little water as possible. Use only water that has been boiled for two minutes to expel all oxygen. This will keep vitamin C loss to a minimum. The amount of water clinging to washed spinach or Swiss chard is sufficient for cooking. In general use 60 to

80 mL (¼ to ⅓ c) of boiled water per .45 kg (1 lb) of root and tuber vegetables. Frozen vegetables require less water than most packages suggest, but you may be guided by the package directions until you find the right amount for your taste and equipment. Dried beans, peas, and lentils require 720 mL (3 c) of water per 240 mL (1 c) of dried food, except when a pressure saucepan is used. In the latter case, use 480 mL (2 c) of water per 240 mL (1 c) of food.
4. Cover the pan. Bring the water to a boil quickly. Then lower the heat until bubbles just form and break. Water boils at a temperature of 100 °C (212 °F). It remains at 100 °C (212 °F) no matter how much more heat is

Table 6-1 Approximate times for cooking vegetables (minutes)[1]

VEGETABLE	BOILING	STEAMING	PRESSURE SAUCEPAN (7 kg [15 lb] pressure)	BAKING
Artichokes, Jerusalem, whole	25–35	35	4–10	30–60
Asparagus, tips	5–15	7–15	½–1½	
Beans, lima, green	20–30	25–35	1–2	
Beans, snap, whole, or 2-cm (1-in) pieces	15–30	20–35	1½–3	
Beets, new, whole	30–45	40–60	5–10	40–60
old, whole	45–90	50–90	10–18	40–60
Broccoli, stalk and buds	10–15	15–20	1½–3	
Brussels sprouts, whole	10–20	15–20	1–2	
Cabbage, green, quartered	10–15	15	2–3	
shredded	3–10	8–12	½–1½	
Cabbage, red, shredded	8–12	10–15	½–1½	
Carrots, young, whole	15–20	20–30	3–5	35–45
mature, whole	20–30	40–50	10–15	60
sliced	15–25	25–30	3	
Cauliflower, whole	15–25	25–30	10	
flowerets	8–15	10–20	1½–3	
Celery, diced	15–18	25–30	2–3	
Chard, Swiss	10–20	15–25	1½–3	
Collards	10–20			
Corn, on cob	6–12	10–15	½–1½	
Eggplant, sliced	10–20	15–20		
Kale	10–15			
Okra, sliced	10–15	20	3–4	
Onions, small, whole	15–30	25–35	3–4	
large, whole	20–40	35–40	5–8	50–60
Parsnips, whole	20–40	30–45	9–10	30–45
quartered	8–15	30–40	4–8	
Peas, green	12–16	10–20	0–1	
Potatoes, white, medium, whole	25–40	30–45	8–11	45–60
quartered	20–25	20–30	3–5	
Rutabaga, diced	20–30	35–40	5–8	
Spinach	3–10	5–12	0–1½	
Squash, Hubbard, 5-cm (2-in) pieces	15–20	25–40	6–12	40–60
Squash, summer, sliced	8–15	15–20	1½–3	30
Sweet potatoes, whole	35–55	30–45	5–8	
quartered	15–25	25–30	6	
Tomatoes	7–15		½–1	15–30
Turnips, whole	20–30		8–12	
sliced	15–20	20–25	1½	

Adapted from *Handbook of Food Preparation* (Washington, D. C.: American Home Economics Association, Terminology Committee of the Food and Nutrition Division, 1975).
[1] The time for any method cannot be given exactly, because it depends on the variety and maturity of each vegetable and the size of the pieces into which it has been cut. Use the shortest time possible to obtain the desired results.

applied, so don't waste fuel. Cook the food until it is just tender, and serve it at once.

Retaining nutrients

The outside leaves and skins of vegetables and fruits contain the greatest amount of the food's vitamins, minerals, and amino acids.

Use all the remaining liquid. Some people enjoy dipping bread in the "pot liquor." This habit helps them retain many of the nutrients released from the food into the liquid. To achieve the same results, the cooking liquid can be used as the base of a soup or a sauce, or in a gelatin salad. and flavor. Whenever possible, cook fruits and vegetables in their skins. If you must peel or trim them, use a peeler or pare thinly with a sharp knife. The less surface exposed, the greater the retention of vitamins and minerals. Table 6-2 shows the amounts of nutrients lost in preparing and cooking fruits and vegetables.

The **panning** method of cooking is well-suited to the following fruits and vegetables: green beans, green peas, summer squash, spinach, cabbage, endive, eggplant, onions, fresh apples, pineapple, and peaches. Place a small amount of fat in a firm, shallow, broad-bottomed pan. You may use a skillet (with a lid), a wok, a chicken fryer, or an electric skillet. Add the fresh or frozen vegetable. Season it and stir until each piece is coated lightly with fat. Little or no water is needed. The thin coat of fat helps the vegetable retain its flavor and vitamins. Cover the pan. Cook only until the vegetable

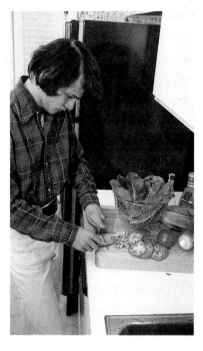 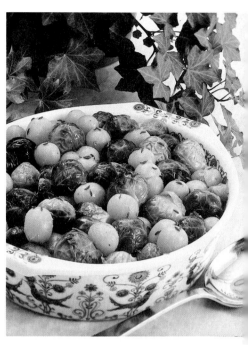

Left: The less surface exposed in cooking, the better vegetables and fruits retain nutrients. *Right:* Cook vegetables briefly with a small amount of water in a tightly covered pan.

is just tender (3 to 5 minutes). Stirring at intervals hastens cooking on all sides and prevents loss of color.

Crock pot cooking is not recommended for vegetables, although crock pots have other advantages. One advantage is that you can put your meal on in the morning and it is ready at night. Another advantage is that tough meat is tenderized. However in crock pot cooking vegetables lose more minerals and vitamins than

Table 6-2 **Loss of four vitamins during preparation and cooking of vegetables and fruits (percent)**

FOOD	THIAMIN	RIBOFLAVIN	NIACIN	VITAMIN C
Citrus fruits, tomatoes	—	—	—	15
Leafy green and yellow vegetables	45	40	40	50
Potatoes, sweet potatoes	25	20	20	35
Other vegetables and fruits	20	20	20	25

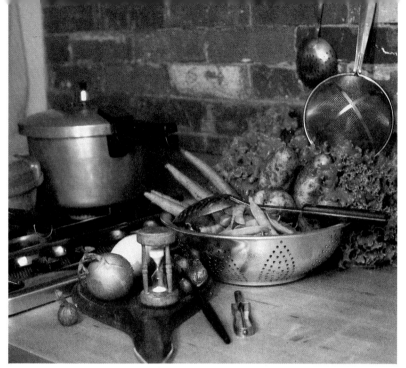

Pressure cooking is a good way to retain color in cooking vegetables and fruits. Microwave cooking is another time-saving method that retains color in vegetables.

with other ways of cooking. If you use the crock pot method of cooking vegetables, be sure to use all of the liquid. This way you regain some of the lost nutrients.

Retaining color

Green vegetables lose their color easily. Heat from cooking may decompose the green chlorophyll. Acids, though harmless, may turn a deep green color to a drab olive. Yet, a deep green color still appeals to your appetite and sense of beauty. How can you retain it?

Adding soda to green vegetables helps preserve the green color but it destroys some of the B vitamins and vitamin C. It is not recommended.

A better way to preserve the green color is simply to cook the vegetable properly. Cook green

vegetables quickly until they are just tender. The pressure saucepan is the best piece of equipment for reaching this goal. Stop the cooking in a pressure saucepan by running cold water from the tap over the lid of the pan. Remove the lid to let volatile acids escape. Serve green vegetables immediately. If you use a regular pan with a lid, leave the lid slightly ajar after cooking. This will free the volatile acids and help retain the green color.

Panned vegetables should be cooked just before serving. Otherwise, they may lose the green color while waiting.

Wrap peeled potatoes tightly in plastic and store them in the hydrator of the refrigerator until you are ready to cook them. This prevents darkening. To retain the whiteness in white potatoes and in other white vegetables such as cauliflower, onions, celery, turnips, white cabbage, just add one teaspoon of vinegar to the cooking water.

When vinegar is added to red cabbage or beets, the acid deepens the color. Alkaline (hard) water turns red foods a blue-purple color.

Light fruits such as pears, peaches, apples, bananas, avocados can darken when peeled. To prevent this, dip them in lemon or lime juice. Or use a commercial color preservative that contains vitamin C.

Seasoning

No amount of seasoning can make up for poorly cooked vegetables. But good seasoning can make well-prepared vegetables a gourmet's delight. Basic seasonings for vegetables are salt, fat, and pepper.

Fruits are so delicate in flavor that seasoning may detract from their taste. Few fruits require sugar, even when eaten uncooked.

Vegetables may taste flat without salt or a salt substitute. Worcestershire sauce, celery salt, onion salt, garlic salt, dried parsley, soy sauce, and prepared mustard all bring out flavor. Salt substitutes are now available for people who are on a low-sodium diet for health reasons.

Fats used for seasoning are vegetable oil, margarine, butter, pork or other meat drippings, and sweet and sour cream. The kind of fat used greatly affects the taste of the vegetable. For example, green vegetables may get a nice, tangy flavor from the drippings of chops, ham, bacon, or a roast. To avoid using animal fat but to keep meat flavor, remove all the animal fat from the brown meat drippings and combine the drippings with vegetable oil.

Butter was once considered the aristocrat of seasonings for vegetables. Less butter is used today for two reasons. One reason is its high price. A second reason is our knowledge of the saturated fatty acids in butter. Modern research is showing that the most healthful fat to use in seasoning is vegetable oil which is high in linoleic acid (For details, see Chapter 14.)

Sour cream has only 30 calories per 15 mL (1 T). A small amount is often used to top baked potatoes, cabbage, cauliflower, and other vegetables, as well as salads.

Pepper may be hot or sweet, black, white, green, or red. It is favored as a seasoning for many cooked vegetables and for salads. The amount you use depends on your taste. In some parts of the world, especially in hot, tropical countries, a great deal of pepper is used. In the days before refrigeration, spices were used to hide the unpleasant flavor of spoiled foods. Today, pepper is used to bring out the flavor of food, not to hide it.

Onion is universally prized for adding savor to a dish. It enhances the flavor of vegetables, meats, soups, stews, casseroles, and salads. Fresh onions can be used. You can use onion salt, dried onion flakes, or frozen onions also. Over two billion pounds of onions a year are used in the United States.

Garlic in fresh cloves, garlic salt, dried flakes, or juice is used with vegetables in small amounts to give a distinctive flavor. A light touch is needed in its use.

Herbs and spices make the flavor of cooked vegetables and fruit dishes more interesting.

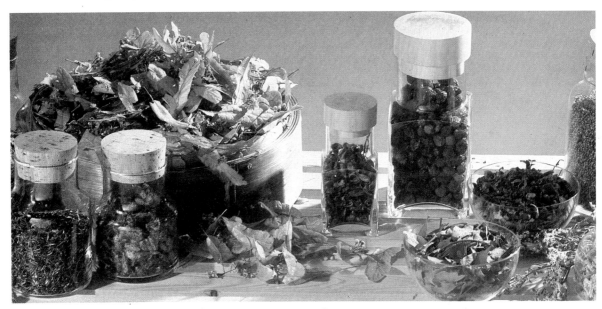

Other spices give a gourmet taste to some fruits and vegetables. Try a few whole allspice in lentil soup for an elusive, mellow flavor. Nutmeg added to carrots with a little honey makes them especially delicious. Cinnamon sticks added to homemade French dressing lend a tantalizing flavor. Nutmeg, cinnamon, clove, or ginger enhances pineapple chunks or pieces of orange or melon. Try different spices or herbs with beets, parsnips, turnips, pumpkin, tomatoes, and other vegetables. (Table 10-7 lists spices and herbs to use for seasoning foods.)

Herbs may be grown in pots in a sunny window. They may also be grown in a border or corner of the yard. Freshly cut herbs can add delightful flavors to fruits and vegetables. Experiment and discover the fun of growing and using fresh herbs.

SALADS

A green salad is important to your daily diet. It can help improve your appearance and increase your vitality.

A fruit or vegetable salad in a meal adds contrast in texture, flavor, and color. Another purpose of a salad is to balance the meal nutritionally. Salads can help in controlling overweight because they add fiber but few calories to the diet. Calories range from 5 to 15 for a salad with lemon dressing. They vary according to the kind of salad and the type and amount of dressing used. In Chapter 14 vegetable oil as an important part of a meal is considered.

Kinds of salads

Salads may be used as a separate course, as the main course, or as dessert in the meal. Select the salad to suit the rest of the menu. If you are having fresh fruit and cheese for dessert, serve a tossed salad. For a festive meal, serve a colorful salad that is low in calories. This is a good idea for everyday meals, too.

The tossed green salad may consist of one kind of green, leafy vegetable or several kinds combined. A variety of fresh or canned fruits may be used on a bed of green lettuce or watercress

The ingredients for green salads are limited only by imagination.

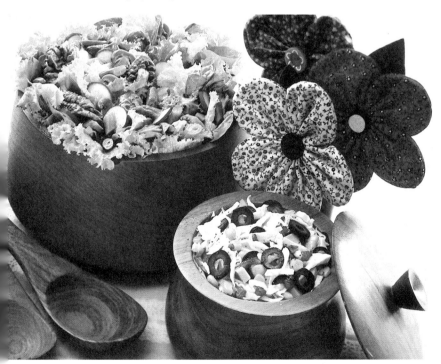

with a mound of cottage cheese in the center. Avocado adds flavor, texture, and color contrast.

Strawberries circling a slice of pineapple make a fruit salad that is moderate in price when both fruits are in season. This combination is beautiful to look at and delicious as a dessert. Chopped or ground cranberries, orange, and apples make a seasonal accompaniment to a holiday meal. Melon balls or cubes make an attractive summer salad. Taking advantage of seasonal fruits is economical and adds variety to your salads.

Chef's salad can be used as a main dish. It consists of tossed greens and 80 mL (⅓ c) of meat, poultry, or seafood per serving. The meats should be cut in pieces large enough to be recognizable. Diced sharp cheese may also be used. Egg sections or slices are used to garnish the salad. For best flavor the meat may be prepared ahead of time and allowed to marinate with the dressing. Greens may also be prepared in advance, ready to toss, and stored in the refrigerator in a plastic bag. Potato salad, hot or cold, may also be used as a main dish when a source of protein is added. The protein source could be cooked ham, frankfurters, eggs, or cheese.

Gelatin salads may be served as a salad or as a dessert. Small pieces of vegetables, fruits, meats, fish, cheese, or poultry or a combination of these may be molded into the gelatin. An advantage of a gelatin salad is that it seals in the other foods. Thus there is no loss of vitamins from oxidation. It is well-suited to the diets of small children and some elderly people.

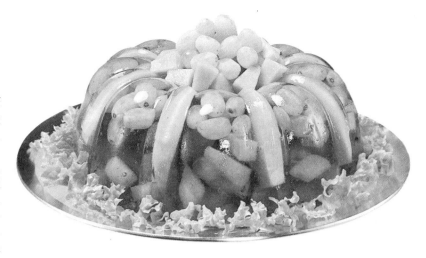

Fruit and gelatin salads may be served as desserts.

Imagination turns fruits and fruit sherbets into fanciful desserts.

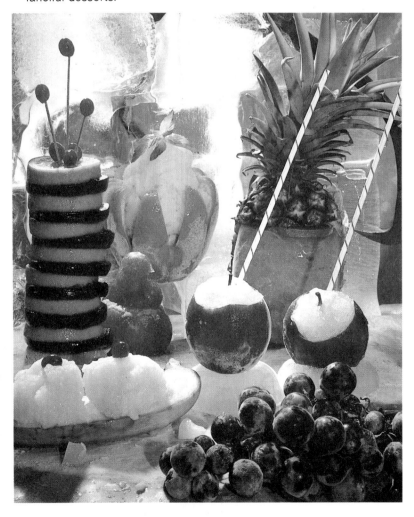

Preparing salads

There are four basic points to remember about salad ingredients. They should be fresh, clean, cold, and crisp. A salad is no better than the quality of its ingredients.

Assemble your equipment and ingredients before you begin. Just before serving, tear the greens in bite-size pieces. Do not cut the leaves with a knife or they will show bruises. As with all foods, pieces should be large enough to keep their shape, but not so large as to be unmanageable for eating.

Making salad dressings

Salad dressings cannot hide poor-quality ingredients. They can, however, bring out the flavor of good ingredients. There are three kinds of basic dressings:

1. French dressing: oil, vinegar, and seasoning
2. Mayonnaise: oil, egg, and seasonings whipped to a smooth, stiff emulsion
3. Cooked or boiled dressing

Each of the three basic dressings may include other ingredients for variety. Favorite herbs and spices, bleu or Roquefort cheese, or chili sauce may be added to dressings. Many ready-to-use or ready-to-mix dressings are available. When you are in doubt, French dressing is always a good choice. Making your own French dressing is less expensive than buying commercial brands, and you can add your own touches. You can choose an oil high in linoleic acid for greater nutritive value. Lemon and lime juice add vitamin C as well as flavor. Wine and tarragon vinegars alter the flavor, too. Oil contains 125 calories per 15 mL (1 T). By using two parts vinegar or lemon juice to one part oil you can reduce calories in French dressing by two-thirds.

Add chili sauce to mayonnaise and you have Russian dressing. Add diced pickle or horseradish to mayonnaise for a tartar sauce to use with fish.

Tossing salads

The tossing of a salad is as satisfying to watch as the carving of a fine roast. Fine restaurants dramatize it. Tossing the salad at the table can add a professional touch to meals at home.

Mix seasonings ahead of time. Experiment with mint, chives, and rosemary in fruit salad. Try chives, parsley, basil, or tarragon in a salad of greens. For added flavor, consider using freshly ground pepper, garlic-flavored toast cubes, bits of cheese, or crumbled bacon.

When you bring the bowl of salad ingredients to the table, pour the seasoning mixture over the ingredients. Then add the dressing. Bring a fork and spoon from the bottom of the bowl up through and over the ingredients. Toss very gently until all the ingredients are moist and glistening but still firm. Use only enough dressing to coat the salad, leaving very little in the bottom of the bowl. Spoon the salad lightly onto salad plates and serve.

RECAP

Economy of fruits and vegetables

Quality in fresh fruits and vegetables

Processed fruits and vegetables

Processing methods   *Canning   Freezing   Drying*
Advantages of processed fruits and vegetables   Drawbacks of processed fruits and vegetables

Shopping for fruits and vegetables

Fresh fruits and vegetables   Processed fruits and vegetables

Storing and using fruits and vegetables

Fresh fruits and vegetables   Canned and dried foods

Cooking fruits and vegetables

Reasons for cooking   Goals for cooking   Techniques for cooking vegetables   Retaining nutrients   Retaining color   Seasoning

Salads

Kinds of salads   Preparing salads   Making salad dressings   Tossing salads

THINKING AND EVALUATING

1. In general, what are the signs of quality in fresh fruits and vegetables?

2. What are the economic advantages of using fresh fruits and vegetables in the diet?

3. What is meant by the term "processed food"?

4. Discuss the advantages of processed fruits and vegetables to a nutritionally adequate diet. The disadvantages?

5. Explain why cooked fruits and vegetables can be beneficial to the diets of older people.

6. Describe how to store the following kinds of fruits and vegetables: fresh, frozen, canned, dried.

APPLYING AND SHARING

1. Invite the produce manager at a local supermarket to explain to the class how he buys fresh fruits and vegetables for his department. What are the differences and similarities between his purchasing techniques and those of the average consumer?

VOCABULARY

aseptic
blanching
crock pot
descriptive label
electronic heating
flash canning
freeze-drying
pectin
pressure canning
protopectin
sulfuring
volatile acids

2. Select and make a list of three fruits and three vegetables. Visit your local supermarket and make note on your list of the various forms in which these foods are sold, and the price of each. Now calculate the cost per serving. Discuss the results in class.

3. Examine vegetables on cafeteria steam tables and in restaurants. How do you rate them in color and texture, from the best to poorest? Give reasons for your rating. Do the same with salads. Compare your ratings with your own home-prepared vegetables.

4. Observe the vegetables and fruits other shoppers select and buy. Do you think they understand how to use their money wisely? Explain. Do you think they show poor manners in handling foods? What are good manners in shopping for these foods?

5. Suppose you wanted to serve a balanced diet each day on a low food budget.

> **a.** Plan the daily menus for one week to meet your total nutrient needs, provide variety in fruits and vegetables, maintain desirable weight, and stay within your budget.
>
> **b.** Underscore once the foods rich in vitamin C in each meal; underscore twice the foods rich in vitamin A; underscore three times those under 50 calories per serving.
>
> **c.** Give two or more ways to prepare each vegetable and fruit in each meal. Indicate which seasonings you would use.
>
> **d.** List other vegetables that would provide you with the same nutrients as spinach.

6. Divide the class into groups. Let each group plan balanced menus that you can prepare at school using fruits and vegetables. Have a tasting session for comparison.

> **a.** First try different methods of cooking the same leafy vegetable, yellow vegetable, white and sweet potatoes, beans, and another vegetable in season.
>
> **b.** Try different forms (fresh, canned, frozen) of the same vegetable, each group using a different form. Compare results.
>
> **c.** Try different seasonings with the same vegetable, varying the amounts. Compare results. Record what you liked best.

CAREER CAPSULES

Produce department manager Works in large grocery store or supermarket; supervises purchasing, storing, inventory, display, pricing of fruits and vegetables and related products. Required education varies; on-the-job training essential.

Small grocery store supervisor Works in district office of chain of small stores; supervises managers of stores, day-to-day operations, budgets. Required education varies; knowledge of business administration essential.

RELATED READING

Day, Avanelle S., and Lillie Stuckey. *The Spice Cookbook*. New York: David White, 1964. Contains excellent recipes for vegetables, salads, pickles, relishes, jams, and jellies, along with sound cooking directions.

Princess Pamela's Soul Food Cookbook. New York: The New American Library, 1969. Section II gives flavorful, nutritious ways to prepare fresh vegetables.

Packard, V. S. *Processed Foods and the Consumer: Additives, Labeling, Standards and Nutrition*. Minneapolis: University of Minnesota Press, 1976. Discusses processed foods knowledgeably and objectively.

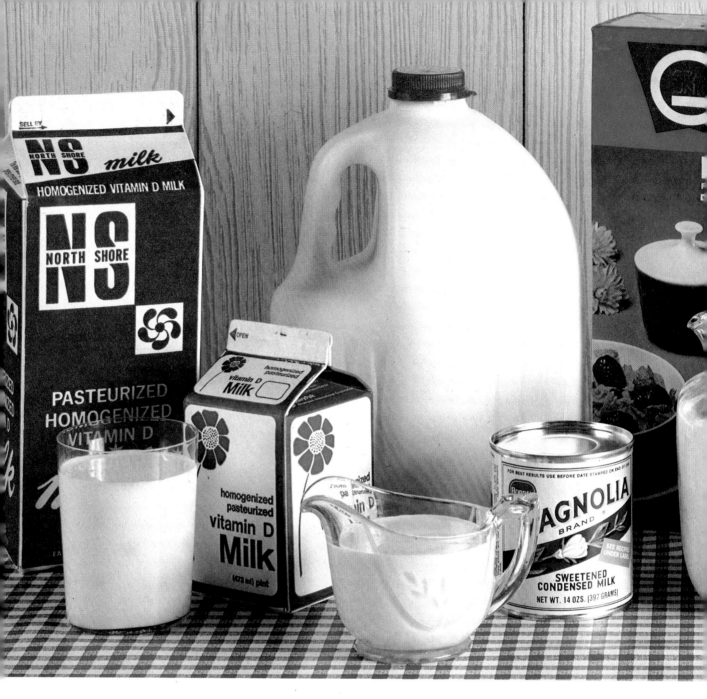

CHAPTER 7

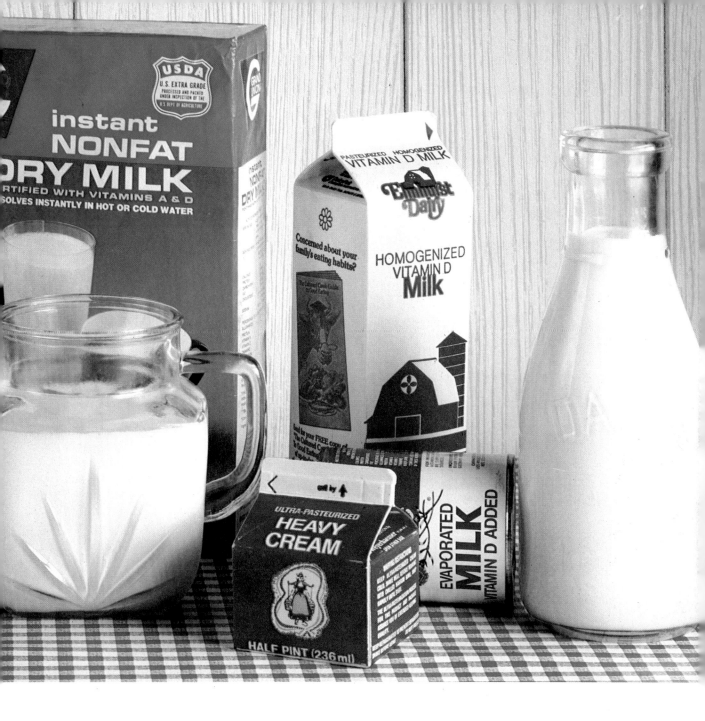

Milk

FACTS ABOUT MILK

When we are born, the only food we have to nourish us is milk. The offspring of other mammals also begin life on a milk diet. There is good reason for this. Milk contains a wide variety of nutrients in generous amounts. The nutrients in milk help us to maintain life and resist disease, and they promote growth.

Many Americans do not use the amount of milk that they need. That was one of the findings of the 1965 National Dietary Survey. The survey found that the diet of all girls and women 9 years of age and over failed to provide the recommended amount of calcium. The diet of boys between 9 and 17 and men 35 years old and older also had too little calcium. The survey also revealed that the average U.S. family used 10 percent less milk in 1965 than in 1955. Figure 7-1 shows that this downward trend continues into the 1970s. One reason for the decline is the greater use of soft drinks, and other beverages, and processed snack foods.

Some people think that milk is harmful. This chapter will show why this is a mistaken belief. When you know the facts, you can judge how much milk and what kind of milk to include in your daily diet.

Milk and nutrition

Calcium, riboflavin, and protein are the primary nutritive contributions of milk. A daily amount of .96 L (1 qt) of milk supplies all the calcium and riboflavin and half the protein needed in the diet. It contains about a fourth of the thiamin and a third of the vitamin A recommended for adults. The fat in whole milk or cheese or in a low-fat milk makes possible the absorption of the fat-soluble vitamins A, D, E, and K.

But even milk, the most nearly perfect food, is not quite perfect. It is low in iron, although the iron that it does contain is absorbed and utilized well by the body. (For a discussion of iron in the diet, see Chapter 9.)

Another weakness of milk is that its fat is mostly saturated. Recent research shows this kind of fat is less desirable than the polyunsaturated kind. However, milk has had to bear an unfair portion of the blame for the excess of saturated fat in our diets.

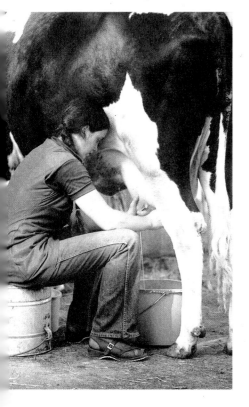
Milk is the almost perfect food.

Figure 7-1   Price and consumption indexes of dairy products.

% of 1960

Retail price

Deflated retail price [1]

Per capita consumption

1960   1963   1966   1969   1972   1975

USDA Economic Research Service, Report 138. Price data from Bureau of Labor Statistics.

[1]All items deflated by consumer price index.

People of all ages need milk.

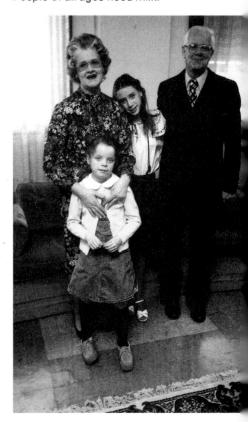

Nonfat milk in any form has all the benefits of fresh whole milk when fortified with vitamins A and D. It also has fewer calories.

Milk and acne

In the United States, acne is probably the most common skin disease. It is most frequently found among young people as they change from adolescence to adulthood.

Many people in the United States have mistaken ideas about the effect of milk on acne. Dr. Philip White, secretary of the Foods and Nutrition Council of the American Medical Association, tells of a letter he received stating that teenagers in the writer's county were encouraged to eliminate all dairy products from their diets. It was believed that milk causes acne, and the writer wanted to know if this were true. Dr. White's answer was that dairy products were too important as sources of nutrients to be eliminated from the diet. It would be difficult, he said, to find other foods that could supply so well a person's needs for calcium, vitamin D, and riboflavin. Dr. White added that it would be foolish and hazardous to deviate from an adequate diet in an attempt to clear up acne.

Doctors tell us that acne is caused primarily by overactive oil glands in the skin. The glands retain secretions and become inflamed. This occurs most frequently on the face and neck and across the back of the shoulders.

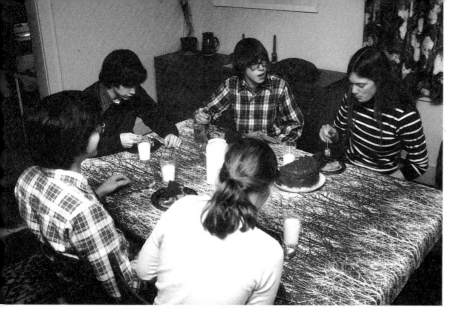

Fried foods, chocolate, nuts, and excess sweets are more likely to contribute to acne than milk.

During a person's teenage years, there is an increase in the amount and variety of hormones secreted into the bloodstream. This may explain why young people are especially prone to acne. Physicians usually advise people with skin problems to avoid eating fatty or fried foods, chocolate, candy, cola-type drinks, nuts, pastries, and excess sweets. Many nutritionists and dermatologists agree that a highly nutritious diet helps to prevent and treat acne.

Far from harming the skin, milk actually helps it. This is because the many nutrients in milk

Table 7-1 Comparison of calories in milk with those in some other foods

FOOD	MEASURE	CALORIES PER SERVING
MILK		
Whole fluid, 3.3% fat	240 mL (8 oz)	150
Low fat, according to % of fat	240 mL (8 oz)	100–125
Nonfat (skim)	240 mL (8 oz)	85
Chocolate	240 mL (8 oz)	210
Chocolate malted, home-prepared	240 mL (8 oz)	235
Lemon meringue pie	100 cm² (16 sq in)	305
Apple pie	100 cm² (16 sq in)	345
Cherry pie	100 cm² (16 sq in)	350
Mince pie	100 cm² (16 sq in)	365
Doughnut, cake type	1	125
Plain cupcake, made from mix	1	
with icing		130
without icing		90
Plain cake	7 cm² (1 sq in)	
with icing		400
without icing		315
Pizza	125 cm² (19 sq in)	145
Hamburger, no roll	84 g (3 oz)	245
Beer	360 mL (12 oz)	150
Cola-type drink	360 mL (12 oz)	145
Potato chips	10	115
Peanut butter	30 mL (2 T)	190
Fudge or caramel candy, no nuts	28 g (1 oz)	115
Plain gelatin dessert	240 mL (1 c)	140

Adapted from *Nutritive Value of Foods,* Home and Garden Bulletin No. 72 (Washington, D.C.: USDA, rev. 1977).

120

nourish the body. And when the body is nourished, the skin is clear.

Milk and weight

Have you ever heard someone say, "Oh, I don't drink milk because it is so fattening"? What are the facts? A chemical analysis of whole milk shows that it contains only 3.5 percent fat. The rest consists of 87 percent water, 3.5 percent protein, 5 percent milk sugar, 0.7 percent minerals, and a wide variety of vitamins.

Table 7-1 shows how milk compares in calories per serving with many other foods. A serving of 240 mL (8 oz) of whole milk contains 150 calories. A serving of skim milk or plain cultured buttermilk contains only 90 calo-

ries. Compare these servings with a piece of chocolate cake (445 calories), an ounce of potato chips (250 calories), or a piece of apple pie (345 calories).

You may ask, "What am I getting in addition to calories in a glass of milk?" You are getting extremely important nutrients, as the rest of this chapter shows.

CALCIUM

Calcium is the most abundant mineral in the body. It composes 1.5 to 2.0 percent of an adult's body weight.

Function of calcium in bones and teeth

The body needs large amounts of calcium for building bones and teeth. In fact, 99 percent of the calcium in the body is contained in bones and teeth.

How is the calcium in milk changed to make bone? Calcium and phosphorous together form tiny crystals called trabeculae. The crystals are arranged in the shape of a honeycomb. They are surrounded by a special fluid. As

the blood circulates, this special fluid traps needed nutrients such as protein, magnesium, and vitamins D, C, and A. By this means, growth takes place and tissue is repaired and maintained.

As bones grow, two important changes occur. Nutrients are laid down on the outside of the long bones—the leg bones, for example. At the same time, material from the inside of the bone cavity is absorbed. This provides a wider hole for the bone marrow. It makes the bone lighter and enables us to move more easily. (See Figure 7-2.)

Teeth are formed in the same way as bone, except that the crystals are larger on tooth enamel. Teeth are composed of the hard-

Figure 7-2 Calcium is important in the formation and maintenance of healthy bones like this femur (human thigh bone).

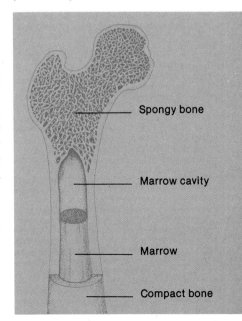

Spongy bone

Marrow cavity

Marrow

Compact bone

est tissue in the body. (See Figure 7-3.)

When the body does not have enough calcium for its various needs, growth is stunted. In nations where little or no milk is used, people's bodies adapt to low calcium in the diet by remaining short in stature.

When a diet is deficient in calcium, a person's posture may be poor. The jawbones and teeth may be poorly formed. This affects appearance and personality. Curvature of the spine occurs in young and old.

Osteoporosis is a crippling bone disease of middle-aged and older people. It is associated with a low calcium intake over a long period of time. It is also associated with other factors, such as overuse of cortisone. A person with osteoporosis loses calcium from the bones. The bones then become fragile, porous, and begin to disintegrate.

Inactivity is another factor that can interfere with proper absorption of calcium. For example, astronauts Gordon Cooper and Charles Conrad were confined for eight days on space flights. They consumed normal amounts of calcium. And yet, after returning to earth, tests showed that they had lost bone calcium amounting to 12 to 15 percent. This surprising case prompted a study of persons confined to bed. The study showed that people lose more bone calcium when they are inactive. It also showed that with increased amounts of calcium in the diet, less bone calcium is lost.

Functions of calcium in bodily processes

Building bones and teeth is not the only function of calcium. A constant level of calcium in the blood helps to keep bodily processes functioning.

Calcium helps control the heartbeat. It triggers the contraction that sends the blood pulsing through every tissue.

Calcium serves as a comember of a team to clot the blood. WHen the blood does not clot, even a small cut can be serious.

Calcium promotes the passage of fluid between cells. This enables them to absorb nutrients and oxygen and give off waste.

Calcium and phosphorous are required for normal functioning of nerves and muscles. When the calcium level in the blood drops, nerves are more irritable. Muscle spasms and leg cramps can also occur when the calcium level drops.

Calcium and phosphorous help maintain the alkaline-acid balance. This keeps the chemistry of the body functioning properly.

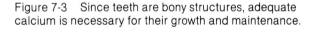

Figure 7-3   Since teeth are bony structures, adequate calcium is necessary for their growth and maintenance.

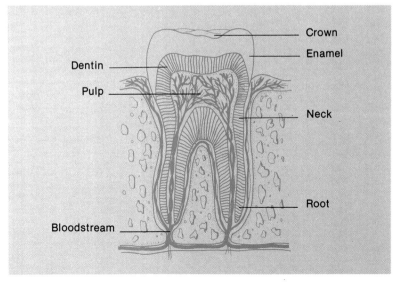

Maintaining calcium level

The parathyroid glands (Figure 7-4) control the level of the calcium in the bloodstream. This tiny pair of glands lies astride the thyroid gland. They secrete a hormone that gives the signals to maintain calcium at a steady, normal level. When there is too little calcium in the diet, they send the message to "rob the bones." When there is too much calcium after all immediate needs and reserves are met, the excess is eliminated in the urine.

When we don't get calcium with our meals in the amount needed, the body adapts to the lack. It does so by taking the calcium it requires from the calcium reserve in the bones. If that "cupboard" is "bare," like the one in the nursery rhyme, our body then takes calcium from the bone structure itself. Thus bones are weakened to keep the body functioning as a whole. The eventual result of this process is premature aging.

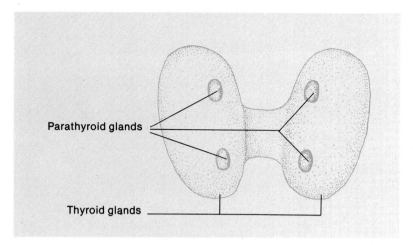

Figure 7-4   The parathyroid glands control the level of calcium in the bloodstream.

Even cheese is not a good substitute for milk as a source of calcium. In making cheese, the calcium stays mainly in the whey, which is drained off. The whey is the clear, watery part of milk. You would need to eat more than 155 g (5½ oz) of firm cheese such as Cheddar or Swiss or 2250 mL (9c) of cottage cheese to get the amount of calcium supplied by just one quart of milk.

Calcium and strontium 90

Atomic explosions pollute the atmosphere all over the world. Radioactive strontium 90 is one of the more worrisome atomic pollutants. It is released into the upper atmosphere and eventually settles down on plants, soil, and water. Animals eat the plants. Humans eat plants and animals.

Daily requirement of calcium

For most young people, .96 L (1 qt) of milk daily provides the recommended amount (1.15 g) of calcium. Two glasses is the recommended amount for most adults, four for people with osteoporosis. (See the RDA table on pages 402-403.) Table 7-2 shows how much of other common foods it would take to equal the amount of calcium in .96 L (1 qt) of milk. Imagine trying to eat 115 hamburgers to get the calcium you need in one day, or 576 ears of corn, or 144 medium-size apples!

Table 7-2   **Amount of other foods required to equal calcium content in 1 quart of milk**

QUANTITY	FOOD
115	hamburgers
115	servings lean roast beef (84 g; 3 oz)
115	potatoes, boiled in jackets
24	servings cooked carrots (224 g; 8 oz)
31	servings cooked green peas (224 g; 8 oz)
4	servings cooked turnip greens (224 g; 8 oz)
576	cooked ears of corn
18	servings cooked green beans (224 g; 8 oz)
12½	servings cooked dried beans (224 g; 8 oz)
115	medium-size bananas
144	medium-size apples
21	oranges
3	servings sardines, with bones (84 g; 3 oz)
300	servings tuna (42 g; 1½ oz)

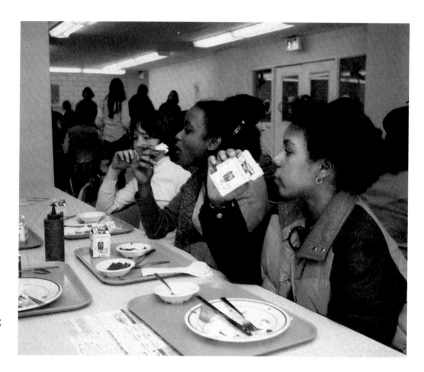

The easiest way to get most of the daily requirement of milk is to drink a glass of milk with each meal.

Strontium 90, like calcium, is deposited primarily in the bony structures of the body. Large amounts in the body may cause bone cancer and leukemia. Leukemia is cancer of the blood that starts in the bone marrow. All the people on earth now have some strontium 90 in their bodies. The younger a child, the more the child's body contains in proportion to its weight.

Authorities tell us that thus far the amounts of strontium 90 found in people are quite small by comparison with what can be tolerated. Fortunately, strontium 90 is less effectively absorbed than calcium. It is also excreted more quickly.

Experimental animals whose diets contain the most calcium retain the least strontium 90. In one study, two groups of white rats were fed diets containing the same amount of strontium 90. There was only one difference in their diets. One group's diet contained 2 percent calcium. The diet of the other group had 0.5 percent, or a fourth as much. What happened? The animals with the larger amount of calcium in the diet retained 75 percent less strontium 90 than the other group.

Chemists who have measured strontium 90 in foods have concluded that milk contains the least. They reported 90 percent less strontium 90 in milk than in the feed that cows eat. The cow seems to act as a filter for her milk. R. F. Holland of Cornell University reports that the calcium in milk has the lowest strontium-90 content of all food sources of calcium. Therefore, the more we use milk as a source of calcium, instead of other foods, the less strontium 90 enters the body.

Milk contains a large amount of the vitamin riboflavin. Riboflavin was discovered in 1879 by isolating a yellowish-green fluorescent substance from the whey of milk. But it was not until 1935 that it was synthesized by scientists. Riboflavin is also known as vitamin B_2, vitamin G, and the "growth-promoting vitamin."

Riboflavin is soluble in water. Heat will not destroy it, but it is easily destroyed by sunlight, daylight, or even artificial light. Thus milk should be kept out of the light. Opaque containers are better than clear glass. When cooking milk in foods, the pan should be covered, if possible. The food should be served immediately or kept covered until serving time. The larger the surface area of foods containing riboflavin exposed to light, the more riboflavin is lost.

Functions of riboflavin

Growth. Riboflavin is an essential vitamin in the B-vitamin group. It is needed from the moment life begins, and the need for it is constant throughout life. Growth is stunted when there is not enough riboflavin in the diet.

Skin and hair. When the diet contains too little riboflavin, the skin and hair become oily. A severe deficiency brings on facial dermatitis, a skin inflammation. The tongue becomes red and sore. The lips crack at the corners and sometimes crust over.

Reproduction. Riboflavin is essential for normal reproduc-

tion. In lower animals shortage of riboflavin causes such deformities as clubfeet, harelip, and cleft palate. Spontaneous abortion may occur. In test studies, animals who had borne deformed young were given a diet rich in riboflavin. Their next litters were normal.

Human babies too may develop abnormally if their mother's diet has too little riboflavin. The problem is common among teenage mothers with a history of poor eating habits. It is also common among mothers in developing countries where the average diet is too low in riboflavin.

Vision. A deficiency of riboflavin causes the eyes to become extremely sensitive to bright light. Many people then feel the need to wear colored glasses.

A deficiency of riboflavin may also cause cataracts. Cataracts are cloudy white growths over the eyes. In extreme cases, cataracts have resulted in blindness in monkeys, mice, white rats, and chicks. One experiment with riboflavin involved a white rat that had developed a cataract in the left eye. When it was given large amounts of riboflavin, the right eye was saved.

Many older people have cataracts. With research, more may be learned about the role of riboflavin in maintaining good vision over a lifetime.

Aging. Riboflavin is part of all cell tissues. Its chief function is to act as a coenzyme with other nutrients in the oxidation in cell tissue of carbohydrates, amino acids, and fats.

Dr. H. C. Sherman of Columbia University studied the effects of riboflavin on the aging of rats. He found that a diet higher than usual in riboflavin promoted better development in the rats. They had more vitality as adults, less disease at all ages, a longer life span, and a longer prime of life. Sherman points out that what he found in lower animals in this respect is undoubtedly true for human beings. In other words, enough riboflavin in the diet can probably increase the chances for a longer and healthier life.

Daily requirement of riboflavin

Only a small number of foods contain significant amounts of riboflavin (Table 7-3). The richest sources are beef liver and beef heart. But the easiest and most practical source to use when planning daily meals is milk. Those who do not use milk in the daily diet are likely to be lacking in riboflavin. In terms of cost and convenience, no food can compare with milk as a source of both calcium and riboflavin.

The need for riboflavin varies with body weight. More is needed during periods of growth because new tissues are being built.

One quart of milk provides 1.6 mg of riboflavin. This is enough to meet the recommended amount for most people of all ages. The RDA table (pages 402-403) shows how much riboflavin is required for different age groups and for both sexes.

Table 7-3 Riboflavin content of some foods (mg)

FOOD	MEASURE	RIBOFLAVIN
Beef liver, fried	84 g (3 oz)	3.56
Nonfat instant milk	240 mL (8 oz)	1.19
Sweetened condensed milk	240 mL (1 c)	1.27
Heart of beef, braised	84 g (3 oz)	1.04
Evaporated milk	240 mL (1 c)	.80
Cheddar cheese	240 mL (1 c) grated	.42
Baked custard	224 g (1 c)	.50
Chocolate milk	240 mL (1 c)	.41
Skim milk	240 mL (1 c)	.37
Buttermilk	240 mL (1 c)	.38
Whole Milk	240 mL (1 c)	.40
Cottage cheese, creamed	120 mL (½ c)	.18
Pork, roast	84 g (3 oz)	.78
Roast beef, relatively lean	84 g (3 oz)	.18
Salmon, canned	84 g (3 oz)	.16
Sirloin steak	84 g (3 oz)	.15
Chicken	84 g (3 oz)	.16
Eggs, raw	1 whole, without shell	.15
Ice cream	84 g (3 oz)	.12
Turnip greens, cooked	120 mL (½ c)	.17
Collard greens, cooked	120 mL (½ c)	.19
Broccoli, cooked	120 mL (½ c)	.16

Nutritive Value of Foods, Bulletin No. 72 (Washington, D.C.: USDA, rev. 1977).

OTHER NUTRIENTS IN MILK

Protein

Milk can supply a large part of the protein needs of all age groups. Only 3.5 percent of milk is protein. But .96 L (1 qt) of milk yields 36 grams of protein. This is more than half the daily need. Milk also contains all the amino acids required by the body, and each in about the daily required amount.

The protein in milk is also found in milk products. It is not lost as milk is made into cheese and other dairy foods.

Phosphorus

Milk and cheese are good sources of **phosphorus,** an essential mineral. Phosphorus is a part of each living cell. It is required by the body in about the same proportion as calcium. It is found in many foods besides milk—meats, organ meats, fish, poultry, cereals, legumes, and nuts. Diets are unlikely to be deficient in phosphorus.

Current research indicates the possible danger of having too much phosphorus, especially if the calcium content of the diet is too low. In 1968, in an experiment at Cornell University, dogs were fed a diet high in phosphorus and low in calcium. The dogs developed trouble with their teeth, jaws, and gums. The research team suggested that many people today have diets that are

126

high in meat and low in milk. This means a diet high in phosphorus and low in calcium, like that in the experiment. Such a diet, the scientists say, may produce loss of teeth and gum disease in human beings. See the RDA table on pages 402-403 for recommendations on the amount of phosphorus needed daily.

Magnesium

Milk contains another mineral that is required in your daily diet. That mineral is **magnesium.** It is essential for all plant and animal life. People who lack this mineral become extremely nervous and unusually sensitive. Their blood vessels dilate, and their heart beats so rapidly it may cause convulsions. It is not likely that you will have too little magnesium if you eat a balanced diet.

Good sources of magnesium are wheat germ, wheat bran, whole wheat, soy beans, peas, nuts, and green, leafy vegetables. Bananas are the best source among fruits. Meat, milk, and eggs are fair sources of this mineral. See the RDA table on pages 402-403 for recommended daily intake of magnesium.

Magnesium is a part of the bone framework. Seventy percent of it works with calcium, phosphorus, and other nutrients in building bones. It is also present in the soft tissues of the body and in the blood. When a diet is deficient in magnesium, the body draws on the magnesium reserve in the bones. When magnesium is not in proper balance, the bones do not form normally. It is therefore needed for normal growth.

Magnesium acts as a coenzyme in building amino acids into body protein. It is thought that magnesium activates enzymes, contributes to muscle-nerve contractions, and helps regulate body temperature.

Milk sugar

Milk makes yet one more important contribution to our diet. It contains **lactose** or milk sugar. This is the most desirable form of sugar found in any food. Only one step is required to digest lactose. Even so, it is digested slowly. As it is being digested, it helps a healthful type of bacteria to grow in the intestinal tract. It also checks the growth of less desirable bacteria. Furthermore, lactose makes calcium more soluble and more easily absorbed. No other sugar does this. Finally, lactose helps the body make some B-complex vitamins right in the intestines.

RECAP

Facts about milk

Milk and nutrition   Milk and acne   Milk and weight

Calcium

Functions of calcium in bones and teeth   Functions of calcium in bodily processes   Maintaining calcium level   Daily requirement of calcium   Calcium and strontium 90

Riboflavin

Functions of riboflavin   *Growth   Skin and hair   Reproduction   Vision   Aging*   Daily requirement of riboflavin

Other nutrients in milk

Protein   Phosphorus   Magnesium   Milk sugar

VOCABULARY

calcium
cataracts
lactose
magnesium
osteoporosis
parathyroid gland
phosphorus
riboflavin
strontium 90

THINKING AND EVALUATING

1. List some common misconceptions about milk. Have you believed any of these? Do you believe them now? Explain your feelings about milk. Are they based on fact or fallacy?

2. Summarize in your own words the reasons that milk and its products are outstanding foods.

3. What is the difference between whole milk and skim milk? How do they compare in terms of calories, nutrition, and cost? When would you use each? Why would you use milk in a weight-control diet?

4. Explain how bones and teeth are formed. Why is milk so important to good posture? Healthy jaws? Strong teeth? In prolonging the prime of life?

5. How does the body store calcium? What happens when the diet is low in calcium?

6. Explain the importance of milk in terms of its riboflavin content.

7. Of what value is milk in relation to strontium 90?

8. Do you consider the money spent on milk a good investment? Why?

APPLYING AND SHARING

1. Using the table of nutritive value of foods on pages 404–430, figure out how much calcium, riboflavin, protein, vitamin A, and fat is provided by

    a. 240 mL (1 glass) whole milk

    b. 240 mL (1 glass) nonfat milk

    c. 120 mL (½ c) cottage cheese, creamed

    d. 120 mL (½ c) ice cream

    e. 28 g (1 oz) Cheddar cheese

2. Select three beverages and six foods that you like and eat. Compare them with milk in calories, nutritional contribution, and cost per serving. What is your conclusion?

3. Plan a balanced dinner in which you use cheese as a meat substitute. Compare the nutritional contribution of the meal with that of a similar meal using meat.

4. Create a new snack idea using any dairy product you wish. The snack should be nutritious, creative, and enjoyable.

CAREER CAPSULES

Dairy farm herder Works on large farm under a manager; assists in breeding, feeding, and milking. High school education required; further education in dairy science and animal husbandry helpful.

Food broker Works for food brokerage firm as a field sales representative; sells a variety of grocery products to markets, processors, hotels, restaurants, school systems, or the military. High school education required; on-the-job training essential.

RELATED READING

Meister, Harold E., and Jennie L. Brogdon. "Versatility, Inc., with Milk and Our Other Dairy Foods." *Food for Us All: Yearbook of Agriculture, 1969.* Washington, D.C.: USDA, 1969. Emphasizes the kinds of milk, methods of caring for milk, cooking with milk, and using milk foods such as cheese.

Speck, Martin. "Safeguarding Our Milk." *Protecting Our Food Supply: Yearbook of Agriculture, 1966.* Washington, D.C.: USDA, 1966. Describes steps taken to provide consumers with safe, clean milk.

White, P. L., and Nancy Sekvey, Eds. *Let's Talk About Food: Answers to Your Questions About Foods and Nutrition.* Acton, Mass.: Publishing Sciences Group, 1974. Includes 21 questions and answers on different aspects of milk; includes a diet liberal in calcium.

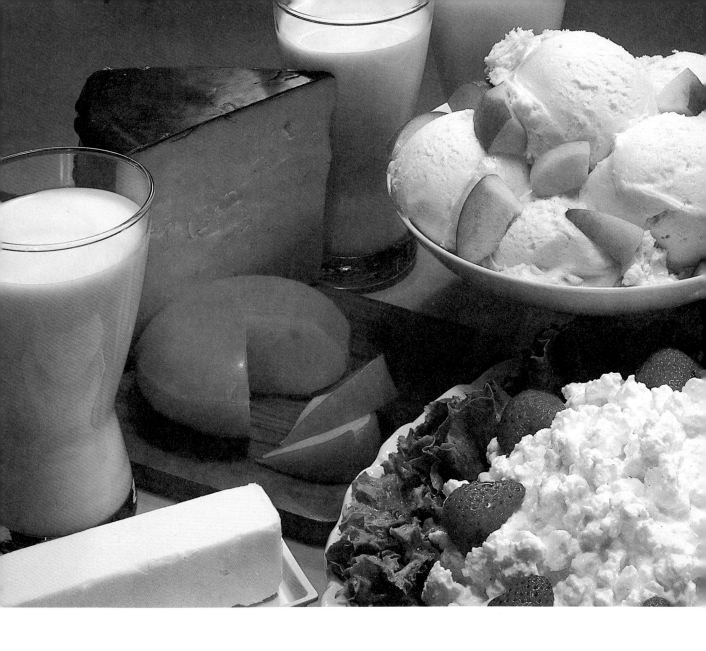

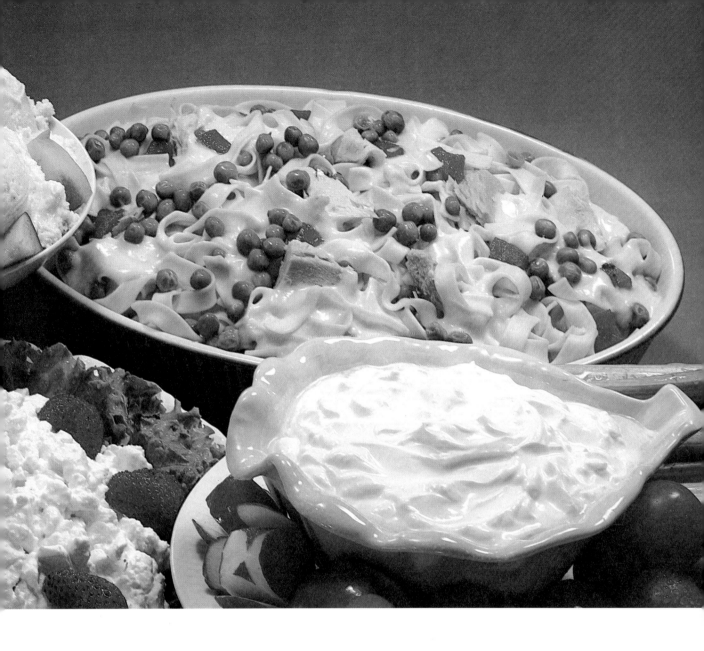

CHAPTER 8

Milk in meals

After studying this chapter, you will be able to

- choose the form of milk best suited to your dietary needs.
- apply your knowledge of milk and milk products in shopping, storing, and preparing meals and snacks using these foods.
- identify sanitary standards that protect our milk supply during handling and processing outside and inside the home.
- plan and prepare balanced meals in which cheese is used as a meat substitute.

MILK PRODUCTION

Standards for cleanliness

Clean, wholesome milk is made possible through the observance of high standards at every step of production. Milk requires sanitary handling at all times. Herds of cows are carefully checked for cleanliness, disease, and infection. They are fed a well-balanced diet and kept in clean barns. After the cows have been milked, the milk is quickly cooled to 10 °C (50 °F). It is transported in refrigerated trucks or railway cars and is kept refrigerated until it is sold. Then its care is up to the consumer.

Pasteurization

Less than a hundred years ago, people drank raw milk taken directly from the cow. Milk in this form was highly perishable. It often became contaminated with bacteria that caused diseases and infections.

In 1895, a French chemist named Louis Pasteur made a discovery that has greatly improved our lives. He discovered a process for destroying harmful bacteria in milk by partial sterilization. Pasteurization, as this process is called, has made milk a safe and healthful drink and has also made food canning possible.

Milk products—cream, butter, ice cream, and cheese—are also

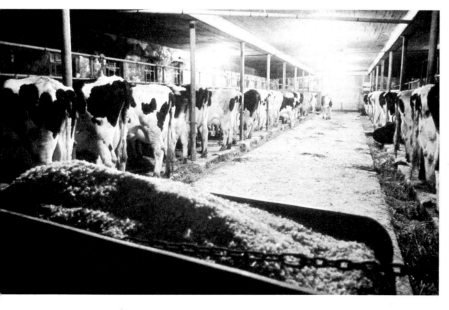

High standards of cleanliness are observed in producing, storing, processing, packaging, and warehousing milk.

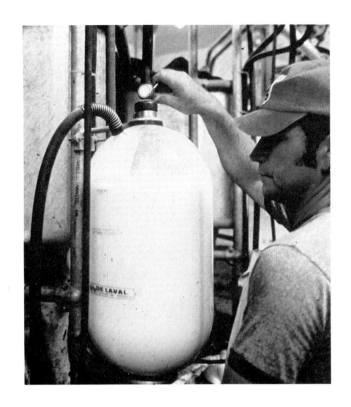

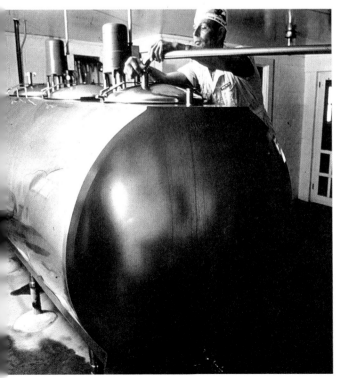

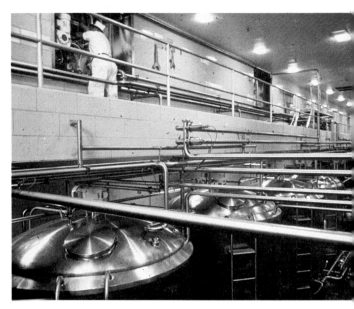

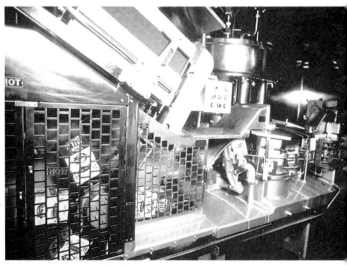

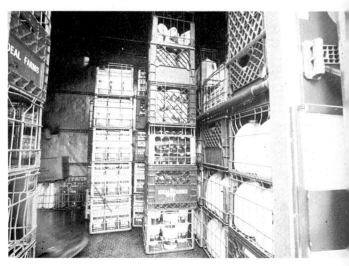

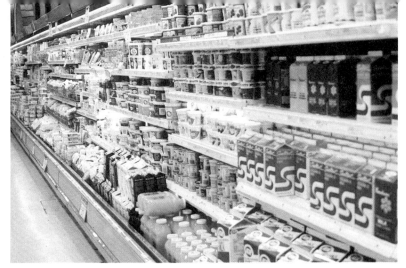

Whole and skim milks, buttermilk, and forms of cream are perishable and are refrigerated from the time they are produced to the time they are consumed.

pasteurized. Fortunately, pasteurization does not destroy the main nutrients of these foods—calcium, riboflavin, protein, and vitamin A. There is some loss of

vitamin C and thiamin, but the protection of health far outweighs this slight loss.

Pasteurization consists of rapidly heating milk. In a process called the hold method, milk is heated to 62 °C (143 °F) and held at that temperature for 30 minutes. In the quick method, milk is heated to between 73 and 79 °C (163 and 175 °F) and held for 15 seconds. In each case, the milk is cooled at once. Families who use milk from their own cows can pasteurize it very simply by bringing the milk quickly to a boiling temperature, cooling it quickly, and refrigerating it.

FORMS OF MILK

Our markets contain a remarkable variety of milk and milk products. Whole milk, nonfat milk, and low-sodium milk are available. Milk can be frozen, canned, condensed, concentrated, fermented, or dried. Milk may be certified, fortified, and homogenized.

A wide variety of food products are made from milk. They include yogurt, flavored milk drinks, ice cream, and cheeses. The prices vary considerably. So do the flavors and nutritional value of these products. Their use in the United States is described in Table 8-1.

Ready-to-drink milks

Milk may be drunk raw, or it may be processed in a variety of ways and packaged for direct consumption.

Raw milk. Raw milk is not pasteurized. It is often used by people who own their own cows and by those who are opposed to pasteurization. Cows must be inspected regularly to be sure they are in good health if their milk is not pasteurized. Raw milk is not sold commercially on a wide scale.

Table 8-1 **Per capita sales of milk and milk products in the United States, 1964–1974**

PRODUCT	1964	1974
Fluid whole milk	118.4 L (123.3 qt)	89.3 L (93.0 qt)
Skim milk, low-fat milk	14.1 L (14.7 qt)	35.0 L (36.5 qt)
Evaporated and condensed whole milk	10.9 L (11.4 qt)	5.2 L (5.4 qt)
Nonfat dry milk	2.2 kg (4.8 lb)	1.7 kg (3.8 lb)
Whole-milk cheese	3.9 kg (8.6 lb)	5.4 kg (14.2 lb)
Cottage cheese	2.1 kg (4.7 lb)	2.1 kg (4.6 lb)
Ice cream	8.5 kg (18.6 lb)	8.0 kg (17.8 lb)
Ice milk	2.9 kg (6.3 lb)	3.5 kg (7.8 lb)
Cream	3.5 L (3.7 qt)	2.6 L (2.7 qt)
Butter	2.7 kg (5.9 qt)	1.9 kg (4.3 lb)

Milk Facts 1975, Milk Industry Foundation. Original data mostly from the USDA.

Certified milk. Certified milk is a form of raw milk that has been inspected and found to have a low bacterial count. It meets the high standards set by the American Association of Medical Milk Commissions. Because of its high cost, it is not a practical food. Also, it deteriorates quickly. Pasteurized milk is often certified also.

Whole milk. Whole milk has all the nutrients of milk. The milk we buy is "pooled" from different herds. The milkfat content is set by state law. The proportion of milk solids is also set by law. Milk solids are the total dry nutrients in milk. The law usually states that milk should contain at least 8.5 percent milk solids. The label on milk containers tells whether or not milk solids have been added.

Skim milk. Milk with nearly all the fat removed is called skim milk. One important difference among the various milks is their fat content. Consumers have been drinking low-fat milk in increasing amounts. According to the Milk Industry Foundation, we used 439 percent more fluid low-fat milk per person in 1974 than in 1964. The consumer wants and needs to know the amount of fat a milk or milk product contains. Unfortunately, the percentage of fat is usually not given on the labels of milk containers.

Homogenized milk. The fat globules in whole milk and low-fat milk can be broken up into a fine emulsion. Fat is then evenly suspended throughout the milk and does not rise as cream. The process of treating milk in this way is called homogenization. Homogenized milk has a creamy color and smooth texture.

Fortified milk. Fortified milk is made by adding to milk such nutrients as 400 IU of vitamin D per liter (quart). Vitamin A and milk solids may also be added. This adds little to the price but much to the nutritional value.

Concentrated milks

Milk may be processed and packaged in ways that allow it to be stored for long periods of time.

Evaporated milk. In 1856 dairy farmer Gail Borden discovered a way to evaporate the water in milk, thus reducing its volume. Civil War soldiers found evaporated milk so helpful that its use quickly spread. Today it is produced by heating pasteurized homogenized whole milk in vacuum tanks to draw off 60 percent of the water in vapor. The milk is then canned, sealed, and immediately sterilized by heat. The milk loses no major nutrients in the process, but vitamin C and thiamin are reduced. Vitamin D is added to the milk to aid the body's absorption and use of calcium.

When an equal amount of water is added, evaporated milk is used in the same manner as whole fresh milk. When used in concentrated form in such dishes as mashed potatoes, scalloped vegetables, creamed meats, and gravies, it increases their nutritional value.

Evaporated milk is sterile and has a soft curd. It is emulsified and easy to digest. It is therefore well-suited to infant feeding. Cans are easily stored on the shelf. However, once a can is opened, the contents should be refrigerated.

Condensed milk. The processing method for condensed milk is the same as that for evaporated milk, with one difference. After the water has been removed, sugar is added to the milk before the cans are sealed. The final product is about 42 percent sugar. It is no substitute for other forms of milk, but it is useful for making desserts, candy, ice cream, and beverages.

Dry milk. Dehydrated milk (dried milk) is produced by a process that removes all the water, leaving essential nutrients in concentrated form. Dry milk is marketed in several forms. These include whole milk, nonfat milk,

Evaporated milk, condensed milk, and dry milk may be stored unrefrigerated for long periods of time.

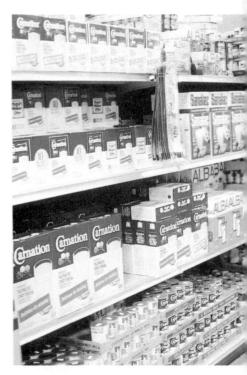

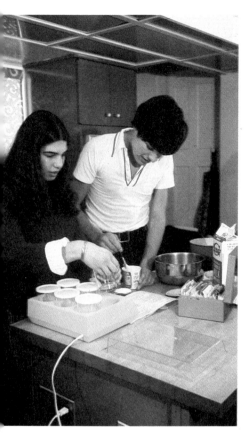

Yogurt, which may be made inexpensively at home, helps to prevent excessive putrefaction in the intestines.

instant milk, cream, and buttermilk. They may or may not be fortified with vitamins D and A.

Dehydrated milk has many advantages. Dry milk is the least expensive form of milk per serving unit. It is also the easiest to store, as it does not require refrigeration. It contains all the nutrients of whole pasteurized milk except vitamin A. And it costs only about one-third as much. It can be added to other foods as a milk substitute or as half-and-half with fresh fluid milk. It may be reconstituted by mixing with water according to directions on the package. Dry milk is sterile, nutritious, and easy to digest. When reconstituted it has a pleasant flavor as a beverage.

In addition, dehydration increases the number of ways milk can be used. Nonfat dry milk may be added to the foods of invalids, children, people who are dieting to lose weight, and people with poor eating habits. The nutrients in a snack, a meal, or the day's diet are thus increased without changing the flavor of the food and without adding many calories.

Fermented milks

Healthful bacteria may be added to milk to change the texture and taste.

Buttermilk. Buttermilk is usually made from skim milk. Several steps are involved in changing skim milk into buttermilk. First, a culture of lactic acid bacteria is added. Then the mixture is fermented at about 21 °C (70 °F) until milk sugar (lactose) is converted to lactic

acid. This makes the flavor tart rather than sweet. Some of the lactic acid unites with a protein in the milk called casein. This forms a thick curd or gel called clabber. Babies and others who can't tolerate milk sugar can tolerate buttermilk or yogurt. Many enjoy the sour taste and thick texture of buttermilk. When prepared commercially, buttermilk may be slightly salted to bring out its flavor. Sometimes a gum is added as well to prevent the whey from separating.

Yogurt. Yogurt is made from whole homogenized milk, low-fat milk, or nonfat dry milk. Yogurt offers some unusual health benefits. The microorganisms that produce yogurt also change the type of bacteria in the intestinal tract. This helps to prevent excessive putrefaction in the intestines. It also helps to form some B vitamins. Sometimes physicians recommend yogurt after a patient has been given antibiotics. The yogurt helps to restore useful intestinal bacteria the drugs may have destroyed.

Yogurt does not have to be bought commercially. You can make it at home with nonfat dry milk at low cost (see the recipe on page 366).

Flavored milk drinks

The introduction of flavorings to milk creates interesting tastes but often adds calories.

Chocolate. Starch, gelatin, and gums go into chocolate-flavored milk. These ingredients produce a thick texture and prevent the cocoa from separating from the liquid. It is higher in sugar and calories and is less nutritious than plain milk. The milk-fat content is usually about 2.3 percent. A 240-mL (8-oz) serving contains 190 to 245 calories.

Fruit. Fruit-flavored milk drinks are also available. Read the labels on all flavored milk drinks, as some are artificially flavored. Some are made from skim milk, with water added.

You can make your own milkshakes using fresh mashed fruit and milk. You then know what is in the drink. It may also cost less. To make it thicker and more nourishing, add 80 mL (⅓ c) of nonfat dry milk to 240 mL (1 c) of low-fat or evaporated milk.

Cream

Cream is milkfat. Measure for measure, cream contains far more calories and vitamin A than milk. Several classifications of cream are available.

Heavy cream. Heavy cream is usually 35 to 40 percent fat. It may be whipped and used to top desserts. Whipped cream is also used as part of frozen and chilled desserts such as ice cream or mousse.

Light cream. The fat content of light cream is usually 18 to 20 percent. It is used as pouring cream for coffee and cereals.

Half-and-half. The combination of half milk and half cream has a fat content of about 8 percent. It is more popular as pouring cream than light cream.

Sour cream. Cream mixed and fermented with lactic acid is called sour cream. It is usually 12 to 18 percent fat. It is used in seasoning vegetables and meat, as an alternate for whipped cream, and in salad dressings.

Milk substitutes

Economical and nutritious substitutes for milk are still being developed.

Filled milk. Filled milks are now sold as substitutes for milk. Filled milks contain nonfat milk solids that may or may not equal those in natural milk. These "milks" are promoted as substitutes for real milks. Yet they do not always contain exactly the same nutrients as real milk. For example, some kinds of filled milk do not contain vitamins A and D.

Filled milks contain vegetable oil instead of milk fat. In the past, coconut oil was used as the fat in this product. Over 90 percent of coconut oil is saturated, as compared with 60 percent saturated fat in whole milk. For this reason, some manufacturers now produce filled milk with oils containing polyunsaturated fats such as corn, soy, cottonseed, or safflower oil. (Fat is discussed in detail in Chapter 14.)

Imitation milk. Imitation milk contains water, vegetable oil, and sodium caseinate (a milk protein) or soybean protein. The vegetable oil is frequently coconut oil. In 1975, imitation milk had 1.5 percent protein. This compares with 3.3 percent in whole milk. It is a poor substitute for milk.

MILK PRODUCTS

Milk is versatile. From cream butter is made (discussed in Chapter 14). Both milk and cream can be mixed with other ingredients and frozen. The solid parts of milk may be isolated and aged to become cheese.

Frozen desserts

Probably the most popular dessert all over the world is ice cream in its various forms. Ice cream is not only flavorful. It is nutritious as well.

Ice cream. Some claim that the Romans originated ice cream for the Emperor Nero and his court. It was said to have been served in the royal dining salons of seventeenth-century France. In 1796 it was first advertised for sale in the United States. It is now among the favorite desserts of Americans. Vanilla is the first choice of flavors, with chocolate next, and strawberry third.

Ice cream made with safflower oil instead of dairy fat is on the market today. Ask for it, but remember that it contains about 12 percent fat. Like regular ice cream, it is high in calories. But like ice milk, it is high in a healthful fat.

Ice milk. Ice milk contains 2.6 to 4.3 percent fat, while ice cream contains 11 to 16 percent.

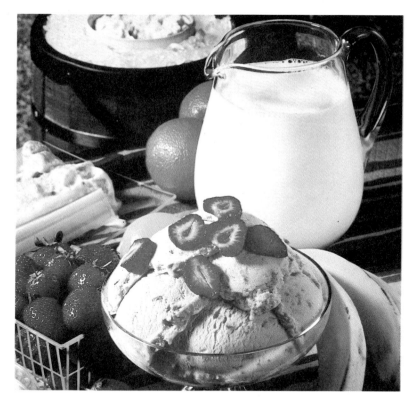

Ice cream, ice milk, and sherbet are probably the world's favorite desserts.

Ice milk has fewer calories, 92, compared to 135 in ice cream. And it has less than half the fat of ice cream, 3 g instead of 7 g. Consumer demand has led some firms to substitute other, less saturated oils for the coconut oil in their ice milk.

Sherbet. Sherbet may be made with fruit, fruit juice, or coloring and fruit flavoring. It contains 1 to 2 percent fat and 2 to 5 percent milk solids. This compares to 20 percent milk solids in ice cream and 11 to 15 percent in ice milk. Sherbet contains almost twice as much sugar as ice cream and ice milk. A 120 mL (½ c) serving contains 135 calories. There is less fat—only 2g—but more sugar. For this reason, the common belief that sherbert is a wiser choice in weight-control diets is not true.

Many varieties of cheese are produced in the United States or imported from other countries.

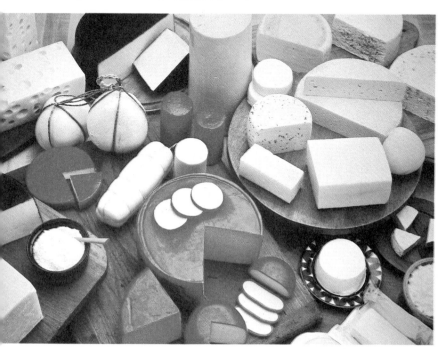

Cheese

Cheese may have been discovered as early as 9000 B.C. Early records show that the Arabs were using cheese about 2000 B.C. How was cheese originally discovered? Perhaps early travelers carried milk in containers made from the dried stomachs of animals. The enzymes in the animal-stomach flasks then acted upon the warm milk and converted it into curd and whey.

Most cheese is made from the curd or solid part of milk. The curd contains most of the protein and fat. It also contains some of the minerals and vitamins. But most minerals and vitamins are water soluble and thus stay with the whey, the watery part of milk.

The most nutritious kinds of cheese go through a special process where the water is evaporated from the whey and the remaining milk solids are returned to the cheese.

Cheese consumption in the United States has steadily increased as our interest in gourmet cooking and dining has increased. Over 2 billion pounds of cheese are made each year. The most popular cheese is American Cheddar, either natural or process.

Over 400 varieties of cheese are produced, and they are known by more than 2000 names. Most cheese is made from cow's milk, although the milk from goats or other animals is sometimes used. Cheese is classified according to its degree of hardness or softness and whether its flavor is mild, medium, or sharp. Table 8-2 shows some of the varieties of cheese popular in the United States.

Process cheese is a molded cheese. It is made up of one or more varieties of cheese and an emulsifying mixture. The mixture is never more than 3 percent of the total weight of the finished product. Process cheese is pasteurized, molded, and sealed in packages that need no refrigeration until they are opened. Many process cheeses contain added milk solids and are therefore especially nourishing. Some consumers prefer this type of cheese for cooking. It costs less per pound, melts quickly, and blends smoothly.

USING MILK AND MILK PRODUCTS

Milk and ice creams are perishable and delicate. They must be refrigerated and used soon after purchase. Cheese lasts longer. Both milk and cheese demand a light touch when used in cooking.

Storage

Milk. As soon as you bring milk home, wash the container and dry it with a paper towel. This removes surface contamination. Then refrigerate milk at 4.5 °C (40 °F). Refrigeration inhibits growth of bacteria and keeps out light, thus protecting the riboflavin content. It insures further protection of flavor and nutritive value.

Milk can be contaminated in the home by bacteria from sneezing or coughing, or from dirty hands. Every member of the family should cooperate to keep milk and milk products clean, covered, cold, and out of the light.

Ice cream. Commercial ice cream and sherbet should be stored in their containers in the freezer section of the refrigerator. Homemade ice cream should be stored in tight freezer containers in the freezer. All frozen milk desserts should be used within a week after storage. It should not be refrozen when it melts, unless it has just been freshly made.

Cheese. Cheese and cheese foods should be stored in closed containers, in the refrigerator. For best flavor, they should be served at room temperature.

Cooking with milk and cheese

Techniques. Proper cooking of milk and milk products preserves their flavor and nutritive value. Milk scorches easily because of the sugar it contains. To avoid scorching, and to keep out light, cook milk and cheese at a low temperature in a covered pan. The fastest method is to place a thick-bottomed pan di-

Cheese browns easily at a low cooking temperature.

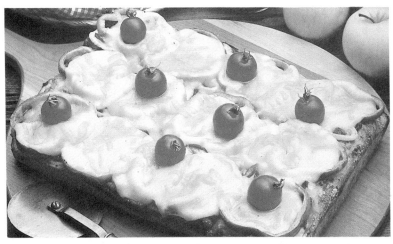

Table 8-2 **Kinds of cheeses in our markets**

CLASS	NAME	COUNTRY OF ORIGIN	FLAVOR AND USE
NATURAL For grating Ripened by bacteria	Parmeasan Romano Sapsago	Italy Italy Switzerland	Sharp flavor; used as seasoning, for topping dishes Pungent flavor; used in cooking Aromatic; clover leaves added; made from skim milk, used in cooking
HARD To eat as is or use in cooking Ripened with bacteria	Cheddar American Cheddar Caciocavalle Edam Gouda Swiss (Emmenthaler) Gruyère Provolone	England U.S. Italy Netherlands Netherlands Switzerland Switzerland Italy	Mild, medium sharp, or very sharp flavor; used as is, in sandwiches, in cooking Flavor mild to very sharp; our favorite cheese; same uses as cheddar Sharp, according to age; used as is, and as seasoning Cannonball shape, red cover; mild flavor; used as is, with fresh fruit, with crackers Cannonball shape, red cover; mild flavor; mealy texture; same uses as Edam Medium flavor; has large eyes or gas holes; alternate use for Cheddar Tiny gas holes or eyes; flavor milder than Limburger; used for dessert Mild to sharp flavor; stringy texture in cooking; used in cooking
SEMISOFT To eat as is Ripened with bacteria	Brick Muenster Monterey Jack Port du salut Gammelost	U.S. Germany California, U.S. France Norway	Flavor mild to sharp; used for buffet and sandwiches Mellow flavor; used for buffet and sandwiches Mild flavor; used for buffet and sandwiches Flavor mild to sharp; used for buffet and sandwiches Mild flavor; used for buffet and sandwiches
SEMISOFT MOLD Ripened by bacteria Blue mold produced by *Penicillium Roqueforti*	Roquefort Gorgonzola Bleu Stilton	France Italy France England	Sharp flavor; used for salad, buffet, dessert Sharp flavor; made in cylinders 30 cm (12 in) in diameter; used for salad, buffet, dessert Sharp flavor; used for salad, buffet, dessert Sharp flavor; used in salad, buffet, dessert, cooked foods
SOFT Ripened	Bel Paese Camembert Brie Neufchatel	France France France France	Rich flavor; used for dessert Rich flavor; used for dessert, served with crackers and fruit Rich flavor; used for dessert, served with crackers and fruit Mild flavor; flavored with pineapple or other condiments; used as appetizer, in spreads
SOFT Unripened Made from skimmed milk but may have cream added	Cottage Ricotta Mysost Gjetost Cream	Universal— Holland claims to have originated, but origin not certain Italy Scandinavia U.S.	Bland flavor; a cottage or home-made cheese of all nations; used plain, for salads, cooking Mild flavor; used in cooking similar to cottage Light brown color; sweet, mild flavor; made of whey; buttery texture. Local name is *primost*. Used as is, on crackers Mild flavor; used in spreads, sandwiches, appetizers

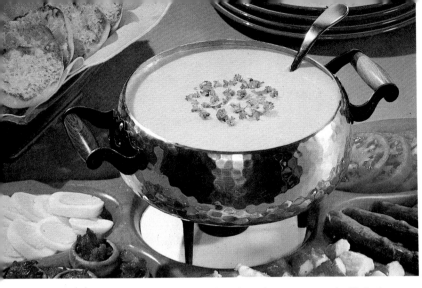
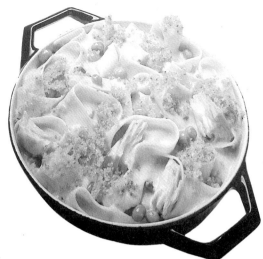

Left: Welsh rabbit, a main dish using cheese, can substitute for meat. *Right:* A tuna casserole is a popular and economical main dish using milk as a sauce base.

rectly over heat. Another method is to use a double boiler. This avoids the danger of scorching, boiling over, or toughening the protein. It also assures good flavor and a simple clean-up job.

Covering the pan not only helps retain the riboflavin. It also prevents a "skin" from forming on top of the milk. If a skin should form, beat it back into the milk. It is a good protein food.

Meals using milk. You know the contributions that milk makes to a meal and to the day's diet. You also know its weaknesses. In planning meals, use milk along with other foods for a tasty and healthful diet.

The easiest way to get the recommended amount of milk is to drink some with a meal or snack. But this is not always desirable. Other ways of getting the benefits of milk are plentiful.

There are many ways to use milk for breakfast besides drinking it or eating it with cereal. Scramble an egg with one-third cup of nonfat dry milk or cottage cheese. Or melt a slice of cheese on a fried egg. Make a cheese omelet or a toasted cheese sandwich.

Main dishes using foods from the milk group are usually inexpensive and easy to make. Macaroni and cheese, Welsh rabbit, and creamed chicken are some examples. A cooked vegetable and a vitamin C-rich salad or a citrus fruit for dessert served with the hot dish balance the meal in nutrients.

Foods cooked with milk augment a meal that may be low in milk's nutrients. Fish may be poached in milk and delicately seasoned with onion, parsley, black pepper, and lime juice or tarragon vinegar. Pork chops become tender and brown when

Many sweet desserts, especially puddings and custards, include milk as a main ingredient.

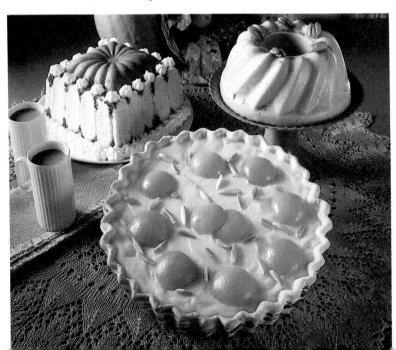

141

baked in milk. White sauce may be used as a base for creamed eggs, meat, fish, or ground meat.

Milk makes yeast breads and hot breads nourishing and moist. Spoon bread contains the most milk. It is an excellent main dish for breakfast, lunch, or dinner. It is unusual in flavor and easy to prepare.

Cheese with crackers or fresh fruit is a wholesome ending for a good dinner. Ice cream and milk puddings have unlimited possibilities as desserts. They may be served alone, atop a piece of plain cake or pie, or with fresh, stewed, or canned fruit.

A cup of fruited yogurt is a popular and nourishing snack. You can make your own by buying plain yogurt and adding fresh or frozen fruit.

There are many other ways of using milk and milk products for all your meals and snacks. Use your ingenuity and your nutritional knowledge to make milk and milk products an important part of your daily diet.

RECAP

Milk production

Standards for cleanliness   **Pasteurization**

Forms of milk

Ready-to-drink milks   *Raw milk*   *Certified milk*   *Whole milk*   *Skim milk*   *Homogenized milk*   *Fortified milk*   **Concentrated milks**   *Evaporated milk*   *Condensed milk*   *Dry milk*   **Fermented milks**   *Buttermilk*   *Yogurt*   **Flavored milk drinks**   *Chocolate*   *Fruit*   **Cream**   *Heavy cream*   *Light cream*   *Half-and-half*   *Sour cream*   **Milk substitutes**   *Filled milk*   *Imitation milk*

Milk products

Frozen desserts   *Ice cream*   *Ice milk*   *Sherbet*   **Cheese**

Using milk and milk products

Storage   *Milk*   *Ice cream*   *Cheese*   **Cooking with milk and cheese**   *Techniques*   *Meals using milk*

THINKING AND EVALUATING

1. What is pasteurization? How old is the process of pasteurization?

2. What kinds of milk are on the market? Which kinds of milk would you recommend for a low-fat diet? Why?

3. How are cheeses classified?

4. What is process cheese?

5. Explain how milk and its products should be stored in the home to insure sanitation and to retain flavor and nutrients.

VOCABULARY

casein
certified milk
clabber
curd
fermented milk
filled milk
fortified milk
homogenized milk
imitation milk
milk solids
pasteurization
raw milk
whey
whole milk

6. What precautions should you take when cooking with milk and milk products?

7. Besides drinking a glass of milk, how else might you use milk in your meals?

1. Divide the class into groups. Each group is to make a trip to the supermarket. Find and list the different forms of milk and milk products and the cost per serving for each. Be prepared to discuss in class which forms you would use on low and moderate budgets.

2. What standards have been set up in your community to assure consumers safe, clean milk of acceptable quality? Do you consider the standards adequate? (If a summary of standards is not available in your library, apply to your local or state public health department.)

3. Plan menus for five days using various forms of milk in each meal.

4. Visit a dairy farm or pasteurizing plant in your community, if possible. Discuss what you learned there.

5. Research the differences in nutritional and ingredient content between Cheddar cheese, cottage cheese, and cream cheese. How do they compare? Which would be best for a weight-control diet? Discuss your findings in class.

CAREER CAPSULES

Public relations account executive Works for a public relations agency on accounts of food companies that do not maintain their own public relations departments; disseminates press releases, informational and educational materials, new product announcements. Four-year college education usually required; knowledge of home economics helpful.

Home economics consultant Works for food company; develops educational programs, training materials, consumer communications, food demonstrations. Four-year college education in home economics required.

RELATED READING

Given, Meta. *Modern Encyclopedia of Cooking*, rev. ed. New York: Doubleday, 1955. Contains many excellent recipes for milk (among other types of foods), with charts, tables, and menu sections.

White, Ruth Bennett. *You and Your Food*, 4th ed. Englewood Cliffs, N.J.: Prentice-Hall, 1976. Unit Two concentrates on the uses of milk and milk foods, with emphasis on nonfat types of milk and on the cost, care, and use of milk in different forms.

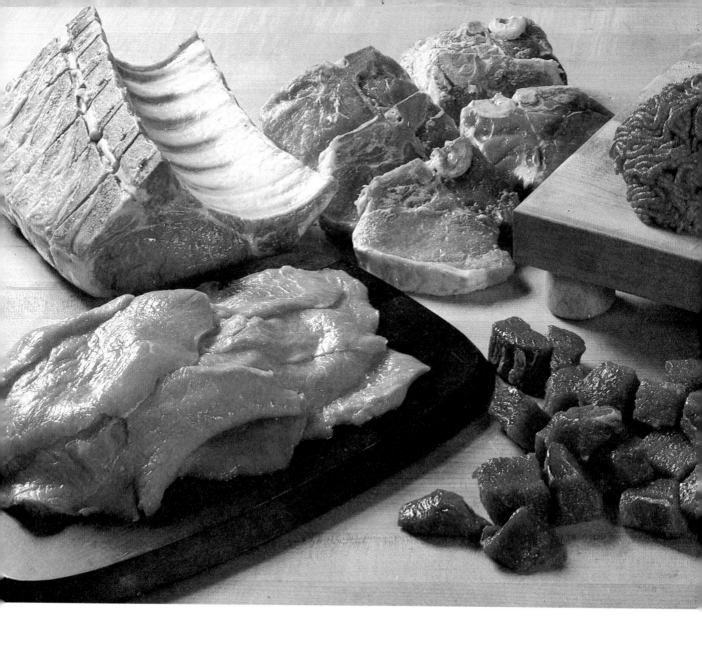

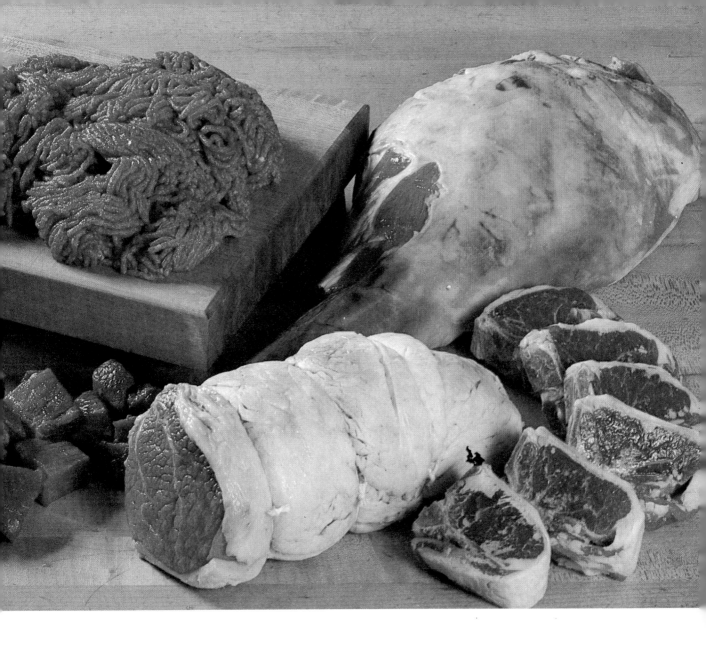

Meat

After studying this chapter, you will be able to

- compare the advantages and disadvantages of meat in the diet.
- explain the types of protein available and list their sources.
- illustrate how the body uses iron, and plan and prepare iron-rich foods for your diet.
- compare the benefits of meat, eggs, and legumes as protein sources.
- describe the body's need for B vitamins and list their sources.

We spend more money for meat than for any other food. This is partly because meat is so enjoyable to eat. The juicy flavor and mouth-watering aroma of meat form the center of interest in many meals. Meat is also valuable to us for nutritional reasons.

Foods in the meat group provide the proteins that are essential to a balanced diet.

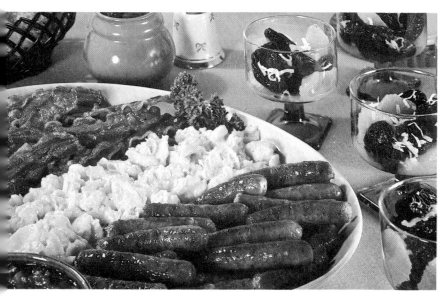

Advantages of meat

Nutriments. Meat has high-quality protein that gives us strength and energy, helps us to grow, and helps to maintain vigor. Meats—especially liver—contain many of the B vitamins necessary for the development of healthy red blood cells. Meats also contain minerals. Iodine (in saltwater fish), phosphorus, magnesium, and traces of many other minerals add zest to life and aid full growth.

Like meats, eggs are a source of complete protein. The protein in eggs is so perfectly balanced in amino acids that the egg is used as the standard for protein in other foods. The white contains water, protein, sodium, and riboflavin but no fat and no cholesterol. The egg yolk contains some degree of almost every known nutrient except vitamin C. The hen passes on to us one of the neatest calorie packages of nutritional balance found in foods. An egg can make up for

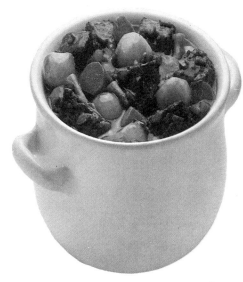

Although all meats lose many of their nutrients in cooking, stews retain some of the lost nutrients in the liquid.

the protein deficiency of vegetables, fruits, and grain products. It also balances milk in iron content.

Digestion. Another advantage of meat is that it can be almost completely digested. This is not true of most plant foods. Some of their protein is bound to the indigestible fiber. Thus only 70 to 80 percent of the protein in vegetables can be digested.

Disadvantages of meat

Cost. The chief disadvantage of meat is its high cost. If we use too much of our food budget on meat, we may shortchange ourselves in milk, vegetables, and fruits. Our diet will not be balanced.

Nutritional weaknesses. Meats are low in calcium and vitamin C. Most meats, except liver, are low in vitamin A. These are major nutrients that are often lacking in our diets.

Experimental studies show that meats lose nutrients in cooking. Thiamin loss ranges from 60 percent in roast meat to 70 percent in broiled meat. Stewed meat loses 75 percent of thiamin, but much of this is retained in the liquid. When meat is pan-fried, however, about 90 percent of the thiamin is retained. Experimental studies show that most riboflavin and niacin are retained during cooking. These nutrients drip with the juice into the brown drippings, which may be used as gravy.

Putrefaction. Another disadvantage is that the bacteria in meat are putrefactive in the intestinal tract. Putrefaction is counteracted when we include fruits, vegetables, and milk in the meal.

Fat. The amount of fat in meat is a serious problem for two reasons. First, the total amount of fat is usually high. Fat content varies with the kind of animal and also with the cut and grade of meat. The amount of fat may be as low as 10 percent or as high as 40 percent. Fish, chicken, and turkey contain less fat than goose, duck, and red meats. Young animals and poultry contain more lean and less fat per pound than older ones.

Second, the fat in meat is saturated. Fat in fish and poultry is less saturated. Research shows that the kind and amount of fat in the diet are associated with some types of heart and circulatory disease (Chapter 14).

The fat in meat often contributes more calories to the diet than the lean contributes. Look at the table of nutritive values on page 409. Notice that there are 34 g of fat but only 17 g of protein in an 84-g (3-oz) serving of roast beef. Consider too that there are 9 calories in every gram of fat but only 4 calories in every gram of protein. Now multiply the fat grams in a serving of roast beef by 9 and the protein grams by 4. You will

Chicken and turkey contain less fat than goose or duck.

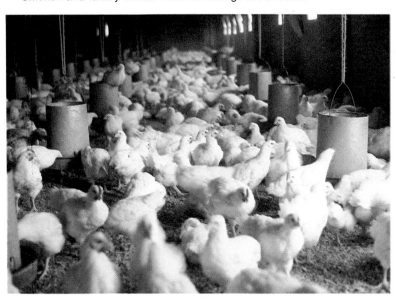

find that there are 306 calories in fat but only 68 calories in protein. In other words, fat in roast beef yields over four times as many calories as does protein.

Commercial cold cuts are a good example of how fat creeps into the diet. A frankfurter appears to be solid lean meat. It may actually contain 7 g of protein and 15 g or more of fat. The protein yields 28 calories and the fat yields 135. Four slices of bologna yield 24 calories from protein and 126 calories from fat. Two ounces of "dry" salami yield 56 calories from protein and 198 calories from fat. Four grams (1¾ oz) of liverwurst (not smoked) yield 32.4 calories from protein and 109 calories from fat. Of the cold meats, however, liverwurst is a more nutritious food. It has far more iron in proportion to weight than any fresh meat—except liver itself. It also has more vitamin A and riboflavin.

Fortunately scientists are now able to breed animals and poultry that produce more lean meat and less fat. Scientists have also reduced the amount of saturated fat and increased the more healthful type of fat in cattle. This advance is of great importance to beef-eating nations.

PROTEIN

A Dutch physician and chemist, G. J. Mulder, found a substance in plants and animals that was essential for life. He named it protein, a Greek word meaning "of first importance."

Protein forms the nucleus (center) of all cells. It is essential for the growth and repair of all tissue. Proteins consist of small units called amino acids. Amino acids are sometimes called the building blocks of protein. They contain carbon, hydrogen, oxygen, and nitrogen. Some also contain sulfur or other elements.

There are about 22 amino acids, some of which the body can manufacture. Those the body cannot make, and which are needed for life processes, are called essential amino acids. These must be obtained from the foods we eat. Adults need nine essential amino acids; children need at least nine, possibly ten. The body requires amino acids in combinations in its tissues and many processes.

Plants synthesize protein out of the energy of the sun, the oxygen in the air, and the water and nitrogen in the soil. One group, legumes, can take nitrogen from the air, as well as from the soil. Animals can make protein from plants. Since we eat both plant

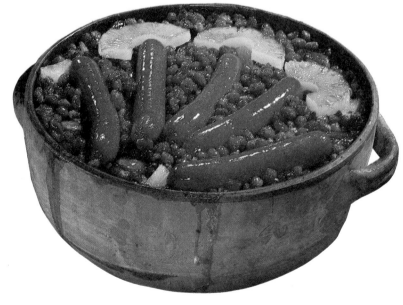

Legumes, such as these baked beans, are good sources of protein, especially when supplemented with a little meat, milk products, eggs, or cereal grains.

and animal foods, we get protein from both sources. But the proteins in plants lack some essential amino acids completely or lack the amount that human beings must have. The milk and meat groups are best protein sources.

Types of protein

Complete proteins. Foods contain different amounts of amino acids. Those that contain all the essential amino acids in amounts necessary for growth and repair of cells are called **complete proteins.** Every meal should contain some of these.

Less complete proteins. Foods in which one or more of the essential amino acids are not present in large enough amounts to meet our needs are called partially complete, or less complete protein. These are the proteins found in plants—legumes, seeds, vegetables, fruits.

The body's use of protein involves many factors. One factor is that the nine or ten essential amino acids are present in different quantities in foods. In plant protein some of these may be present in small amounts. But for all to be used for growth and cell repair, other amino acids must be available. There are two ways this can be done: First, the less complete protein foods can be supplemented. When you eat protein-rich animal foods with plant foods, the less complete protein of plant food is used well. So modern science has found a sound basis for the historic custom of eating some bread with meat, milk, or eggs and having vegetables and fruits in a meal.

Second, if two or more foods which together contain enough of all the essential amino acids are eaten at the same meal, they provide the body with the same nutrients as a complete protein food. Such protein foods are called complementary proteins. Beans and rice are examples of these.

Functions of protein

Normal growth. When infants, growing children, and adolescents do not have enough high-quality protein in the diet they cannot grow normally. Their growth is stunted. Adults too can suffer from protein deficiency. Older people without enough protein may become weak and feeble. Muscle tissue becomes soft and flabby and lacks strength for normal activity. Poor posture results.

What happens when the body does not receive enough high-quality protein from the diet? It "steals" protein from itself. First, it takes amino acids from the liver. The liver is a depot for most nutrients. But the protein reserve there is low. When the liver reserve is used up, the body then takes amino acids from the muscles or other tissues. When the body begins to take protein from our tissues to maintain the processes of life, we begin to look old and tired prematurely. We may develop other symptoms of aging, ill health, or starvation.

Body processes. Amino acids are needed to build new cells and repair worn ones in the muscles, organs, nervous system, blood, skin, hair, and nails. They are used in enzymes that spark chemical re-

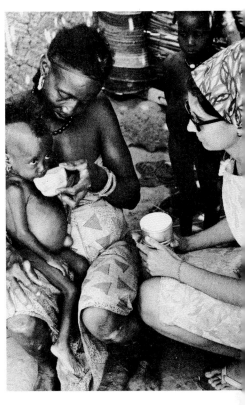

Protein deficiency can result in kwashiorkor, a disease characterized by stunted growth and a swollen abdomen.

actions in cells and in hormones that regulate body processes. Normal fetal brain cell development depends upon adequate protein in the mother's diet. For all these needs to be met, two things are required: enough complete protein and enough calories in the diet. If no other source of energy is available, the body burns protein. Then the amino acids can't be used.

Resistance to disease. Our bodies need high-quality protein to resist infections and viruses. Antibodies need protein to fight bacteria and give us immunity to some diseases.

American babies do not get kwashiorkor, a protein-deficiency disease. But many young children in developing nations

Table 9-1 Meeting the recommended daily allowance of protein

Recommended daily protein allowance

GROUP	AGE	GRAMS
CHILDREN	1–3	23
MALES	11–14	44
	15–22	54
	23 +	56
FEMALES	11–14	44
	15–18	48
	19 +	46
PREGNANT WOMEN		+ 30
LACTATING WOMEN		+ 20

Protein provided by Recommended daily balanced diet

MEASURE AND FOOD	APPROX. GRAMS	
ANIMAL PROTEIN		
1 L (1 qt) milk	36	
1 egg	6	
1 serving cooked lean meat, poultry, or fish	17–23	
Total animal protein		59–65
PLANT PROTEIN		
4 slices bread, or 3 slices bread plus 1 serving cereal	8	
4 servings vegetables and fruits, including potato but not legumes	4	
1 serving dried beans or peas	7	
Total plant protein		19
TOTAL PROTEIN FOR DAY		78–84

Computed from *Nutritive Value of Foods,* Home and Garden Bulletin No. 72 (Washington, D.C.: USDA, rev. 1977) and *Recommended Daily Dietary Allowances* (Food and Nutrition Board, National Research Council, National Academy of Sciences, 1974).

have it after they are weaned and placed on the adult diet. A virtual miracle takes place when they are fed a protein-rich diet. Dry milk, imported into their countries and fed to children, is especially helpful in fighting kwashiorkor.

Scientists are now helping all people meet their protein needs by researching and developing acceptable forms of protein-rich foods. They have produced a food made out of corn, cotton-seed meal, sorghum, and yeast. It is called incaparina. Children who eat this food or other multipurpose foods do not develop kwashiorkor.

How the body uses protein

There is more protein in the body than any other nutrient. It makes up half the dry weight. A tenth is in the skin, a fifth is in the bones, and a third is in the muscles. The thick part of the blood is 95 percent protein. Protein also is an important part of body fluid.

Let us look closely at what happens to protein in the body. During the digestive process, enzymes break up the protein and form amino acids. These are absorbed and travel in the bloodstream. Each tissue in the body needs a specific combination of amino acids. For example, the hair, skin, and nails need amino acids that contain sulfur. As the amino acids circulate through the microscopic capillaries, each cell traps the combination it needs. All the amino acids a cell needs must be present at one time to make body protein. The cell cannot take what amino acids are there, hold on to them, and wait until the other amino acids it requires come along. Thus it is imperative to have the balance of protein foods we need in every meal.

Daily requirement of protein

The daily need for protein relates to growth. The faster the growth, the greater the need of protein. The larger a person is, the more body tissues have to be maintained. Pregnancy, lactation, and disease are special conditions requiring more protein.

The recommendations for the daily amount of protein needed by each age group are given in the RDA table on page 402. One-half to one-third the daily protein should come from animal foods—meat, eggs, milk, and cheese. The other half or two-thirds of the protein should come from bread, cereal foods, and vegetables (Table 9-1).

Research has disproved an old belief that the more a person exercises, the more protein he or she needs. Exercise requires more calories to burn as energy. It does not require more protein,

unless muscle growth takes place during the exercise. Athletes need a balanced diet like the rest of us.

Protein is better used by the body when it is about equally divided among the three meals of the day. This principle was demonstrated in an experiment with college girls at the University of Nebraska. The girls were placed on a controlled diet that was adequate for the day as a whole. But when they drank two glasses of milk with dinner and no milk at breakfast, they did not retain the protein as well as when they drank one glass with each meal.

IRON

Unfortunately, many of the foods that people enjoy eating are low or lacking in iron (Table 9-2). Of the iron that does occur in food, the body absorbs only about 10 percent. Iron is more easily absorbed from animal foods than plant foods. Liver is richer than any other food in iron. It is a source of some quantity of almost every nutrient in the body, except calcium. It is low in fat and richer than any other food in vitamins A and D and the B vitamins. A 112-g (4-oz) serving of liver has as much vitamin A as 1.4 kg (3 lb) of butter or fortified margarine. Soybeans are the only plant food that contains iron that is easily absorbed.

For iron to be effectively absorbed and used, the following are needed: copper, vitamin C, protein, the intrinsic factor in hydrochloric acid in the stomach, a large number of B vitamins, and other nutrients.

Function of iron in red blood cells

The meat group provides nutrients important to the formation of healthy red blood cells. Iron is essential for building red blood cells. It combines with protein and vitamins, especially B vitamins, to make hemoglobin. The body contains only four to five grams of iron. That is only about enough to make one straight pin. But the value of iron in the diet far outweighs the small amount needed. Iron is required for the formation of enzymes. It has been found in minute amounts in all cells.

Hemoglobin is a compound of iron and protein in red cells. The iron attracts oxygen, giving red blood cells their color, and these cells carry oxygen to all the body cells. Iron is needed for the body to make hemoglobin.

The red blood cell is known technically as an erythrocyte. It

is commonly called the red corpuscle. It is shaped like a biconcave disc and is flexible like a bag. It can squeeze through narrow capillaries that have diameters the size of a hair. This enables us to receive oxygen in every cell. Growth and tissue repair proceed normally when blood is normal.

Blood consists of red and other blood cells and plasma the fluid which carries them.

Blood makes up about 7 percent of the weight of an average adult. In volume, this amounts to 3.8 to 4.7 L (4 to 5 qt). An adult man has more than 5 million red blood cells per cubic millimeter of blood. A woman averages about 4.5 million per cubic millimeter. An adult's body contains an estimated 25 to 35 trillion red blood cells.

The normal hemoglobin content of the red cell is 16 g per 100 mL of blood for an adult man and 14 g for a woman. If the he-

Liver is the food richest in iron. It is important to regularly include foods with iron in the diet.

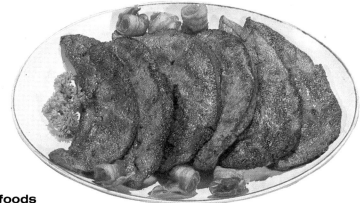

Table 9-2 **Iron content of various foods**

FOOD	MEASURE	APPROX. MG IRON	FOOD	MEASURE	APPROX. MG IRON
MEAT, FISH, POULTRY, EGGS			Banana	1	0.8
			Avocado	½	0.7
Pork liver, raw	98 g (3½ oz)	19.2	Grapefruit	½	0.5
Lamb liver, raw	98 g (3½ oz)	10.9	Orange, navel	1	0.5
Calf liver, raw	98 g (3½ oz)	8.8	Apple	1	0.4
Beef liver, raw	98 g (3½ oz)	6.5	Endive, green, raw	56 g (2 oz)	1.0
Chicken liver, raw	98 g (3½ oz)	7.9	Spinach, cooked	120 mL (½ c)	2.0
Liverwurst	98 g (3½ oz)	5.9	Turnip greens,		
Lamb kidney	84 g (3 oz)	7.6	cooked	120 mL (½ c)	0.8
Beef heart	84 g (3 oz)	5.0	Collards, cooked	120 mL (½ c)	0.6
Oysters, raw	120 mL (½ c)	6.6	Broccoli, cooked	120 mL (½ c)	0.6
Clams, raw	84 g (3 oz)	5.2	Brussels sprouts,		
Shrimp, canned	84 g (3 oz)	2.6	cooked	120 mL (½ c)	0.9
Beef, loin, broiled	84 g (3 oz)	3.0	Sauerkraut	120 mL (½ c)	0.7
Hamburger			Coleslaw	240 mL (1 c)	0.4
lean	84 g (3 oz)	3.0	Carrots	120 mL (½ c)	0.5
regular	84 g (3 oz)	2.7	Pepper	1	0.5
Pork roast	84 g (3 oz)	2.7	Potato, peeled, boiled		
Ham, cured	84 g (3 oz)	2.2	white	1	0.8
Lamb roast	84 g (3 oz)	1.4	sweet	1	1.0
Chicken, ½ breast					
and bone	92 g (3.3 oz)	1.3	**CEREAL- BREAD**		
Chicken, drumstick,			Oatmeal, cooked	240 mL (1 c)	1.4
fried	59 g (2.1 oz)	0.9	Bread, white,		
Eggs	1	1.1	enriched	1 slice	0.6
VEGETABLES, FRUITS			**MILK, MILK PRODUCTS**		
Beans, dried, cooked	240 mL (1 c)	4.9	Milk	240 mL (1 c)	0.1
Peanuts	120 mL (½ c)	1.5	Cheese, American		
Peanut butter	30 mL (2 T)	0.6	Cheddar	2.5-cm³ 1-in.	
Peas, green	120 mL (½ c)	1.5		cube	0.1
Figs, dried	2 whole	1.2			
Apricots, cooked	120 mL (½ c)	2.6	**SWEETS**		
Prunes, cooked	120 mL (½ c)	2.3	Sugar, white	15 mL (1 T)	trace
Tomato juice, canned	240 mL (1 c)	2.2	Molasses		
Blueberries	240 mL (1 c)	1.4	light	15 mL (1 T)	0.9
Cantaloupe	½	0.8	blackstrap	15 mL (1 T)	3.2

Adapted from *Composition of Foods,* Agriculture Handbook No. 8 (Washington, D.C.: USDA, 1963) and *Nutritive Value of Foods,* Home and Garden Bulletin No. 72 (Washington, D.C.: USDA, rev. 1977).

moglobin falls far below normal or if it has too few red cells, anemia develops.

Red cells are made in the bone marrow. All bones are involved in making red cells until the age of 20. At that time, the marrow of the long bones becomes too fatty. Then, only the bones of the vertebrae, the sternum, and the ribs make red cells.

Red cells are not made to last for a lifetime. A red cell lives only about four months. Its membrane gets old and falls apart. The spleen is the chief organ that destroys the cells. About 80 percent of the iron in the hemoglobin of dying cells is salvaged and stored in the liver, the spleen, and the bone marrow for future use in constructing cells.

Types of anemia

Anemia, a physical condition caused by too few red blood cells, is one of the major dietary deficiency diseases and is closely related to insufficient iron in the diet. It occurs all over the world. Teen-age girls and adult women, older people, infants, and children are especially affected in the United States.

Iron-deficiency anemia. Nutritional anemia, another name for iron-deficiency anemia, has four common causes. One cause is a long-term diet too low in iron. A second cause is the regular loss of blood in menstruation. A third cause is occasional long or excessively heavy menstrual periods. Fourth, excessive loss of blood at childbirth can cause iron-deficiency anemia. Anemic mothers

usually produce babies that have too low an iron reserve. The infants use up this reserve quickly. They become anemic, unless their diet is intelligently managed. Avoiding anemia during pregnancy is extremely important and is discussed in Chapter 20.

Hemorrhagic anemia. As a result of severe bleeding, bleeding ulcers, frequent nosebleed, or severe loss of blood at childbirth, hemorrhagic anemia may occur. Blood transfusions are usually used to treat this type of anemia. It is important that both the patient and the donor of the blood eat an iron-rich diet. They will be better able to combat loss of blood if the blood contains the correct amount of iron. Donors may develop nutritional anemia if they give as many as five blood donations a year, unless their diet is iron-rich.

Pernicious anemia. Pernicious anemia is a disease in which red blood cells are too few in number and far too large. Once fatal, it is now controlled by vitamin B_{12} (see the section in this chapter on B vitamins).

Macrocytic anemia. Macrocytic anemia is discussed in Chapter 5. It especially affects pregnant women and infants. Macrocytic anemia is caused by a deficiency in folic acid.

Daily requirement of iron

To build stamina, males age 11 to 18 and females from age 11 to 50 need 18 mg of iron in the daily diet. After age 18, the daily requirement for males drops to 10 mg.

Top: Magnified 450x, healthy red blood cells (stained brown) and white blood cells (purple). *Bottom:* Iron-deficient red cells magnified 1,000x.

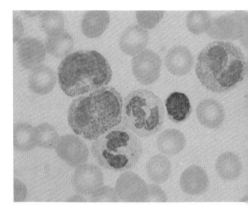

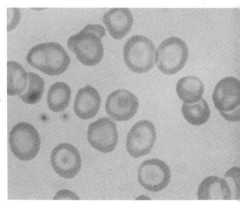

Girls and women need more iron daily in their food because they regularly lose blood—and iron with it—through menstruation. Studies have found that the loss of iron during menstruation is about 1 mg per day.

Sufficient iron is important for people on reducing and low-fat diets, pregnant and lactating women, and growing children. It is also important for many people following an illness (unless prohibited by the physician), especially people who tend to be anemic.

Iodine is needed to make thyroxin. **Thyroxin** is a hormone secreted from the thyroid gland. It regulates the cells' use of energy. Sometimes a person does not get sufficient iodine from the diet to enable the thyroid gland to make the necessary thyroxin. The gland strains to meet the body's need. It then becomes overstimulated and enlarged, resulting in simple goiter.

Saltwater fish and shellfish are excellent sources of iodine.

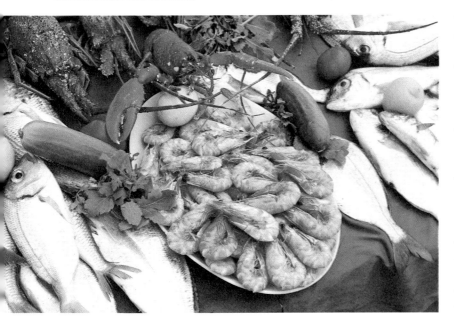

An experiment in Akron, Ohio, in 1920 proved that a lack of iodine causes goiter. Nearly 2500 girls took part in the experiment. About 2000 of them had slightly enlarged thyroid glands. Moderately enlarged glands were noted in 246 girls. Toxic goiters occurred in 39. A small amount of sodium iodide was given in drinking water to the 2000 girls with enlarged thyroid glands. Of these, only 5 developed further thyroid enlargement. This compared with the 500 in the control group who did not take the treated water.

Through research in nutrition, we have learned why people who eat seafood and plants that grow near the sea do not have goiter. Saltwater fish, shellfish, dried seaweed, and cod-liver oil are rich in iodine.

Iodized salt has proven effective in preventing simple goiter. Studies showed that goiter increased in the United States from 1955 to 1975. They also showed that the use of iodized salt dropped from 80 to 40 percent. Iodized salt costs no more than plain salt and is available in food markets throughout the country.

Vitamin B$_{12}$

The history of vitamin B$_{12}$, an important nutritional contribution of meat and eggs, is long and important. In 1920, Dr. G. H. Whipple of the University of Rochester, in his studies of pernicious anemia, discovered a principle known as the **intrinsic factor**. The intrinsic factor is a function of the gastric juice that enables food to be digested. In people with pernicious anemia, the intrinsic factor is absent.

A second crucial discovery was made six years later by Dr. G. R. Minot and Dr. W. P. Murphy of Boston. They found that pernicious anemia could be cured by feeding patients 111 to 224 g (¼ to ½ lb) of liver every day. Patients placed on such a diet could produce red blood cells again. For their work, Dr. Whipple, Dr. Minot, and Dr. Murphy were awarded a Nobel Prize in 1934.

Finally, in 1948, vitamin B_{12} was discovered by scientists in both England and the United States. Within the same month, universities in both countries announced that they had discovered a red crystalline substance that was identified as vitamin B_{12}. It was also called the extrinsic factor because it comes from food or from outside the body. Further experiments disclosed that the extrinsic factor must combine with the intrinsic factor before the body can absorb it from the digestive tract.

Vitamin B_{12} is the second largest, second most complex molecule known, next only to protein. When vitamin B_{12} is injected into the muscle, it can restore blood to normal. The vitamin makes the person comfortable, since it eliminates the nervousness associated with pernicious anemia. Vitamin B_{12} also promotes growth and helps the body use amino acids.

The richest source of vitamin B_{12} is liver, but the vitamin is also found in other organ meats, muscle meats, shellfish, egg yolks, and milk. People who eat a balanced diet get all the vitamin B_{12} they need for normal health.

Niacin

The meat group is an excellent source of niacin, another of the B vitamins (Table 9-3). When people have too little niacin, they develop

Table 9-3 Niacin content of common foods

FOOD	APPROX. MEASURE	APPROX. MG NIACIN
Peanut butter	100 g (3½ oz)	14.7
Liver		
beef, raw	100 g (3½ oz)	13.6
calf, raw	100 g (3½ oz)	11.4
Tuna fish, canned, solids	100 g (3½ oz)	11.9
Heart, beef, raw	100 g (3½ oz)	7.5
Salmon, canned, red	100 g (3½ oz)	7.3
Meats, lean muscle, raw	100 g (3½ oz)	4.6
Peas		
dried	100 g (3½ oz)	2.2
fresh	100 g (3½ oz)	3.7
Bread		
whole wheat	100 g (3½ oz)	2.8
enriched white	100 g (3½ oz)	2.4
unenriched white	100 g (3½ oz)	1.1
Beans, dried, cooked	240 mL (1 c)	1.3
Nuts (except peanuts)	240 mL (1 c)	1.7
Fruits, dried (except raisins), or cooked and unsweetened	100 g (3½ oz)	2.3
Cornmeal		
whole, dry	240 mL (1 c)	2.3
degerminated, enriched	240 mL (1 c)	4.8
Corn, sweet fresh, cooked	1 average ear	1.0
Rice, enriched white, cooked	240 mL (1 c)	2.1
Lima beans, fresh, cooked	240 mL (1 c)	2.2
Oatmeal, cooked	240 mL (1 c)	0.2
Broccoli, cooked	240 mL (1 c)	1.2
Leafy vegetables	100 g (3½ oz)	1.1
Fresh fruits	100 g (3½ oz)	0.3
Cheese	100 g (3½ oz)	0.15
Eggs, whole, fresh	100 g (3½ oz)	0.1
Milk, whole, fresh	240 mL (1 c)	0.2
Potato		
white	1 medium	1.7
sweet	100 g (3½ oz)	0.7
Oil and fats		0.0
Sugar		0.0
Carbonated beverages		0.0

Adapted from *Composition of Foods*, Agriculture Handbook No. 8 (Washington, D.C.: USDA, 1963) and *Nutritive Value of Foods*, Home and Garden Bulletin No. 72 (Washington, D.C.: USDA, rev. 1977).

pellagra. This disease attacks the skin, the gastrointestinal tract, and the nervous system.

Dr. Joseph Goldberger of the U.S. Public Health Service proved that pellagra is caused by a poor diet, specifically by insufficient niacin. He fed a group of volunteer prisoners a diet eaten by people afflicted by the disease and the prisoners developed pellagra. He then cured them with a balanced diet that included B vitamins, particularly niacin.

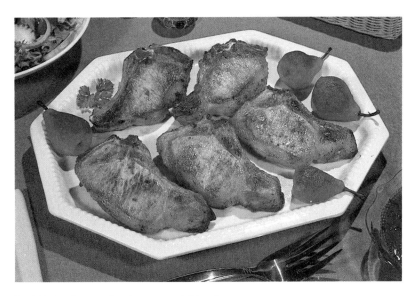

Pork is the best animal source of thiamin.

one-third. This is why milk, for example, can help prevent pellagra. Its niacin content is low, but tryptophane is high.

Foods rich in tryptophane are meat, poultry, fish, eggs, liver, and other organ meats. Peanuts, peanut butter, and brewer's yeast are also good sources. Milk, whole grains, enriched cereals, legumes, potatoes, and some green, leafy vegetables provide fair amounts of tryptophane.

An essential amino acid called tryptophane can produce niacin in the body. With the aid of suitable bacteria and vitamin B_6, tryptophane is chemically changed into niacin in the digestive tract.

Today we know that when the diet contains sufficient high-quality protein, such as that found in meat, eggs, and milk, the body can increase its amount of niacin by

Other B vitamins

Riboflavin, thiamin, and some quantity of most other B vitamins are found in meat, poultry, fish, and eggs. Liver is the richest food source of B vitamins. Pork has been found to be an excellent source of thiamin. A serving of roast pork contains 7 times as much thiamin as roast veal. It contains over 15 times as much as a serving of roast beef (see the table of nutritive values of foods on pages 407 and 409-411).

VITAMIN D

The cause of rickets was a mystery until the twentieth century. In 1909, a Russian physician prescribed cod-liver oil for a four-year-old child who had never walked because of rickets. After taking the cod-liver oil for two months, the child had absorbed and laid down enough calcium and phosphorus in the bones to start walking. Now we know that calcium and phosphorus cannot produce strong bones and teeth unless enough vitamin D is present. Ribs may become deformed, causing a pinched chest with

crowded internal organs. Children with rickets have trouble standing because their leg bones bend. They may become bow-legged or knock-kneed.

Sources of vitamin D

Cod-liver oil, sunlight, and fortified milk are the best sources of vitamin D in our diets. Milk, fortified with 400 IU of vitamin D per liter (quart), has greatly contributed to eliminating rickets in the United States.

When the sun shines directly on the skin, the ultraviolet rays activate a form of cholesterol that then changes into vitamin D. This explains why rickets is seldom found in tropical countries. Clouds, clothing, dust, fog, smog, windowpanes, and even dark pigment in the skin prevent ultraviolet rays from helping to form vitamin D in the body.

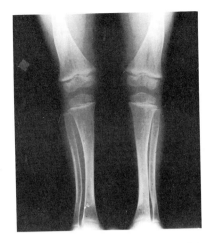 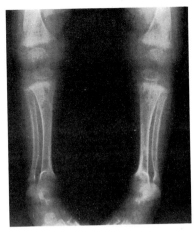

Vitamin D deficiency causes rickets, characterized by a softening and bending of the bones. *Left:* X-ray showing normal leg bones. *Right:* Leg bones afflicted with rickets.

Daily requirement of vitamin D

In the RDA table on pages 402–403 you will note that 400 IU of vitamin D are recommended daily from infancy through age 22. This does not mean that our need stops when we are grown. Calcium and phosphorus cannot do their repair work without vitamin D. However, once the structure of bones and teeth is formed, most adults get enough vitamin D from the diet and from sunshine to maintain bony structures in the body.

An excess of concentrated vitamin D produces a toxic effect. Among the symptoms are loss of appetite, vomiting, diarrhea, and calcification of the walls of the blood vessels, the heart, and the soft tissues. Natural food and milk fortified with vitamin D do not bring on a toxic effect. However, a parent applying the concept that, if a little is good, more is better, can give too much supplemental vitamin D to an infant or young child.

B vitamins

Vitamin B_{12} Niacin   Other B vitamins

Vitamin D

Sources of vitamin D   Daily requirement of vitamin D

VOCABULARY

amino acids
complete protein
erythrocyte
essential amino acids
extrinsic factor
goiter
hemoglobin
hemorrhagic anemia
intrinsic factor
iron-deficiency
   anemia
kwashiorkor
less complete protein
nucleus
pellagra
pernicious anemia
plasma
protein
rickets
thyroxin
tryptophane

THINKING AND EVALUATING

1. Why can eggs be used as a meat alternative? In what ways are legumes good alternatives to meat?

2. Explain what is meant by the terms "complete protein" and "less complete protein." Give examples of both. What is meant by the term, "essential amino acids"?

3. List the ways in which an adequate amount of complete protein in your daily diet can contribute to your well-being.

4. Explain why iron is so important in the diet. What types of anemia can be controlled with proper diet? Which nutrients are especially helpful? Why should young women learn to include iron-rich foods in the diet every day?

5. Discuss the ways in which the discovery of vitamin B_{12} has been important for us. What are its food sources? Which of these foods are most important for niacin content? How does niacin help you?

6. Explain why it is important to include several iron-rich foods in your diet each week.

7. What kinds of fish do you like best? How many different kinds have you eaten? Why are fish, liver, and eggs so important on a weight-control or low-fat diet? In a normal diet?

8. Check the seven-day record you kept of your own eating habits (Chapter 4). Did you have a complete protein in each meal? How much did you have in each meal? In snacks? Compare this record with your RDA.

APPLYING AND SHARING

1. Compare your seven-day food record (Chapter 4) with the food you ate yesterday. Use the table of nutritive value of foods on pages 404-430 to figure out the following problems:

   a. How many grams of protein did you eat in each meal? In each day?

   b. What percent of the day's calories was derived from animal protein? From plant protein? From fat? Discuss the results. Calculate the cost of a serving of each.

   c. How many milligrams of iron did you have? Of niacin?

   d. Compare your intake with the recommended quantities for each nutrient. Which foods helped most in meeting your recommended daily allowance of each nutrient? Were there any weaknesses? Make a plan showing how you can improve.

2. Plan daily balanced menus for your meals and snacks for one week. Show how you would use the variety of meats and meat alternatives studied in this chapter, and stay within the budget of your family at present. How would you change the plan to meet the needs of a lower budget?

3. Write to the Department of the Interior for information on fish as a food and for recipes using various kinds of fish.

4. Using various cookbooks as references, look up ways to prepare liver and fish. Try two different recipes for each of these at school and at home.

CAREER CAPSULES

Veterinarian Works "in the field"; performs animal check-ups, diagnoses and administers to ill animals, delivers baby animals, sometimes carries out government animal health programs. Advanced degree in veterinary medicine required.

Meat packer Works in wholesale meat packing houses; cuts and trims meat, fills orders of distributors or retailers. Vocational education or union training program required.

RELATED READING

Better Homes and Gardens Meat Cookbook. New York: Meredith Press, 1969. Contains many good recipes using a wide variety of meats.

Harlan, Jack R. "The Plants and Animals that Nourish Man." *Scientific American,* Volume 235, Number 3 (September 1976). Points out that of the several thousand species of plants and several hundred species of animals, only a relatively small number has been domesticated; explains the mutual dependency of people, plants, and animals.

Sebrell, William H., Jr., James J. Haggerty, and Editors of *Life. Food and Nutrition.* New York: Time, 1967. Presents in excellent pictorial essays and text world foods and the process of nutrition.

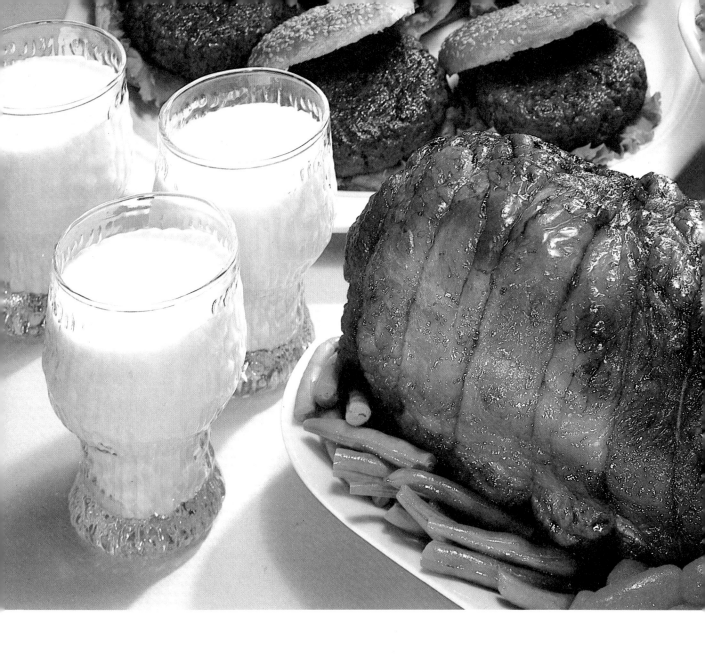

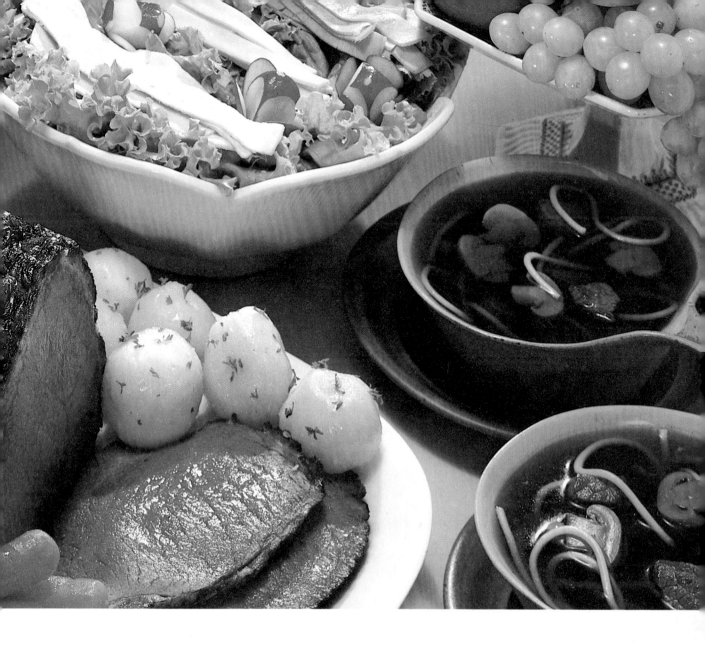

Meat in meals

After studying this chapter, you will be able to

- describe the composition of meat and explain its relationship to nutrition.
- explain the significance of the grade and inspection stamps.
- explain how an understanding of the different grades and cuts of meat can help you save money.
- plan and prepare colorful and flavorful meals using meat or eggs as the protein dish.

Meat is a food that many people enjoy eating; however, it is also one of the more expensive foods to purchase. This can especially be a problem for people who have to support themselves on a low income. Many are accustomed to eating higher-quality, more expensive meat than they can afford on a low budget. You should be able to resolve this conflict when you have completed your study of food. It is possible to serve delicious meats in meals, yet stay within a food budget.

There are many kinds of meat on the market (Table 10-1). What kinds are the best to buy? What is the best way to prepare each kind of meat? To understand how to select and cook cuts of meats, you must know about their composition—lean muscle fiber, connective tissues, bones, and fat—and how to recognize the grades of meat.

Six factors determine the cost of meat: (1) grade, (2) cut, (3) age, (4) method of processing, (5) amount of fat and bone, and (6) kind of meat, fish, or poultry. Calculate the cost of meat on the basis of how many 112-g (4-oz) servings of raw, lean meat you can get from 0.45 kg (1 lb). Four hamburgers can be made from 0.45 kg (1 lb) of lean ground beef. A 0.45-kg (1-lb) fish fillet yields three to four servings. But it takes half a broiler or a plateful of tiny riblets from a young lamb to make a serving because of the bone and fat.

Composition of red meats

Meat is composed of the lean muscle fiber, connective tissues, bone, and fat of animals.

Table 10-1 **Kinds of meats**

RED MEAT	ORGANS (variety meats)	FISH	POULTRY
Beef	Liver	Salt water	Chicken
Veal	Heart	Fresh water	Turkey
Pork, lean (not	Kidneys	Shellfish	Duck
bacon or fatback)	Sweetbreads	Oysters	Goose
Lamb	Brains	Shrimp	Squab
Mutton	Lungs	Crab	Cornish hen
Goat	Tripe	Clams	Pheasant
	Tongue	Lobster	Wild birds
		Scallops	

Muscle fiber. The lean muscles provide most of the vitamins, minerals, and protein.

Connective tissues. Connective tissues are creamy white, threadlike strands that bind the muscle fibers in little bundles. They also bind the muscles to the bones. If the connective tissues are tender, the meat will be tender and enjoyable. If the connective tissues are tough, the meat will be tough. This is an important point to remember in selecting and cooking meat.

Connective tissues are generally tender in fish, young poultry, lamb, pork, and some cuts and grades of beef. They are tough in older poultry, beef, and thin or poorly nourished animals. Old animals and exercised parts of an animal have tougher connective tissues. Tougher connective tissues can become tender during proper cooking.

Bone. Bone in meat, fish, and poultry is an important part of the diet for Eskimos and others who use little or no milk. Among many primitive peoples, bones are cooked until soft and the calcium-rich gristle is eaten. In the United States, however, we do not usually eat bone. You should therefore avoid spending money for cuts of meat that have a lot of bone in them. You will find less lean meat in such cuts and a higher cost of lean per pound.

Fat. Fat surrounds the carcass of animals and poultry just beneath the skin. Well-nourished animals produce meat that is tender, juicy, and interlaid with fat. Poorly fed animals lack fat. Their meat is tough.

Different kinds of meat have different amounts of fat. Veal,

Table 10-2 **Grades of beef in order of quality**

GRADE	CHARACTERISTICS
USDA PRIME	Cherry-red color in fresh beef, darker in "ripened" meat. Fine-grained; firm; lean, with white connective tissue, much marbling of fat in lean portion.
USDA CHOICE	Firm-grained; firm; lean, with white connective tissue, less marbling of fat.
USDA GOOD	Coarser-grained; lean, with creamy-white connective tissue, less fat in lean and around it.
USDA STANDARD OR USDA COMMERCIAL	Darker red color; coarser lean, with darker connective tissue, less fat.
USDA UTILITY	Lowest grade on the market, and usually not seen on meat counters.
CANNER AND CUTTER	Not seen on the market; used for processed meat products.

which is beef three months old or younger, has so little fat that the meat is tough unless properly cooked. Broilers, which are young poultry, have little fat, but their meat is tender. Cooked pork has slightly less fat than similar amounts of beef or lamb.

Grades of red meat

When meat is graded, the quality of the whole carcass is judged. The grade indicates the juiciness of the meat and the tenderness of the lean meat and the connective tissue. It also indicates how the meat can best be cooked to develop its flavor and tenderness. Table 10-2 shows you at a glance the different grades of beef. Prime is the top grade. Each succeeding

grade is slightly lower in quality than the grade above it.

A beef carcass has more tough meat than any other kind. This is one reason beef has more grades than any other meat. Knowing the different grades of beef helps you make the best purchasing decision.

Prime grade is the best grade of meat. It has the most calories per serving. The reason is that thin streaks of fat are intermingled with the lean. This fat is called marbling. Well-marbled meat is exceptionally tender and juicy. It "melts in the mouth." Most prime-grade meat goes to the better restaurants, but it can be specially ordered from local butchers.

Choice grade is the one most used in the home. It costs less

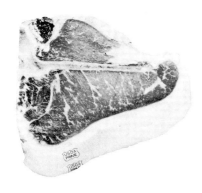

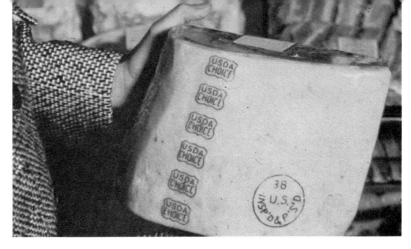

Shields stamped in a harmless purple dye indicate that meats have been federally graded and inspected.

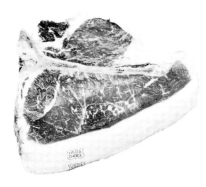

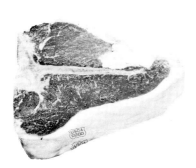

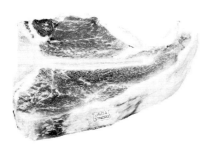

Beef is graded according to color, grain, leanness, firmness, and marbling. *Top:* Prime. *Top center:* Choice. *Bottom center:* Good. *Bottom:* Standard or commercial.

than prime grade because it has less marbling. Choice-grade beef is tasty, tender meat.

Today, we are seeing more good-grade beef in the market. Standard, utility, and canner grades are usually sold to processors for purposes other than human consumption.

Grading. Federal grading is indicated by a shield stamp with the U. S. grade on it. A harmless purple vegetable dye is used to stamp grades of meat on the outside of the carcass. The federal government sets standards for grading meat. Many meat companies do their own grading based on the federal standards. Some meat companies employ and train specialists to grade their meats. There is no U. S. law saying they must grade meat.

Most grading is honestly done according to federal standards. However, in 1977, a retailing chain was discovered to be using "choice" stamps on meat that was only "good" grade. This kind of practice is illegal. The consumer must be able to distinguish grades in order to recognize and act against dishonest grading.

U.S. inspection. Federal inspection of meat carcasses for wholesomeness is mandatory. Carcasses are inspected by government officials. A round inspection stamp is placed on all grades of meat that have been federally inspected and found to be wholesome and to have been processed under sanitary conditions. (See Chapter 2 for the federal safeguards that govern the inspection of meat and poultry.)

Cuts of red meat

Cuts of meat—unlike grades—are not stamped on the meat itself. They must be learned. To get to know the different cuts, study Figures 10-1 through 10-4. Then test your knowledge in the meat markets.

Knowing the cut of a piece of meat will help you to judge how tender or tough it is likely to be. The least exercised portions of the animal are the most tender. They lie along the backbone and upper ribs. The less tender cuts come from the legs and shoulders. The tougher, exercised portions of meat cost less per pound than the tender cuts. The tougher cuts contain less fat and more lean and nutrients. The cut is im-

Figure 10-1   Cuts of beef

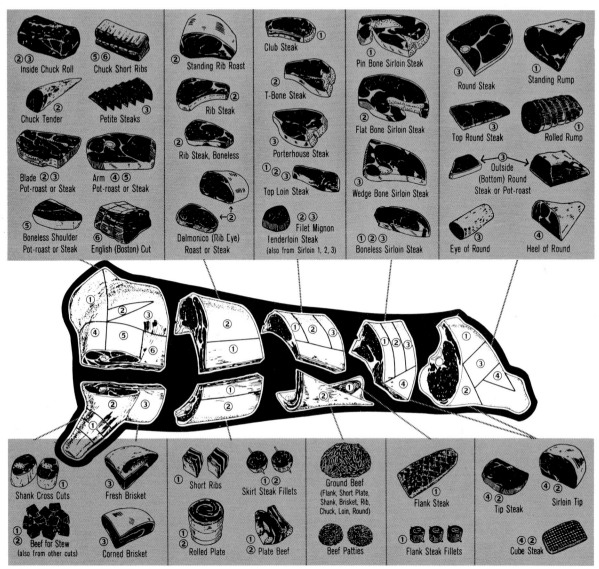

National Live Stock and Meat Board

portant in determining the price to pay and the proper method for cooking.

Other forms of red meat

Meats are prepared for the market in many different ways for many different reasons. They can be ripened, tenderized, cured, canned, frozen, or dried.

Ripened meat. In the process of ripening, meat hangs in a refrigerated warehouse for two to three weeks. This process allows the enzymes to act on the lean and the connective tissues. It makes the meat more tender, juicy, and delicate in flavor, and also more costly. Usually it is the hindquarters, ribs, and loins of beef that are ripened. Lamb may also be ripened.

Tenderized meat. Tenderizing meat improves its tenderness and quality. Meats can be tenderized in many ways. One way is to let the meat sit in brine for about six weeks. A shorter tenderizing

Figure 10-2   Cuts of veal

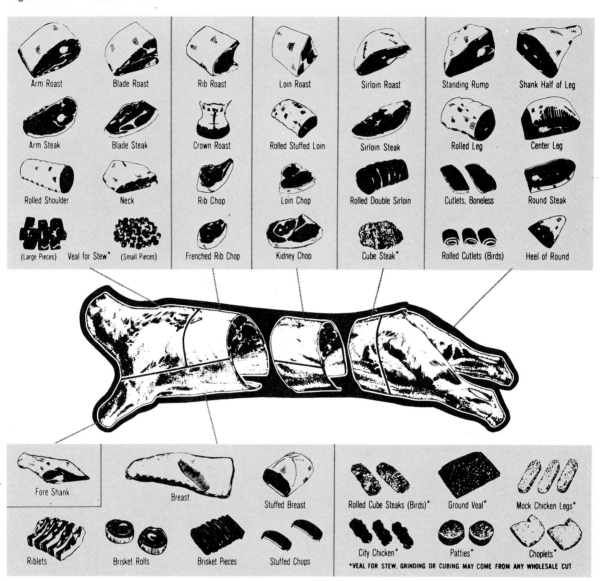

National Live Stock and Meat Board

method takes only two weeks. It is used today for hams. Enzymes and other curing agents are injected into the meat. They circulate through the tissues, making them more tender and moist and softer in texture. Another tenderizing process, used in making Virginia hams, results in a hard, dry cure.

Meat may also be tenderized by breaking or softening the muscle fibers and connective tissues. In markets, a machine is used for this purpose. At home, we pound meat with a spiked hammer. Grinding the meat or using a tenderizing powder are other ways to tenderize low grades and tough cuts. Cooking at low temperature

166

Figure 10-3   Cuts of pork

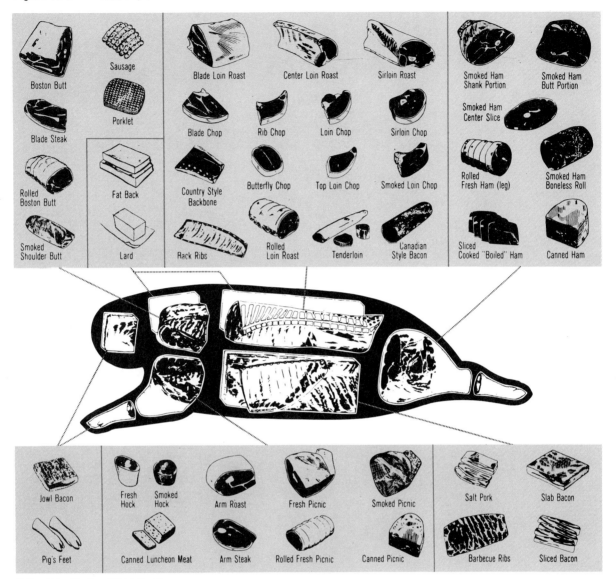

National Live Stock and Meat Board

with moist heat softens tough fibers.

Cured meat. Cured meat is made by heavily salting fresh meat and letting it stand in the brine. The meat most commonly cured is pork. The hind legs of pork are hams. The forelegs are Boston butt and picnic ham. The side is bacon. Bacon is consid- ered a fat rather than a meat. We buy it and enjoy it for its flavor. Canadian bacon comes from the loin and is leaner.

Some cuts of beef, such as the rump, plate, round, and brisket, are cured. Cured beef is called corned beef.

Processed meat. Meats are processed by canning, freezing, freeze-drying, drying, and pick- ling. Cold cuts are the most com- mon form of processed meats and the most expensive. They are made from the lowest grades and toughest cuts of meat. They also contain more fat than many fresh meats.

The freezing of meats, poultry, and fish does not destroy any

Meat in meals   **167**

Figure 10-4   Cuts of lamb

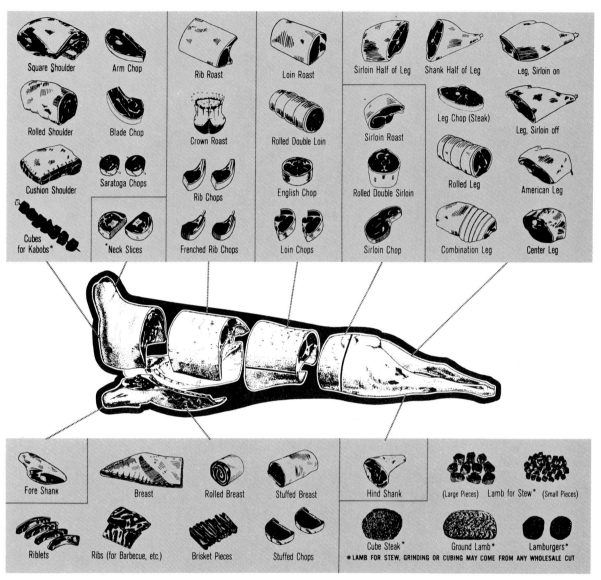

National Live Stock and Meat Board

flavor or nutrients. It does destroy some harmful bacteria. Freezing enables millions of people to enjoy a better diet, throughout the year, no matter where they live.

Frozen meat spoils quickly once it is thawed. Any processed meat, once opened, should be wrapped or covered and stored in the refrigerator.

Beef is the most commonly dried meat in the United States. Dried beef is made from low-grade meat or tough cuts. The meat is cured in brine, dried, thinly sliced, and then sold at a high price. The cost of the labor, time, and equipment used in processing raises the price of processed meats.

168

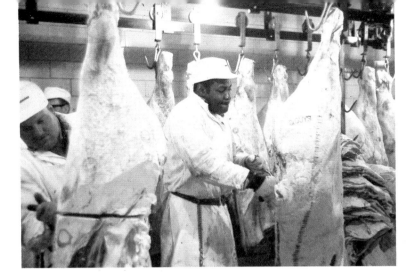

Meat is ripened in refrigerated warehouses.

Most fish and shellfish is cleaned and frozen right after it is caught.

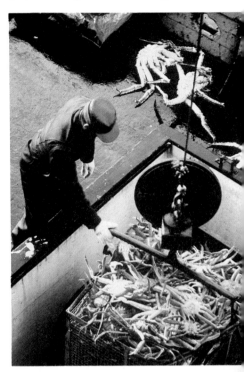

Top: Hams are tenderized and cured pork. *Bottom:* Cold cuts are popular processed meats.

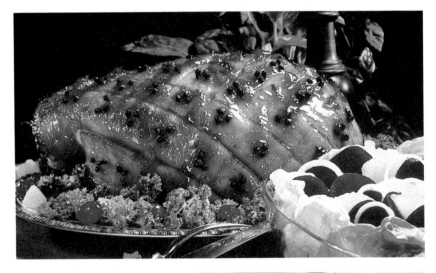

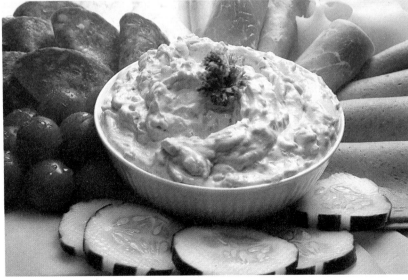

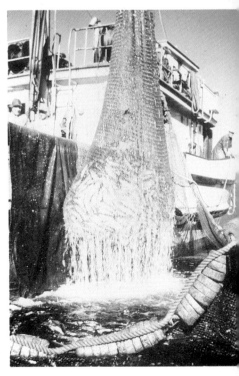

Figure 10-5 Poultry as well as meat is federally inspected and graded.

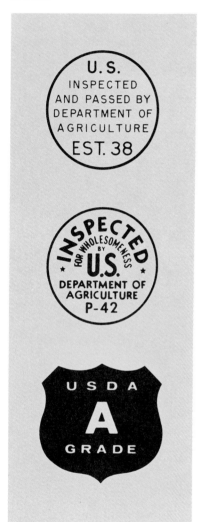

Selecting high-quality fresh poultry and fish is less bewildering than finding the way through the maze of grades and cuts of red meats. A few common-sense rules of sight and smell may be used as guides for buying poultry and fish.

Poultry

When choosing poultry, look for firm, thick flesh. A layer of yellowish fat should be present beneath the skin. Check to see that there are few, if any, pinfeathers and no bruises or blemishes.

High-quality poultry is inspected and graded (Figure 10-5). The inspection indicates that it is clean and wholesome. Poultry is graded by federal government standards as A and B. A is the top grade. Poultry is also graded by characteristics (Table 10-3.)

Fish

The quality of fresh fish is best judged if the fish is bought whole (Table 10-4). Odor is the most important indication of freshness. A fresh fish has little odor. Once the fish begins to deteriorate, the odor becomes strong and offensive.

In fresh fish, the eyes should bulge as in live fish. They should be bright and shining, not dull or slimy. The gills should be firm, red-pink in color, and free from mucus. The scales should have a bright sheen, as if the fish had just been caught. The flesh should be firm and should spring back when touched.

Most fish is frozen as soon as it is caught. Some is canned immediately. Canned fish is of high quality if the label on the can bears the marks of federal inspection.

Large poultry farms have their own plants for plucking, cleaning, and refrigerating carcasses before they are shipped to market.

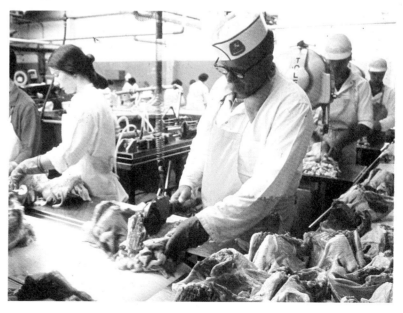

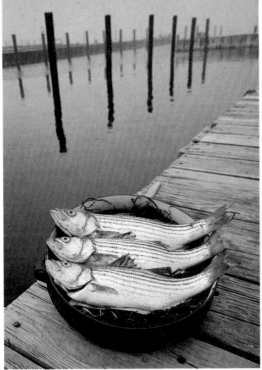
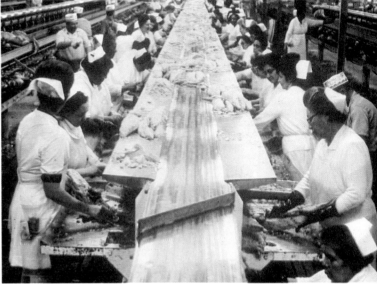

Left: Fresh fish should be as shining and firm as if it were still alive. *Right:* Canned fish improves the diet for those who do not have access to fresh or frozen fish.

Table 10-3 **Guide for selection and use of poultry**

KIND	WEIGHT kg (lb)	CHARACTERISTICS	HOW TO USE
ROASTER Chicken Turkey Capon Goose Duck	1.4–2.7 (3–6) 2.3–11.7 (5–26) 1.4–2.7 (3–6) 1.8–4.5 (4–10) 0.7–1.8 (1½–4)	Firm breastbone; fleshed breasts; pliable, smooth skin; yellowish and evenly distributed fat.	Roasted whole in oven (stuffed, if desired, with bread, cornbread, rice, bulgur); barbecued on spit; roasted in parts
FRYER (whole or parts)	0.9–1.4 (2–3)	Has less fat; breastbone flexible cartilage; short legs; well-fleshed	Broiled; fried disjointed; baked
BROILER	0.3–0.9 (¾–2)	Same as fryers. More pinfeathers on young birds	Split in halves down back and breast; broiled in stove on grill
CORNISH HEN	0.3–0.5 (¾–1)	Breast broad; well-fleshed; flexible breastbone; wings flexible when pulled	Roasted, stuffed as above
FOWL	1.4–2.7 (3–6)	Same as roasting chickens (older birds, tougher)	Stewed; chicken and dumplings; casseroles; salad; sandwiches; fricassee; soup; croquettes; pies; hash

Table 10-4 **Guide for selection and use of fish**

KIND	CHARACTERISTICS	HOW TO USE
FISH		
Mackerel Sardines Shad Eel Herring	Flesh firm, colored, highest in fat Odor: clean, mild, fresh	Broiled, baked, fried (add lime or lemon)
Halibut Haddock Swordfish Snapper Flounder Black bass Trout Cod Salmon Pickerel	Fresh or frozen Low fat; firm flesh—no fingerprint when pressed; white or pink flesh for its kind Odor: for its kind, not strong or offensive	Thaw frozen Broiled, baked, fried, or poached Add seasonings with oil and rub in to improve flavor. Add lime or lemon. Cook at low temperature to destroy odor.
SHELLFISH		
Oysters	Fresh, canned, and frozen Firm, plump, little odor Season: September to April	Stewed, creamed, scalloped, fried Raw as first course (on half-shell) Serve with lemon, lime, or sauce.
Scallops	Firm; almost odorless Season: September to March	Deep-fried, pan-fried, fritters, chowder
Clams	Buy only unbroken shells. Quahogs, little neck—both round shape. Season: All year Soft-shell—long shape. Season: May to October	Chowder; raw, on half-shell; steamed; broiled; boiled; juice, in appetizers
Crab	Fresh, frozen, canned High-quality—back fin, white claw Season: Hard-shell, all year; soft-shell, summer	Cocktail, salad, deviled, casserole, scalloped
Shrimp	Flesh firm, color pink Season: All year	Cocktail, salad, boiled, fried, curried, casseroles, appetizers
Lobsters	Select only live or boiled. If alive, should be very active to touch. Season: fresh—summer; frozen, canned—all year	Broiled, boiled, cocktail, salad
Fish roe (eggs)	Shad, sturgeon (caviar) Fresh or canned	Appetizer, sandwich Shad roe—broiled, poached, casserole

In storing and cooking meats of all kinds, the preservation of freshness will assure good flavor, texture, and color, and retention of nutrients. When shopping, buy meat, poultry, fish, and cold cuts last. The less time they are unrefrigerated, the fresher they will be when eventually cooked.

Storing meats, poultry, and fish

Fresh meats. Store meats, poultry, and fish in the coldest part of the refrigerator. Fresh, unfrozen meats should be loosely wrapped if they are not to be cooked on the day they are purchased. Too-tight packaging increases the growth of microorganisms and hastens spoilage.

Wipe the outside of packaged meat with a damp paper towel before it is placed in the refrigerator. Wrap fresh fish so that no odor escapes into the refrigerator or freezer. Wash it just before cooking. Dry off excess water with paper towels.

Leftover meats. Leftover cooked meat should be cooled quickly and placed in the coldest part of the refrigerator. It should be used within a day or two. For freezing, it should be tightly sealed and placed immediately in the freezer. Stuffing should be removed and frozen in a separate container.

Frozen meats. Frozen precooked meat should be used within the time schedule in Table 10-5. Mark on the package the date the food is put into the freezer. Whether frozen meat is cooked or raw, thaw it gradually in the refrigerator. Save the juice that escapes in thawing and use it in cooking the meat. The juice contains valuable nutrients.

Cooking meats, poultry, and fish

The aim in cooking meat is to produce the best dish possible from the kind of meat chosen. Cooked meat should be tender in texture. It should be juicy and of pleasing aroma, color, and flavor.

How does the cooking process change meat? First of all, the fat begins to melt. The meat loses moisture and changes in color. The proteins coagulate. When moist heat is used, the collagen (gristle) softens and releases gelatin. These changes improve the flavor of meat and make it more digestible. Cooking also destroys harmful bacteria.

Temperature. Meat should not be cooked at high temperatures. The proteins in lean meat coagulate at about 60 °C (140 °F). Above this temperature, protein hardens. This makes

---

Folklore and Superstition

Have you heard that

. . . fish is a brain food?

. . . gelatin is one of the best protein foods?

. . . high-grade meat is more nutritious than lower grades?

. . . expensive cuts of meat are more nourishing than inexpensive cuts?

. . . the protein in beef is better than that in other red meats?

. . . the protein in fish is not as nourishing as that in other meats?

. . . kidney trouble is caused by eating too much meat?

. . . heart trouble is caused by eating too many eggs?

. . . meat and carbohydrate foods, especially starchy ones, should not be eaten in the same meal?

. . . fish and milk are poisonous when eaten in the same meal?

. . . the protein of eggs is not as nourishing as that of meat, fish, or poultry?

. . . pork is the least nutritious of meats, and the most unhealthful?

. . . pork is the most fattening of meats?

. . . high-protein foods are not fattening?

. . . it is better to eat the most meat, fish, or poultry of the day at dinner?

Don't you believe it!

Table 10-5 **Meat storage times**

MEAT	REFRIGERATOR[1]	FREEZER
FRESH		
Beef	2–4 days	6–12 months
Veal	2–4 days	6–9 months
Pork	2–4 days	3–6 months
Lamb	2–4 days	6–9 months
Ground beef, veal, lamb	1–2 days	3–4 months
Ground pork	1–2 days	1–3 months
Variety meats	1–2 days	3–4 months
PROCESSED		
Luncheon meats	1 week	Not recommended
Sausage, fresh, pork	2–3 days	Not recommended
Sausage, smoked	3–7 days	Not recommended
Sausage, dry and semidry (unsliced)	2–3 weeks	Not recommended
Frankfurters	4–5 days	2 weeks
Bacon	5–7 days	2 weeks
Smoked ham, whole	—	60 days
Beef, corned	1 week	2 weeks
COOKED		
Leftovers	4–5 days	2–3 months
FROZEN COOKED		
Meat pies	—	3 months
Swiss steak	—	3 months
Stews	—	3–4 months
Prepared meat dinners	—	2–6 months

Lessons on Meat (Washington, D.C.: National Live Stock and Meat Board).
[1] The range in time reflects recommendations for maximum storage time from several authorities. For top quality, fresh meats should be used in 2 or 3 days. Ground meat and variety meats should be used in 24 hours.

meat tough, rubbery, and dry, regardless of the grade or cut.

Low temperature is the key to cooking meat to make it tender, juicy, and mellow in flavor. Low temperature is preferred for the highest grades and most tender cuts, as well as for the lower grades and tougher cuts. Meat shrinks less when cooked at low temperatures, which means more servings per pound.

As a general rule, red meat should be roasted at a temperature of 150 °C (300 °F), and poultry and pork at 165 °C (325 °F). However, a 1970 study compared beef roasted at 95 °C (200 °F) and 150 °C (300 °F). It was found that the lower temperature yielded more servings per pound, thus bringing down the cost per serving. The meat was juicier, more tender, and more flavorful, and fewer nutrients were lost. It must be remembered, however, that low temperatures require longer cooking times than higher temperatures.

Time. The time required to cook meat depends on the kind, grade, cut, thickness and size, method of cooking, and temperature used. Time is approximate when given in minutes per pound. Use a meat thermometer. It is a sure way of knowing that you are allowing the right amount of time. For example, it will tell you when pork has reached an internal temperature of 85 °C (185 °F). At this temperature you can be sure that all harmful bacteria are destroyed. Using a thermometer will enable you to serve other roasts rare or medium rare without guessing.

Methods. Meats may be cooked with either dry heat or moist heat. To find out what method is recommended for different meats, see Table 10-6.

Dry heat is used in broiling and roasting. It is suited to prime-grade and choice-grade meat and tender cuts, or tenderized lower grades and tougher cuts. Broiling and roasting provide maximum flavor and retain nutrients in red meats, poultry, fish, and organ meats.

174

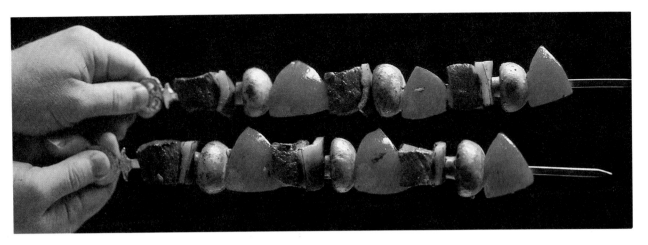

Grilling is a dry-heat method of cooking meats.

Pan broiling is a method of cooking without fat on top of the stove in a heavy skillet or griddle. This method is used for any cut or kind of meat that may be broiled. The meat is browned on one side and turned. Then it is cooked to the desired doneness.

Meat may be cooked in a microwave oven, which saves much time and fuel.

The moist-heat method of cooking is used for lower grades and less tender cuts of meat. The purpose of cooking meat with moist heat is to soften the connective tissue and release the collagen from the gristle of red meat and poultry.

Braising, stewing, or cooking in liquid in a heavy pot with a lid are three kinds of moist-heat cooking. The meat may or may not be dredged in flour, but it is always browned on all sides before final cooking. The meat is usually seasoned before heating. A small amount of water or other liquid is used for braising, and more is added for stewing or making soups. The meat and liquid are covered and simmered at a low temperature until done. The fat is then skimmed off the liquid.

The meat and liquid should occupy no more than half the capacity of the pot. Vegetables may added when the meat is tender and cooked until they are crisp-tender. Most of the vitamins, minerals, and amino acids remain in the liquid. Using a pressure saucepan to cook the meat first saves two hours or more in cooking time.

Deep frying is a quick form of moist-heat cooking. The water inside the food and the heat from the fat cooks the meat. Fat is heated to 175 °C to 210 °C (350 °F to 400 °F). The food is lowered into the hot fat in a basket. The water in the food forms steam that cooks the food.

Because of the high temperature and the danger of splashing,

The nutrients lost in braising meats are retained in the cooking liquid, which may be used in a sauce or soup.

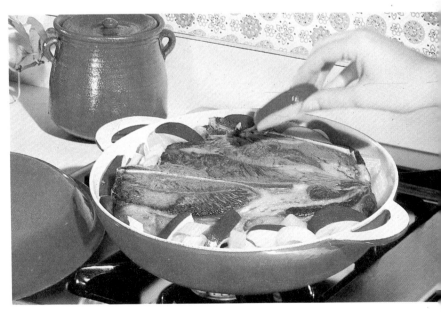

Table 10-6 Basic methods of cooking meat, poultry, fish, and organs

KIND	DRY HEAT			MOIST HEAT	
	Broiling	Roasting	Pan broiling	Braising	Stewing

BEEF[1]	Steaks
	  Porterhouse
	  T-bone
	  Sirloin
	  Tenderloin
	  Filet mignon
	  Club
	  Rib
	  Top round
	  Loin tip
	  Ground
		Rib
		  Standing
		  Rolled
		  Rump
		  Sirloin
		  Loaf
			Steaks
			  Round
			  Ground
			  T-bone
			  Rib
			  Club
			  Filet mignon
			  Sirloin
				Pot roast
				Steaks
				  Lower round
				  Arm
				  Blade
				  Flank
					Soups and stews
					Brisket
					Short ribs
					Shank
					Plate
					Neck
					Flank
					Heel of round
					Corned beef
					Cross-cut shank

VEAL[2]		Loin Leg Rack Shoulder	Cutlet Chops Steak Cube steak Ground	Breast Steak Loin Chops Kidney Cubes Ribs	Neck Riblets Breast Flank Shank Heel of round

PORK[3]	Canadian bacon
	Bacon
	Ham slice
	Smoked shoulder
		Loin
		Sirloin
		Ham, fresh or
		  cured
		Spareribs
		Ham loaf
		Picnic ham,
		  fresh or
		  cured
			Ham, fresh or
			  cured
			Bacon
			Candian bacon
				Chops
				Spareribs
				Shoulder steaks
				Tenderloin
					Ham
					Picnic ham
					Shoulder butt
					Shank
					Hocks
					Tenderloin

LAMB[4]	Chops Loin Rib Sirloin Shoulder Steaks Ground	Leg Shoulder Loaf	Chops Loin Shoulder steak Ground	Chops Shoulder Breast Neck Shank	Neck Flank Shank Riblets Breast

[1]Latest research shows that 92 °C (200 °F) is the most desirable temperature at which to roast beef for economy, juiciness, tenderness, and flavor. Use a meat thermometer to achieve the following internal temperatures.

Rare (red to pink inside)	60 °C (140 °F)
Medium (pink)	70 °C (160 °F)
Well done (brown)	77 °C (170 °F)

[2]Rub veal roasts with oil to prevent them from drying out. Veal is too lean to be broiled.

[3]Fresh pork should be roasted to an internal temperature of 84 °C (185 °F). Cook it at 106 °C (225 °F). Timing will depend on the size and shape of the roast. The same advantages of low-temperature cooking hold for pork and lamb. No fresh pork should be broiled.

[4]Lamb may be roasted or otherwise cooked medium or well done, to internal temperatures of 68 to 75 °C (150 to 165 °F).

Table 10-6 (cont.)

| KIND | DRY HEAT | | | MOIST HEAT | |
	Broiling	Roasting	Pan broiling	Braising	Stewing
ORGANS	Liver (lamb, veal, or chicken) Kidneys Sweetbreads		Liver (lamb, veal, chicken, pork, or beef) Brains	Liver Kidneys Heart Sweetbreads Brains	Brains Kidney Tongue Sweetbreads
POULTRY[5]	Broilers	Broilers Young hens Hen turkeys Young tom turkeys Ducks Geose	Fryers Broilers	Hens Fowls	Hens Fowls Old roosters Old tom turkeys
FISH	Fish is so tender that any kind may be cooked in any fashion that you like.				

[5]Poultry is roasted or cooked well done, to an internal temperature of 86 °C (190 °F).

use care when deep frying. The high temperature of the fat can raise quite a steam inside the food. Water should never be used to put out a fire caused by fat. Instead, use salt or baking soda to put out the fire.

Seasonings. Part of the skill of turning an ordinary piece of meat into a flavorful dish lies in using herbs and spices (Table 10-7). Herbs and spices should be used so delicately that the specific seasonings cannot be identified. A small amount of herbs and spices enhances flavor, while a large amount overpowers it. Vary the quantities slightly until you find the amount that is just right to your taste.

Garnishes. Garnishes add color and flavor to various kinds of meat dishes. Parsley, watercress, lettuce, and pepper rings are common green garnishes. Cherry tomatoes, broiled or stuffed tomatoes or mushrooms, browned potatoes and onions, or attractively arranged strips of vegetables are more likely to be eaten. Sliced or whole green or black olives complement some meat dishes. Mint, radish roses, pickled peaches, or pickled pears are appropriate to lamb. With fresh or cured pork, baked apples, crabapples, apricots, or pineapple do well. Fish is traditionally garnished with lemon or lime slices. Sliced oranges may accompany poultry.

Place garnishes carefully on the meat or around it just before serving. Use just enough to enhance the meat, not to hide it.

Onions, herbs, and lemon slices may be used to season and garnish lamb.

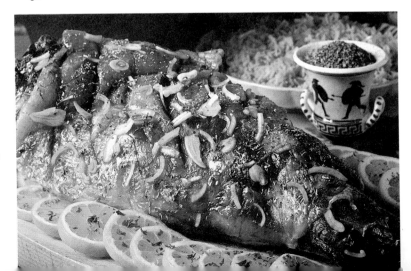

Table 10-7 Use of herbs and spices in meat, poultry, fish, and egg dishes

SPICE OR HERB	RED MEAT	POULTRY	FISH	EGGS
ALLSPICE	Pot roast, stew, patties, loaf, glaze on roast	Stew, pie, fricassee	Poached	Eggnog
ANISE	Stew	Braised, roast, pilaf		
BASIL	Lamb, beef, or veal roast, stew, chops, pies, balls	Fried, boiled	Broiled, baked, poached	Deviled, sandwich, scrambled, soufflé
BAY LEAF	Lamb, beef, or veal stews, pot roast, soup, organ meats	Fricassee, stew, soup	Shellfish, bisque, poached	
CARAWAY SEEDS	Roast, stew, sauerbraten	Goose	Broiled, poached, stuffed	Scrambled, omelet, spread
CARDAMOM SEED	Curry	Curry	Curry	
CAYENNE	Curry, croquettes, soup, sausage	Curry, barbecued, broiled	Curry, broiled, soufflé	Deviled, omelet, soufflé
CELERY SEED CELERY SALT	Pot roast, loaf, stew, broiled, soup	Roast, fricassee, stew	Chowder, baked, broiled	Omelet, soufflé, sandwich
CHILI POWDER	Chili con carne, stew, loaf, pie, meatballs	Casserole, barbecued, broiled, fried	Broiled, baked, poached, chowder	Omelet, soufflé, deviled, sandwich, scrambled
CINNAMON	Stew, sauerbraten, glaze on roast			
CLOVES	Corned beef, stew tongue, ham			
CURRY POWDER	Curry, meatballs, loaf, broiled	Curry, broiled, stuffing	Curry, shellfish, salad, soufflé	Scrambled, omelet, soufflé, deviled
DILL	Chops, stew, roast	Creamed, pilaf	Broiled, pilaf	Deviled, spread
MACE	Meat loaf, veal	Fricassee	Bisque	

Table 10-7 (cont.)

SPICE OR HERB	RED MEAT	POULTRY	FISH	EGGS
MARJORAM	Lamb, beef, or veal roast, stew, pot roast, loaf	Roast, fried, fricassee, stuffing	Poached, salad	Scrambled, omelet, soufflé
MINT	Lamb stew, sauce			
MUSTARD	Pork, loaf, meatballs			Sandwich, deviled
NUTMEG	Pot roast, stew, patties, loaf, glaze on roast	Stew, pie, fricassee	Poached	Eggnog
PARSLEY	Beef, veal, or lamb, hamburgers, loaf, meatballs, stew, soup	Fricassee, salad, pie, soup, stuffing	Garnish, soup, poached, stuffing, creamed	Creamed, omelet, scrambled, deviled
PEPPER PAPRIKA	All kinds	All kinds	All kinds	All kinds
POULTRY SEASONING	Casserole, stew, stuffing	All dishes	Broiled, baked, stew, stuffing	
ROSEMARY	Liver, lamb, shish kabob, pot roast	Broiled, roast, stew, casserole, salad, stuffing	Loaf, salad, croquettes, stuffing	Loaf, salad, croquettes, stuffing
SAGE	Pork, sausage	Roast, casserole, fried, stuffing	Chowder, stuffing, baked, broiled	
SAVORY	All roasts, pies, loaf, meatballs	All dishes	Broiled, stuffing	Omelet, scrambled
SESAME	Garnish	Broiled, roast, fried	Fried, roast, broiled	Scrambled
TARRAGON	All lamb and veal	Fricassee, fried, stew	Salad, broiled	Scrambled, all dishes
THYME	All roasts, stew, loaf, croquettes, liver, organs	Roast, broiled, fried, stew, stuffing	All dishes	Scrambled, shirred, deviled

Using leftovers

It is economical and convenient to prepare larger quantities of meat and save some for future use. By buying larger quantities during "specials", you save fuel, time, and money.

Planned leftovers enable you to make your own convenience meal with a minimum of preparation time. Even single people or small families can eat a large roast, fowl, or ham over a period of time if they plan meals around the leftovers.

EGGS

Eggs are easy to buy, often because they are produced locally. They store well in the refrigerator. Cooked, they make attractive and nutritious main protein dishes. They may be used as ingredients in other foods for purposes of thickening, leavening, and emulsifying.

Buying eggs

Make the best use of your food dollar by selecting eggs according to the use you wish to make of

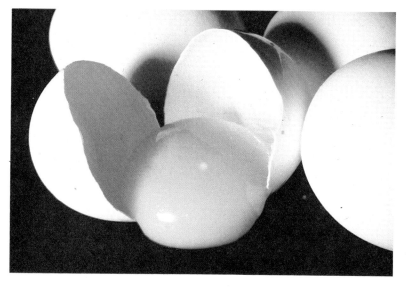

Eggs are graded by the quality of their yolks and whites.

them. Fresh eggs cost the most. The higher the grade and weight, the higher the cost.

Grades. Eggs are placed in front of a strong light beam to determine the grade. This is called **candling.** Grade is determined by the quality of the white and the yolk.

Eggs are graded AA, A, and B. The highest grade is AA. A-grade eggs have high, firm yolks and thick, firm whites. AA-grade eggs are the firmest. In B-grade eggs, the yolk doesn't stand quite as high and the white is thinner and spreads out more. Use top grades for poaching, boiling, and frying. Use lower grades for various cooked dishes, including scrambled eggs and omelets.

Standards for fresh eggs are set by federal and state authorities. The shield on the carton indicates the grade of the eggs at the time the shield was placed there.

Size and weight. When selecting eggs, consider their size and weight. Extra-large eggs weigh 756 g (27 oz) a dozen. Large ones weigh 672 g (24 oz). Medium-size eggs weigh 588 g (21 oz). If the price spread per dozen eggs between one size and the next smaller size in the same grade is not larger than 7 cents, buy the larger size. To illustrate, if extra-large eggs cost 92 cents a dozen and large ones cost 88 cents, the extra-large size is the best buy for your money.

Color. The color of the shell does not relate to nutrients. It does relate to the breed of chicken. The color of the egg yolk depends on the kind of feed given the bird. A deep-yellow color indicates that the hen has had carotene-rich food. Hens eat green grass and can convert carotene from it into vitamin A. Since vitamin A is colorless, the light yolk may contain more preformed vitamin A. Yolk of either color is a good food source for vitamin A.

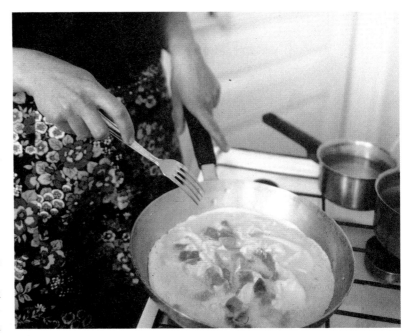

Omelettes are quick and easy to make and show off eggs to their best advantage.

Storing eggs

Store eggs in the refrigerator in a covered container with the large end of the egg up. The air sac will then be at the top. Research shows that eggs stored in the refrigerator for three weeks deteriorate less than eggs stored at room temperature for three days.

Leftover yolks should be covered with water and stored in the refrigerator in a covered jar. Yolks should be used within one or two days. Egg whites will keep in the refrigerator for a week. Yolks or whites may be stored frozen at −18 °C (0 °F) or lower. Thawed eggs may be used in the same ways as fresh ones.

Cooking with eggs

Thickening. Eggs may thicken soups, sauces, soufflés, custards, creamy pie fillings, and ice cream.

In thickening power, one whole egg is equal to two yolks or two whites.

The protein in eggs coagulates at low temperatures. When using eggs for thickening hot liquids, coagulation often occurs too quickly, causing the eggs to curdle, or form lumps. To avoid curdling, condition the eggs by slowly stirring about 5 mL (1 tsp) of the hot liquid into the eggs. Then gradually stir the remaining hot liquid into the eggs. Cooking the entire mixture in a double boiler controls the temperature and prevents curdling. If an egg sauce does curdle, you can easily beat out the lumps with an egg beater.

The baking of a custard may be hastened by heating the milk before adding it to the custard mixture. To make sure the custard bakes evenly, set it in a pan of hot water. Do not cover custards or

Unbeaten as well as beaten eggs are used for leavening baked goods.

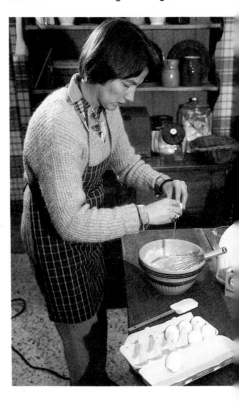

Table 10-8 **Meat, poultry, fish, and egg dishes**

	EGGS	RED MEATS	ORGANS	POULTRY	FISH

BREAKFAST	Boiled
	Poached
	Blindfolded
	Fried
	Shirred
	Scrambled
	Omelet
	French toast
	Popovers
	Spoon bread
	Pancakes
		Canadian bacon
		Ham, cured
		Lamb chop
		Texas steak
		Creamed chipped
		  beef
			Sautéed chicken
			  livers
			Broiled kidney
			Broiled liver
			Broiled
			  sweetbreads
				Fried chicken
				Broiled chicken
				Turkey hash
				Turkey croquettes
				Creamed chicken
					Broiled fish
					  in season
					Creamed fish
					Smoked fish

LUNCH	Quiche Lorraine
	Salad
	Sandwich
	Popovers
	Stuffed
	Soufflé
	Eggs à la
	  goldenrod
	Spoon bread
	Omelet
	Deviled
	In casseroles
	With salads
		Sandwich
		Soup
		Stew
		Casserole
		Hamburger
		Frankfurter
		Salad
		Chili
		Loaf
			Liverwurst
			  sandwich
			Brain salad
			Kidney pie
			Liver casserole
			Any used for
			  breakfast
				Salad
				Sandwich
				Soufflé
				Creamed
				Curried
				Any used for
				  breakfast
					Tuna fish
					  salad
					Crab, shrimp,
					  or lobster
					  salad
					Sandwiches
					Poached
					Chowder
					Broiled
					Casserole

DINNER	Creole eggs
	Ham-and-egg
	  shortcake on
	  corn bread
	Grits soufflé
	Egg and seafood
	  salad
	Soufflé
	Enchiladas
	In casseroles
	With salads
	Any used for
	  breakfast
	  or lunch
		Roasted beef,
		  veal, fresh
		  pork, ham,
		  lamb
		Broiled chops,
		  steaks
		Pot roast
		Braised stew
		  meat
		Barbecued beef
		Barbecued pork
		Shish kabob
		Loaf
		Meat patties
		Chili
			Broiled liver
			Liver pâté
			Liver loaf
			Pan-fried liver
			Liver sausage
			Liverburgers
			Liver-vegetable
			  casserole
			Liver pilaf
			Stuffed heart
			Braised heart
			Heart-vegetable
			  soup
			Broiled kidneys
			Beef-kidney pie
			Sautéed chicken
			  livers
				Roasted
				Oven-fried
				Southern-fried
				A la king
				Casserole
				Stew
				Turkey steaks
				Turkey loaf
				Pie
				Loaf
				Fricassee
				Hash
				Soup or chowder
					Chowder
					Baked
					Roast,
					  stuffed
					Broiled
					Fried
					Casserole
					Cakes
					Canapes
					Sticks
					Salad

egg mixtures in the oven. Browning adds to their flavor.

Leavening. Eggs may be used to leaven mixtures. This means they lighten foods and increase the volume. Angel food, sponge, and chiffon cakes depend on eggs to lighten them. Soufflés made with cheese, chicken, fish, ham, or a vegetable are leavened with eggs. So are sweet dessert soufflés.

Emulsifying. Eggs emulsify or bind together two or more ingredients that separate naturally, such as oil and vinegar. The ingredients in Hollandaise sauce and mayonnaises are emulsified and made smooth with eggs.

Other uses in cooking. Eggs may coat and glaze baked foods. They are used to give firm structure to croquettes and meat loaf and for batters in frying.

PLANNING MEALS USING MEAT, POULTRY, FISH, AND EGGS

Table 10-8 suggests dishes made with foods in the meat group for each of the day's three meals. Although some dishes are accompaniments, appetizers, or first courses, most are main dishes. The serving of meat, poultry, or fish used as a main dish should be at least 56 g (2 oz) without fat or bone. Two eggs are considered a serving.

Naturally any meal using some kind of meat food should contain foods from other groups for nutritional balance. A balanced breakfast should include not only meat and/or eggs but also a citrus fruit or juice or other fruit in season, bread, a spread, and milk. If the diet permits the calories, a dish of cereal and jam or preserves may be added to the basic meal. Coffee or tea are optional at any meal, as they contain no nutrients.

A meat food for lunch should be accompanied by a raw or cooked vegetable, or both, milk, bread and a spread, a simple dessert or fruit. A balanced dinner should include meat or an alternate, a cooked green or yellow vegetable, milk, and a medium-size potato or a serving of corn, macaroni, rice, bulgur, or noodles. A raw vegetable salad with the meal or fresh fruit for dessert should be served. If calories and appetite permit, bread and a spread and a sweet dessert may be added to the basic meal.

Beaten egg is used to make breadings cling to foods that are to be cooked.

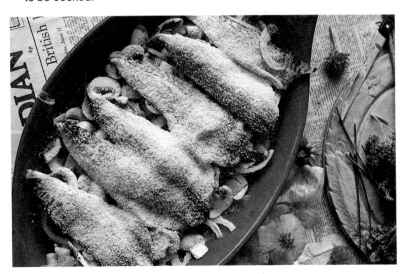

Buying poultry and fish

Poultry   Fish

Using meats, poultry, and fish

Storing meats, poultry, and fish   *Fresh meats   Leftover meats   Frozen meats*   **Cooking meats, poultry, and fish**   *Temperature   Time   Methods   Seasonings   Garnishes*
Using leftovers

Eggs

Buying eggs   *Grades   Size and weight   Color*   **Storing eggs**   **Cooking with eggs**   *Thickening   Leavening   Emulsifying   Other uses in cooking*

Planning meals using meats, poultry, fish, and eggs

THINKING AND EVALUATING

1. Which part of meat contains the most nutrients?

2. Why are fish, lamb, and young poultry more tender than many cuts of meat?

3. Explain what is meant by grades of meat. Which grade costs the most? Which contains the most fat? The most lean? How does an understanding of grades of meat help you save money in buying it?

4. List the different factors that affect the cost of meat.

5. In what forms other than fresh can meat be purchased?

6. Explain how the cooking process changes meat.

7. Give examples of the use of eggs to (a) thicken, (b) leaven, (c) emulsify, (d) glaze, (e) bind, (f) coat, and (g) foam.

APPLYING AND SHARING

1. Visit a large meat department in a supermarket and note the grades, cuts, and prices of beef, veal, pork, lamb, different kinds of liver, poultry, fish, and shellfish. This may be done more efficiently by dividing the class into groups and pooling your information.

2. Do the same for eggs, comparing size, grade, weight, and cost.

3. Evaluate commercials and advertisements for supplementary products to be taken for iron deficiency. How would you use foods in the meat group to help meet the need for extra iron?

4. Develop and apply four different ways to prepare eggs for breakfast. Do the same for lunch.

5. Research the laws on federal inspection of meat, fish, poultry, and eggs. Make a chart to illustrate your findings. Be prepared to explain these regulations to the class.

VOCABULARY

braising
candling
choice grade
collagen
connective tissue
cured meat
deep-frying
emulsify
marbling
pan broiling
prime grade
processed meat
ripened meat
tenderizing

Frozen fish worker Usually works right on the boat as a fisher, as most fish is frozen as soon as it is caught. Required education varies; on-the-job training essential.

Retail butcher Works in supermarket or specialty store; prepares and packages cuts of meat for consumer use, may have purchasing and selling responsibilities. Vocational education required; on-the-job training helpful.

RELATED READING

Batcher, Olive M., and Charles E. Murphy. "All About Meat, That Key Item in Food Buying, Meal Planning." *Food for Us All: Yearbook of Agriculture, 1969.* Washington, D.C.: USDA, 1969. Focuses on beef, pork, lamb, and variety meats, with a discussion of cuts, grades, quality, safety, and methods of preparation for meals.

Crosby, Violet B., and Ashley R. Gulich. "Poultry: A Tasty Anytime Delight that's Popular Dozens of Ways." *Food for Us All: Yearbook of Agriculture, 1969.* Washington, D.C.: USDA, 1969. Points out high nutritional values of poultry in relation to health and weight control; discusses inspection, grading, and kinds of poultry on the market, as well as methods of cooking.

Day, Avanelle S., and Lillie Stuckey. *The Spice Cookbook.* New York: David White, 1964. Contains recipes using eggs, fish, and shellfish, meats of all kinds, and poultry.

Handy, A. Elizabeth, "Eggs—Nature's Prepackaged Masterpiece of Nutrition." *Food for Us All: Yearbook of Agriculture, 1969.* Washington, D.C.: USDA, 1969. Discusses quality, grading, cost, and methods of cooking eggs.

Kerr, Rose G. "Savvy with Seafood in the Store and Kitchen for that Tang of the Deep." *Food for Us All: Yearbook of Agriculture, 1969.* Washington, D.C.: USDA, 1969. Focuses on kinds and forms of fish found in shops, inspection, grades and standards, and methods of cooking.

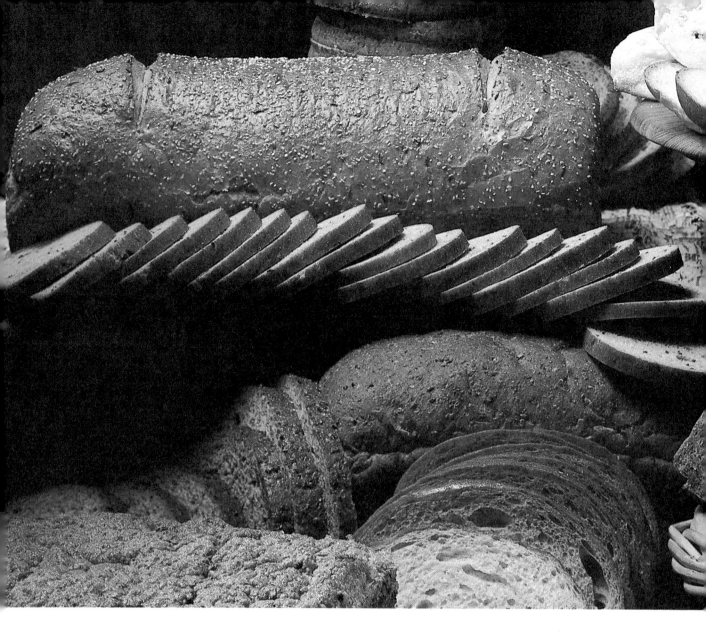

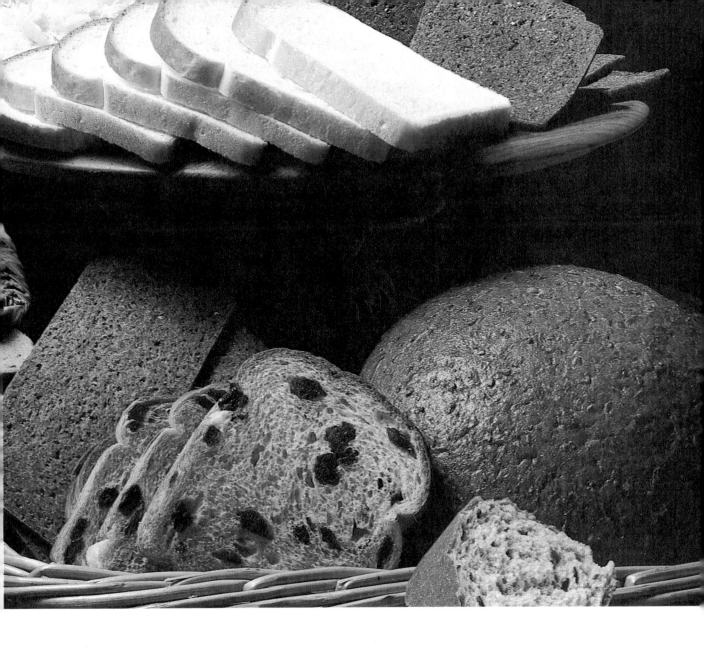

CHAPTER 11

Grain foods

After studying this chapter, you will be able to

- describe the nutritional contributions of grain.
- explain why cereals are important in a low-cost diet.
- list other foods that we need in a meal to balance the proteins from cereal grains.
- understand and explain what is meant by the term *complementary protein*.

Importance of grains to different cultures

Grain or cereal foods are basic to the diets of different cultures throughout the world. The word *grain* applies to the seeds of various grasses that have been processed for human consumption. Corn, rice, and wheat are the grains primarily used in the United States. Rye, barley, and buckwheat are widely used in other cultures, but they do not play a major role in the American diet. All grains are nutritionally similar. They differ in the amount and quality of the nutrients they contain.

Corn. Over three thousand years ago, the Maya Indians in Mexico were growing corn. In the

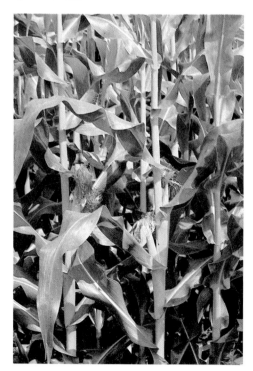
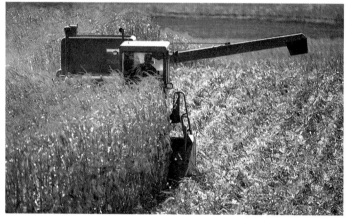
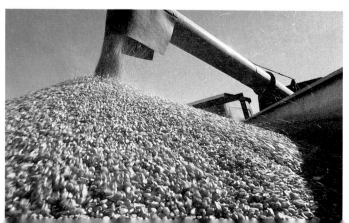

Corn (*left*) is harvested off the stalk (*top right*) and husked (*bottom right*) by combines.

188

National Museum of Anthropology in Mexico City, there is a mural that shows how much the Mayans valued corn. The mural presents corn as well as the sun as symbols of life. In fact, in all the Mexican dialects, the word "corn" means the "source of life." To this day, corn is the preferred grain of Mexico and Latin America.

The Indian peoples of North America also used corn. They taught the first white settlers how to grow corn and cook it. In Europe, people had been used to eating wheat, oats, and rye. When they settled in North America, they had to eat the available grain in order to survive.

By baking corn on hot rocks or hot ashes the pioneers made a bread called corn pone. The Indian word for this bread was *appone* or *apan*. Sometimes the bread was called hoecake, because it would be removed from the hot fire with a hoe. From the Indians, the pioneers learned to mix corn with beans. The Indians called this dish *misickquatash*, which became our word succotash. Succotash, hominy, and corn pone all became standard foods in Mexico and the United States.

Today we grow more corn than any other nation. In fact, we grow 70 percent of the world's supply. Corn leads all our crops in acreage and money value. From it we make many food products.

Rice. Rice, the grain of the Orient, is the world's most abundant cereal. It is the basic food in the diet of over half the world's population. The pharaohs of Egypt ate rice. So did the early Greeks, Turks, and Arabs. When the Moors left Africa for Spain in the Middle Ages, they took rice with them. Its use then spread over Europe. In 1694, a ship from Madagascar, laden with rice, was blown off its course. It landed at Charleston, South Carolina. Thus began the cultivation of rice in North America.

Wheat. Wheat is the cereal grain preferred by most western peoples. It is the best-balanced grain in nutrients. Because of new methods of plant breeding, we now produce wheat that has larger amounts of better-quality protein than ever before.

Foods made from wheat flour include most pastries, sweet baked foods, and macaroni products. But the most important food made from wheat is bread. There is no mystery as to why bread has been called "the staff of life." Nutritionists and chemists have unlocked the secret of the nutritional value of cereal grains.

Nutritional value of grains

As a group, bread and cereal foods provide important nutrients.

Carbohydrates. Foods made from grain are the best sources of carbohydrates. Carbohydrates are the body's preferred source of energy.

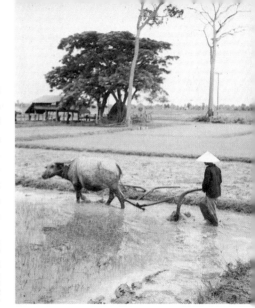
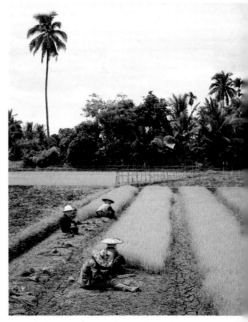
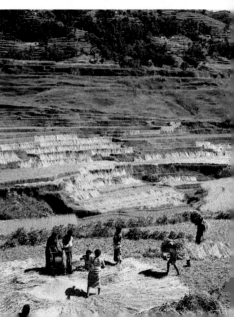

Rice is grown in flooded paddies (*top*), which are drained before the stalks are picked (*center*) and the grain threshed from the stalks (*bottom*).

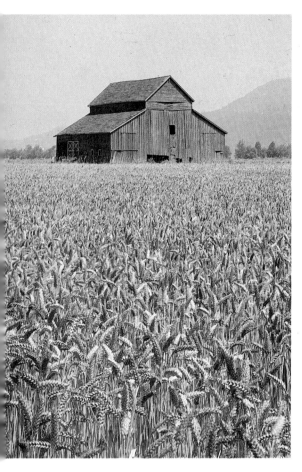
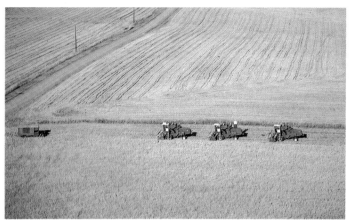
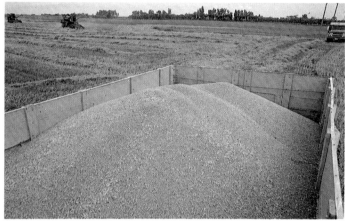

After combines have harvested wheat (*top right*), it is threshed (*bottom right*) before being milled and refined.

Protein. Although the protein in grains is incomplete, bread and cereal foods provide almost a quarter of the protein in American diets. They provide a far greater share in the diet of developing nations.

B vitamins. Whole and enriched grains are good sources of some B vitamins, particularly thiamin and vitamin B_6.

Iron, phosphorus, and other minerals. Iron in the whole grains and in enriched cereal helps each of us meet our daily iron need. A slice of enriched white bread contains 0.6 mg of iron. A 240-mL (1-cup) serving of cooked oats or macaroni contains 1.4 mg. These amounts may seem small. But three slices of bread and 240 mL (1 c) of cereal add up to 3.2 mg, more than one-sixth of a female's daily need from age 11 to 20, or a male's need from age 11 to 18.

Fat. Fat is found in the germ of whole grains. Although the amount is small, it is valuable because it contains linoleic acid, a polyunsaturated fatty acid. (See page 231.)

Practical value of grains

Bread and cereal foods have the following practical advantages.

1. Grains grow quickly and are low in cost. Meat requires a greater investment in land, time, and money to produce.

2. Grains are compact and easy to transport. They store and keep well.
3. Grains may be cooked with a small amount of fuel and equipment.
4. The bland flavor of grain foods enables one to eat them at every meal without monotony.

5. Grains may be used in the diet in many different ways.

With these assets, it is not difficult to understand why cereal grains are the basic foods in the diet of two-thirds of the world today, or why earlier people depended on them so completely.

CARBOHYDRATES

Because of the problems of controlling overweight, we are keenly aware of calories, the units used to measure energy. Some people will not eat bread or potatoes because they think these foods are "too high in calories" and "too starchy." They think that starch is fattening and that if they eat more meat and less starch they will not gain weight. In fact, as you recall, the protein in meat contains the same number of calories (4 per gram) as the starch in carbohydrate foods. The fat in meat contains over twice as many calories (9 per gram).

Carbohydrates are not necessarily fattening. Because we need them for energy, they are too important to eliminate from the diet.

When we feel cold, we shiver. This burns energy. Shivering moves muscles, and the heat that follows the release of energy warms you. You feel hotter when you run hard than when you walk because you are burning more energy. The more energy you use, the more calories you burn.

Heat accumulates more quickly than we can use it, and so our bodies eliminate the excess, or waste. The waste products are carbon dioxide and water. The water may be eliminated through the skin as perspiration. The carbon dioxide may be eliminated through the lungs.

Grain foods are the most important source of carbohydrates..

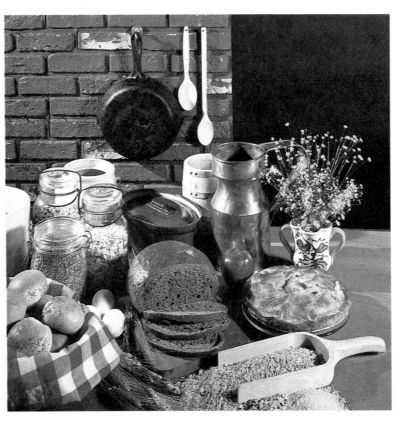

How the body uses carbohydrates

The human body has trillions of tiny cells. Cells are very efficient. They select oxygen and nutrients from the blood's capillaries. With these two ingredients, aided by enzymes and coenzymes (vitamins), a remarkable "explosion" takes place that releases energy and heat.

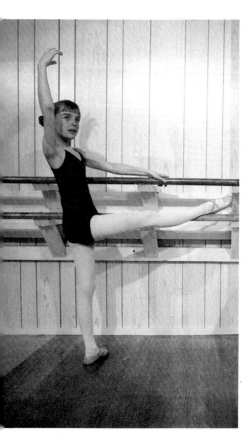

Carbohydrates are the body's preferred source of energy.

Scientists have learned that the nutrient the body prefers to use as a source of energy is carbohydrate. Carbohydrates are broken down during digestion from starch and sugar and are absorbed by the body as glucose. The normal, healthy body maintains a relatively constant level of glucose in the blood. The cells trap glucose, fatty acids, amino acids, and other nutrients. They burn glucose, fatty acids, and even amino acids for energy, though glucose is preferred.

What happens when there are not enough carbohydrate foods in the diet? The body draws on its reserves of carbohydrates in the liver and tissues. These reserves are small. The liver and tissues contain less than a 24-hour reserve supply of carbohydrates. When carbohydrate reserves are exhausted, the body draws on its reserves of fat. Fat is stored in the body as a source of reserve energy. Studies show that carbohydrates are essential for oxidizing (burning) fat.

Protein is the last nutrient to be burned for energy. Most of our reserve protein is in the form of live, working tissue. When fat is exhausted as a source of energy, the body begins to destroy itself by burning tissue protein to maintain the functions essential for life. By including carbohydrates in the diet to burn for energy, protein is spared for use in building tissue.

Carbohydrates burn more easily than fat or protein. They are also more easily digested. Every meal should have some foods that are digested quickly and others that are digested slowly.

Complex carbohydrates

Foods made from cereal grains are complex carbohydrates. They contain starch, cellulose (fiber), pectin, and other substances that are not digested by human beings and thus do not yield energy. Though not digested, they serve human beings in other ways. They help produce healthful intestinal bacteria. They also provide fiber or roughage needed for normal elimination of intestinal waste. Some studies indicate that the fibrous part of carbohydrates may aid in controlling cholesterol levels. Research also indicates that some B vitamins are made in our intestines with the help of plant food fiber.

COMPLEMENTARY PROTEINS

Cereal grains contain different amounts of protein. There may be as little as 6 percent protein in refined cereals and as much as 18 percent in improved types of whole grains (Table 11-1). Grains grown in soil with adequate nitrogen contain more protein than grains grown in soil deficient in nitrogen. Grains grown in a hot, dry climate have more protein than those grown in a humid climate.

Proteins in cereal grains lack one or more essential amino acids. But grains and legumes are complementary proteins. So eaten at the same meal they provide

Table 11-1 **Comparison of nutrients in wheat flour**

.45 KG (1 LB)	PROTEIN g	FAT mg	CALCIUM mg	IRON mg	THIAMIN mg	RIBOFLAVIN mg	NIACIN mg
Unenriched (all purpose)	47.6	4.5	73	3.6	.28	.21	4.1
Enriched (all purpose)	47.6	4.5	73	13–16.5	2–2.5	1.2–1.5	16–20
Whole wheat	60.3	9.1	186	15.0	2.49	.54	19.7

complete protein. Whole wheat bread and peanut butter are examples of **complementary proteins.** Complementary proteins must be eaten at the same meal. Otherwise, the partially complete proteins may be used for energy, and their amino acids lost for tissue repair and other needs.

Foods like milk, eggs, and meat also help to balance the proteins in grain foods. Milk balances the weakness of cereal foods in amino acids. It enables the body to use the protein in grain foods to build and repair body tissues. Hence, milk used in or with bread adds to the protein content of the bread and therefore to the health value of the meal or snack.

Milk is used with breakfast cereal for the same reason. A 240-mL (1-c) serving of oatmeal yields 5 grams of protein when cooked in water. Adding 80 mL (⅓ c) of nonfat dry milk per serving increases the protein value of the oatmeal by 9 grams. If you drink a glass of milk with the oatmeal, you add another 9 grams of protein. The whole adds up to 23 grams of protein. This is a generous amount of protein for breakfast and to start the day. The protein in the cereal will be well used. Add an orange to the meal and you have a well-balanced breakfast containing only 400 calories!

Using bread with egg, meat, chicken, tuna, or peanut butter in a sandwich is a common example of complementing proteins. Other complementary combinations are cheese with macaroni or pizza, meatballs with rice or spaghetti, chicken or fish with noodles, and meat in vegetable soups or stews. To improve the flavor of cereal dishes, people of every nation have used meat, fish, poultry, beans, milk, cheese, eggs, and nuts. As an added benefit, the proteins are also better used.

Incomplete proteins in grain foods can be complemented by the proteins in some legumes and milk, cheese, eggs or meat.

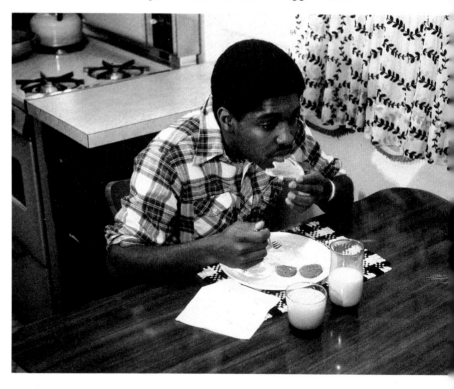

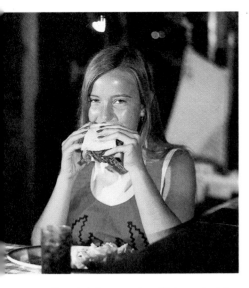

Sandwiches made with bread and meat are a common way of balancing the protein in grain foods.

One reason many people have survived on a diet largely of grain foods is the variety of B vitamins whole grains and cereals contain. Grains are rich in riboflavin, discussed in Chapter 7. They also contain niacin (Chapter 9) and folacin or folic acid (Chapter 5). The primary B vitamins grain foods contribute to the diet are thiamin and vitamin B_6.

Between 1878 and 1883, Dr. B. K. Takaki, a physician in the Japanese navy, proved that white polished rice as the major food in the diet of his men led to the disease known as beriberi. In 1897, Dr. Christian Eijkman, a Dutch physician in Java, noted that his patients who ate white rice got the disease, but that the people whose main food was unpolished brown rice did not get it. By feeding white rice to ducks, chickens, and pigeons, he produced in them the same symptoms as those of his patients. He cured the sick birds by feeding them natural brown rice.

Eijkman misinterpreted his results. Patients who had beriberi had a stiffness in the ankles. They also had neuritis in the feet and legs. In severe cases, this resulted in paralysis, in retention of fluid (edema), in heart disease, and often in death. Eijkman thought these symptoms were due to the larger amount of starch in the white rice. The starch, he believed, "poisoned" the nerve cells. He concluded that the antidote for the poison lay in the materials discarded from the brown rice in the process of producing white rice.

In 1926, two Dutch scientists, C. P. Jansen and W. P. Donath, discovered the vitamin now called thiamin, the first of many B vitamins. They found it in the brown polishings from rice. It is amazing to think that 49 years had elapsed from the time the vital role of thiamin in the diet was discovered to the time it was identified and utilized.

The latter half of his assumption was correct. In 1901 another Dutch physician, G. Grijns, gave the correct interpretation. He said that beriberi was caused by the *absence* of some nutrient found in brown rice that was lost when rice was refined.

Chemists all over the world were excited. They set to work to find this substance. In 1911, the Polish chemist Casimir Funk, working in London, obtained a crystalline product from the brown polishings of the milled white rice. He called this substance the antiberiberi vitamin. He boldly predicted that other diseases might be caused by a shortage of similar substances in the diet. This led others to realize that food could help prevent disease. The realization of the relation between foods and disease stimulated a wave of nutritional research.

Meanwhile, an American, R. R. Williams, was working on the problem. In 1936, Williams and his colleagues worked out the chemical formula for vitamin B_1. The formula made it possible to manufacture thiamin inexpensively, allowing the lost nutrient to be restored to polished white rice.

Functions of thiamin

Thiamin helps us maintain appetite, digestion, waste elimination, and memory. It works with a team of other B vitamins as a coenzyme to help the body burn glucose to release energy. It also is needed for the utilization of protein. It is essential for growth at every age level and has positive benefits for nerve cells and the circulatory system.

Beriberi is no threat in the United States, although deaths from it are sometimes reported. Minor symptoms may be caused by a prolonged mild deficiency of thiamin. The symptoms may be depression, nervousness, poor memory, anger, irritability, low tone of the gastrointestinal tract, fatigue, and general indifference to things that matter.

Chemists have found a test for deficient thiamin by determining the amount of **pyruvic acid** that accumulates in the blood and tissues. When there is enough thiamin in the diet, pyruvic acid does not accumulate. For general good health and well-being, we need thiamin in our diets every day.

Retaining thiamin in food preparation

Like vitamin C and other B vitamins, thiamin is soluble in water, but it is stable in dry form and in the presence of acid in foods. Like vitamin C, it is easily destroyed by alkali. For this reason, we should avoid recipes that call for a large amount of baking soda. Thiamin can be destroyed by high temperatures and prolonged exposure to heat. When bread is toasted or when loaves of bread are baked, the grains lose 15 to 20 percent of their thiamin. The loss is greater in thin, small baked foods. Rolls, for example, lose more thiamin in baking than loaves of bread. Studies show that cooked breakfast cereals retain most of their thiamin.

Daily requirement of thiamin

The daily allowance of thiamin for different age groups is shown in the RDA table on pages 402-403. Table 11-2 gives the amounts of thiamin found in different basic foods.

The amount of thiamin needed daily depends on the number of calories we consume. Naturally, calorie consumption is affected by age, growth rate, and activity. The thiamin requirement increases from infancy to the growth spurt in the teens. During the teen years the body's demand is greatest. When full growth is reached, slightly less is needed because the calorie need has decreased. In a hot, humid climate, more thiamin is required. When a person works or exercises strenuously, more thiamin is needed.

Only a few weeks' supply of thiamin is stored in the liver, heart, muscles, brain, and kidneys. When the body's reserve supply is sufficient, surplus is quickly eliminated in the urine. It cannot be stored for future use. Thus, even though you should plan to include thiamin in every meal, supplementary thiamin probably is not necessary.

When the intake of thiamin is too small, the body calls on its reserves. The muscles give up their reserve of thiamin first. The brain holds its supply to the last. Thiamin is so important to the brain that the body provides built-in safeguards for the brain's thiamin reserves. We can help the body by developing eating habits that provide the nutrients we need in the required amounts.

Many of the nutrients in raw brown rice, including thiamin, are lost in the process of producing white rice.

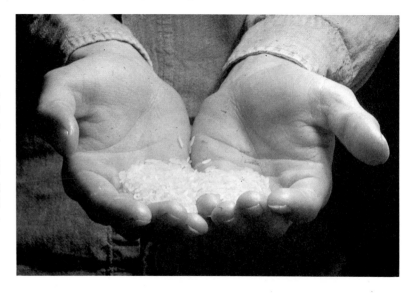

Table 11-2 **Best food sources of thiamin**

FOOD SOURCE	MEASURE	THIAMIN mg
MEATS		
Pork, lean, roasted	98 g (3½ oz)	0.60
Pork liver, fried	98 g (3½ oz)	0.34
Calf liver, fried	98 g (3½ oz)	0.24
Lamb, lean, roasted	98 g (3½ oz)	0.14
Oysters, raw	98 g (3½ oz)	0.14
VEGETABLES		
Green peas, fresh, cooked	120 mL (½ c)	0.28
Green peas, frozen, cooked	120 mL (½ c)	0.27
Soybeans, dried, cooked	120 mL (½ c)	0.21
Asparagus spears, cooked	120 mL (½ c)	0.16
Collards, cooked	120 mL (½ c)	0.14
Navy beans, cooked	120 mL (½ c)	0.14
Lima beans, cooked	120 mL (½ c)	0.13
Okra, cooked	120 mL (½ c)	0.13
Tomato juice	240 mL (1 c)	0.12
FRUITS		
Orange juice, fresh	240 mL (1 c)	0.22
Watermelon	200 cm² (32 sq in)	0.13
GRAIN FOODS		
Rice, brown, cooked	240 mL (1 c)	0.23
Rice, enriched, white, cooked	240 mL (1 c)	0.23
Oatmeal, cooked	240 mL (1 c)	0.19
Wheat cereal, enriched, dry	240 mL (1 c)	0.19
NUTS	16–24	0.18

Composition of Foods, Agriculture Handbook No. 8 (Washington, D.C.: USDA, 1963) and *Nutritive Value of Foods,* Bulletin No. 72 (Washington, D.C.: USDA, rev. 1977).

VITAMIN B$_6$

Vitamin B$_6$ (pyridoxine) was discovered in 1926. But until 1951 we did not know that it was vital. In that year, doctors noticed that some babies in different parts of the country were developing similar strange symptoms. The babies were irritable, and some went into convulsions. Their muscles twitched. There seemed to be no explanation for the condition.

A research worker in the FDA observed that the symptoms in the human babies were just like those in baby rats fed a diet deficient in vitamin B_6. The doctors added this vitamin to the babies' diets and the symptoms were relieved immediately. It was then determined that all the babies had been eating the same canned baby food. Since this discovery in 1951, vitamin B_6 has been added to all canned baby food.

in the milling of white or refined cereals. Highly refined cereals have almost no B_6, unless it is put back. Many food companies fail to replenish B_6 when enriching breads and cereals. The companies that do add B_6 to the product state it on the label. Look for this. Up to 50 percent of vitamin B_6 may be destroyed in cooking.

Daily requirement of vitamin B_6

The recommended daily allowance of B_6 is given in the RDA table on pages 402-403. Table 11-3 shows the best known sources of this vitamin. A balanced diet provides all the vitamin B_6 we need.

Functions of vitamin B_6

When there is not enough vitamin B_6 in the diet, the symptoms are similar to those in other B-vitamin deficiencies. The symptoms include rash and oiliness of the skin, sore mouth, dizziness, nausea, mental confusion, nervous disorders, failure to grow, loss of weight, anemia, convulsions, and kidney stones. All, with the exception of kidney stones, are immediately relieved when enough B_6 is added to the diet.

Vitamin B_6 is a coenzyme in the use of food by cells. Without B vitamins, normal metabolism is upset and nutrients are wasted. Symptoms of illness follow that are often not recognized for what they are. An example of how B_6 works as a coenzyme is in joining with the amino acid tryptophane to make the B vitamin niacin. It is also thought to be important in the body's use of linoleic fatty acid (Chapter 14).

Retaining vitamin B_6 in food preparation

Vitamin B_6 is easily destroyed by exposure to heat, light, and air. Seventy-five percent of B_6 is lost

Table 11-3 **Best food sources of vitamin B_6**

FOOD SOURCE	B_6 CONTENT mg per 100 g
GRAIN	
Wheat germ	1.31
Wheat bran	0.82
Buckwheat flour	0.58
Soya flour	0.57
Brown rice	0.53
Corn	0.48
Wheat	0.41
Whole-wheat cereal	0.40
Barley	0.39
Popcorn	0.37
Whole-wheat bread	0.20
Rice cereal, dry	0.14
Oatmeal	0.12
MILK	
Canned, evaporated	7.50
Cow's, fluid	0.10
MEAT	
Liver	1.42
Ham (cured and fully cooked)	0.70
Salmon, canned	0.28
Frankfurter, cooked	0.16
Beef, ground, cooked	0.10
VEGETABLES AND FRUITS	
Lima beans	0.60
Bananas	0.32
Carrots	0.21
Frozen peas	0.11

Most of these values are taken from M. M. Polansky, E. W. Murphy, and E. W. Toefer, "Compounds of Vitamin B_6 in Greens and Cereal Products," *Journal of the Association of Official Agricultural Chemists,* 47:750, 1964.

Grains lose nutrients in the milling and refining processes that produce the grain products we use. Some of the lost nutrients can be replaced.

Enriched grain products

To enrich a grain product, standard amounts of thiamin, riboflavin, niacin, and iron are added to processed (refined) food, which in part replaces nutrients lost in milling (Table 11-4). Over a dozen other lost nutrients are not returned (Table 11-5). For example, the protein in .45 kg (1 lb) of whole-wheat flour is 60.3 g. Enriched and unenriched white flour have only 47.6 g, an unreplaced loss of 12.7 g of protein in milling.

The enrichment of bread and cereal foods with thiamin, riboflavin, niacin, and iron became mandatory in the United States in January 1943, in order to improve meager wartime diets. The

Table 11-4 **Federal enrichment standards for grain products**

FOOD 0.45 kg (1 lb)	THIAMIN mg	RIBOFLAVIN mg	NIACIN mg	IRON mg
Bread and rolls	1.1–1.8	0.7–1.6	10.0–15.0	8.0–12.5
Flour	2.0–2.5	1.2–1.5	16.0–20.0	13.0–16.5
Cornmeal, grits	2.0–3.0	1.2–1.8	16.0–24.0	13.0–26.0
Macaroni and noodles	4.0–5.0	1.7–2.2	27.0–34.0	13.0–16.5

U.S. National Archives, Code of Federal Register Title 21, Food and Drugs, 1955, with supplement to 1957.

Table 11-5 **Loss of nutrients in the refining of wheat**

NUTRIENT	CONTENT IN WHOLE WHEAT	LOSS IN WHITE FLOUR percent
Thiamin	3.5 ug/gm[1]	77.1
Riboflavin	1.5 ug/gm	80.0
Niacin	50.0 ug/gm	80.8
Vitamin B_6	1.7 ug/gm	71.8
Pantothenic acid	10.0 ug/gm	50.0
Folacin	0.3 ug/gm	66.7
A-tocopherol	16.0 ug/gm	86.3
Betaine	844.0 ug/gm	22.8
Choline	1089.0 ug/gm	29.5
Calcium	0.045%	60.0
Phosphorus	0.433%	70.9
Magnesium	0.183%	84.7
Potassium	0.454%	77.0
Manganese	46.0 ppm[2]	85.8
Iron	43.0 ppm	75.6
Zinc	35.0 ppm	77.7

Adapted from H. A. Schroeder, *American Journal of Clinical Nutrition*, 24:562, 1971.
[1]ug = 1/1000 mcg
[2]ppm = parts per million

ruling was a significant step toward better health through improving the nutrients in a basic food. It is also a fine example of how the government, nutritionists, public health officials, and food industries can cooperate for the benefit of the consumer. The ruling expired in 1946. Enrichment of foods is now voluntary in certain states.

Restored, converted, and fortified grain products

The words restored, converted, and fortified are sometimes confused with the term enrichment. The word restored means that some of the nutrients lost in processing are returned to the refined or processed grain food. The word converted refers only to rice. The rice is steeped in hot water under pressure in a cylinder containing no air. This process forces a large amount of the nutrients into the starchy part of the grain. When

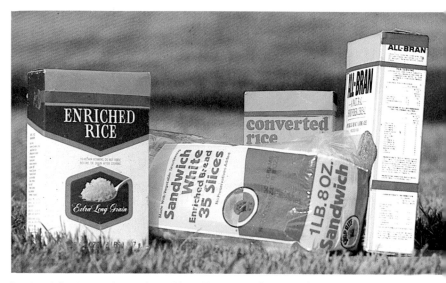

Lost nutrients can be replaced in milled grain foods if they are restored. Enriched foods have had standard amounts of B vitamins and iron added, while fortified foods have had nutrients added that may not have been in the unprocessed food.

the grain is polished, these nutrients are not lost. Conversion of rice has been practiced in India in a simplified form for many decades. Thus beriberi is not a common disease in India, as it has been in other parts of Asia.

The word fortified means that nutrients that may or may not have been in the unrefined food have been added. For example, vitamins A and D are added to nonfat milk. Iron and other minerals, vitamins, or amino acids may be added to fortify a food. Fortifying foods with needed nutrients improves the diet, but does not replace the need for a balanced diet.

RECAP

Value of grains

Importance of grains to different cultures   *Corn   Rice   Wheat*   **Nutritional value of grains**   *Carbohydrates   Protein   B vitamins   Iron, phosphorus, and other minerals   Fat*   **Practical value of grains**

Carbohydrates

How the body uses carbohydrates   **Complex carbohydrates**

Complementary proteins

Thiamin

Functions of thiamin   **Retaining thiamin in food preparation**   **Daily requirement of thiamin**

Vitamin B$_6$

Functions of vitamin B$_6$ Retaining vitamin B$_6$ in food preparation   Daily requirement of vitamin B$_6$

Replacing nutrients in milled grains

Enriched grain products   Restored, converted, and fortified grain products

THINKING AND EVALUATING

1. Did you have any mistaken ideas about starch before reading this chapter? What were they?

2. List the nutritional contributions made by cereal grains.

3. What are the practical advantages of using grain foods in meals?

4. What is the chief function of carbohydrates in the body?

5. Describe how carbohydrates are broken down in the body.

6. Explain how the body maintains its energy level when the diet is low in carbohydrate-rich foods.

7. Why can't we depend on grain foods alone for the protein we need?

8. What is thiamin? How does it benefit us? What precautions would you use in cooking food to retain the most thiamin? Apply the same questions to vitamin B$_6$.

9. If you were trying to reduce, which carbohydrate-rich foods would you include in your daily diet? Explain the reasons for your choices.

APPLYING AND SHARING

1. Record the foods you ate yesterday. What percentage of the total calories was derived from carbohydrates? How many calories were from starch? From sugar? Did you make the wisest choices among these foods? How might you improve your choices?

2. Using this same record, calculate the grams of thiamin provided by the grain foods you ate. Calculate the amount contributed to your diet by animal foods. Does the total conform to the RDA for you? If not, how can you improve your thiamin intake without consuming too many calories?

3. Plan menus for three days using grain foods to help meet the daily recommended allowances in calories, protein, thiamin, riboflavin, niacin, and iron.

4. Plan a balanced menu for each of the following meals using the indicated grain foods:

    Breakfast: Oatmeal cooked with nonfat dry milk
    Lunch: Noodles
    Dinner: Brown rice

Food company sales representative Sells company's products to food stores or vending machine distributors, assists food store personnel with advertising and other promotional efforts. Four-year college education usually required; knowledge of accounting helpful; communications skills essential.

Laboratory technician Assists scientists in plant, animal, or environmental research; carries out experiments. High school education required; vocational training helpful.

RELATED READING

Aykroyd, W. R., and Joyce Doughty. *Wheat in Human Nutrition.* FAO Nutritional Studies, No. 23, 1970. Studies the contribution of grain to the human diet and discusses measures to increase their production and consumption.

Deutsch, Ronald M. *The Family Guide to Better Food and Better Health.* Des Moines, Iowa: Meredith, 1971. Explains nutrition for the lay person based on concepts of body chemistry and food.

Kehr, August E., et al. "50% More Crop Output Seen by 2000." *A Good Life for More People: Yearbook of Agriculture, 1971.* Washington, D.C.: USDA, 1971. Describes development of higher-protein cereal grains and methods of using them with other foods to improve diets.

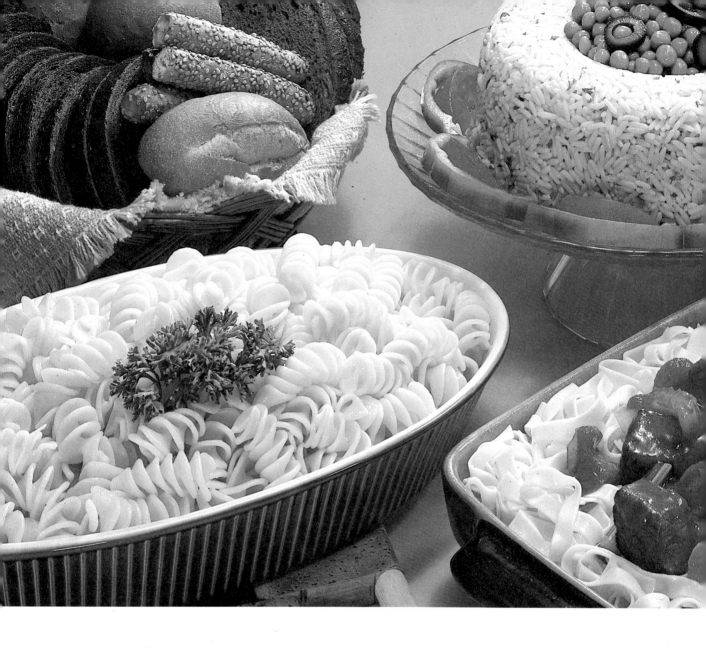

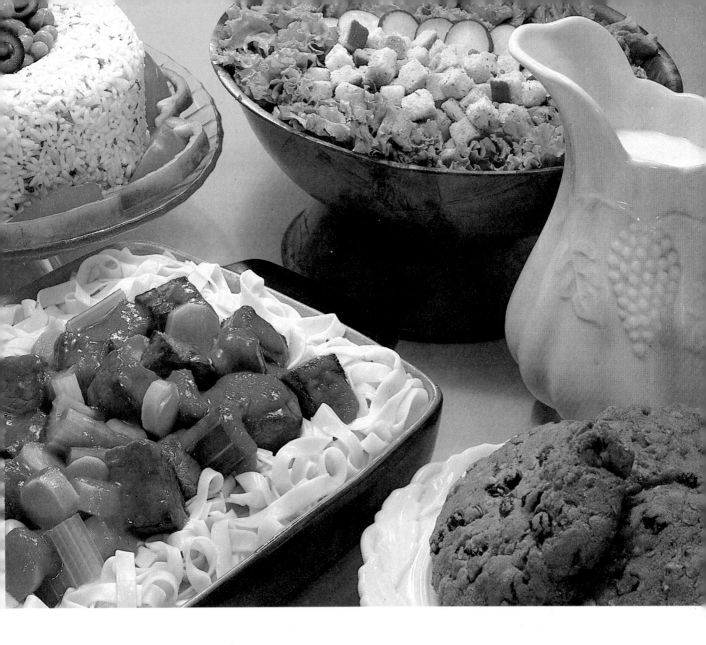

CHAPTER 12

Grain foods in meals

After studying this chapter, you will be able to

- identify the most popular groups of grain products.
- describe ingredients and their functions in baked grain foods.
- explain what information to look for on a breakfast cereal package.
- buy and prepare cereals, breads, and pastas to balance the diet and save money.

POPULAR GRAIN PRODUCTS

How much nutritional value can you expect to get from bread and cereals? That depends on how wisely you select them. There are many varieties to choose from on the market. Some grain products are quite expensive per serving. Others are among the lowest-costing foods. Some help balance the day's meals. Others high in fat, sugar, and calories may throw meals out of balance. The nutritional value of grain foods also depends on how well you prepare them and fit them into your meals and your diet as a whole.

Breakfast cereals

Breakfast cereals come in many different forms. They may be raw (to be cooked), quick-cooking (partially cooked), or ready-to-eat. We are probably most familiar with breakfast cereals as a morning meal, but they serve many other purposes. Breakfast cereals can be used as casserole toppings, meat coatings, or ingredients in cakes, cookies, breads, and candied snacks.

Macaroni products

Macaroni, or noodles, originated in China. Marco Polo discovered them there and brought them back to Italy. From Italy, the use of macaroni spread throughout the world. It became a gourmet dish. An Englishman traveling in Italy in the sixteenth century ate macaroni for the first time. He liked it so much that he later organized a gourmet club. He called

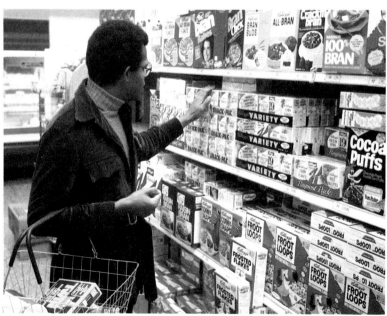

Breakfast cereals are among the most common grain products.

it the Macaroni Club. The fame of macaroni spread to America. It even became part of an American song, "Yankee Doodle."

Flour

We are probably most familiar with flour as the main ingredient in most baked goods. Another important use of flour is as a thickener in sauces, gravies, puddings, and pie fillings. Flour provides starch and **gluten,** a protein. When liquid is added, the starch swells, giving structure and volume to the finished baked product.

Flour is made from grains of wheat (Figure 12-1), buckwheat, rye, corn, rice, barley, and oats. It is also made from the potato, cottonseed, soybean, peanut, and lima bean. Let's examine more closely the most popular types of flours and how they are used.

Whole-wheat flour. Bread made from whole-wheat (or graham) flour has a nutty flavor. Its texture is coarser and its color is darker than that of bread made from white flour. Whole-wheat is the most nutritious flour because it contains all the nutrients of wheat. It has less starch and more **bran**—the outer covering of the grain of wheat—than other kinds. Therefore, it contains 5 to 8 fewer calories per slice.

White flour. White flour (also called plain or wheat flour) contains less protein than whole-wheat flour because the aleurone layer, the bran, and the germ of the grain are all lost in the milling process. The **aleurone** layer, located just beneath the bran, contains the highest-quality protein in

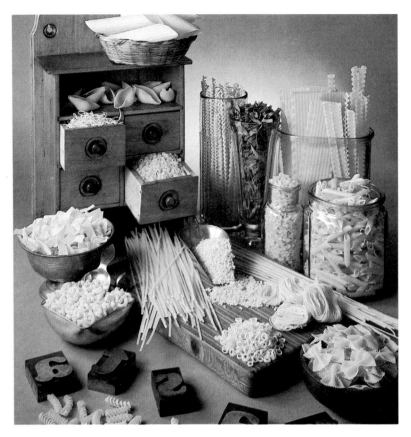

Pasta comes in many different shapes, sizes, and forms, from large, flat lasagne noodles to thin spaghetti, from elbow macaroni to shell macaroni.

wheat. It is almost as good as animal protein. The milling process leaves only the **endosperm,** or starch, of the grain. Endosperm, too, contains protein—but protein of a weaker type. White flour is usually enriched to restore some of the vitamins and minerals lost in milling. Most white flour is also bleached with peroxide, chlorine, and other chemicals. This produces the whiter product consumers commonly prefer.

Cake flour. Cake flour is made from soft wheat—wheat that has a soft kernel—and is lowest in gluten. It is used for the finest-textured cakes. Though less nourishing than other flours, it costs more.

Figure 12-1 Whole-wheat flour uses the entire grain of wheat, while white flour lacks the aleurone, the bran, and the germ of the grain.

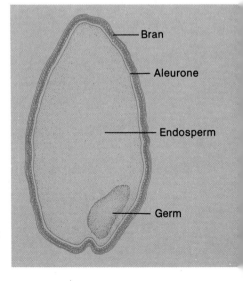

Bran

Aleurone

Endosperm

Germ

All-purpose flour. All-purpose flour is a blend of hard- and soft-wheat white flours. It is used for any purpose. It absorbs less liquid than bread flour but more than pastry flour. For cake-making, less all-purpose flour is required—30 mL (2 T) less per 240 mL (1 c)— than low-gluten cake flour.

Self-rising flour. Self-rising flour is soft-wheat or all-purpose flour with added salt and baking powder, and sometimes soda. We buy it in all types of mixes. We also buy it as self-rising flour.

BAKING WITH FLOUR

Cooked flour-based foods are of two basic kinds. Leavened baked goods contain an ingredient that makes them rise, or expand. Unleavened flour products contain no rising agent.

In ancient times, leavenings were not known. People would gather grains, crush them, and mix them with water and vegetables. They would boil or bake the mixture on heated stones. Today, people still eat some kinds of unleavened products. Matzos and tortillas are two popular types of modern unleavened bread.

Leavening agents

About three-fourths of the grain products we eat are leavened breads. The most common leavened breads are loaves and rolls. Also familiar to most of us are quick breads, muffins, biscuits,

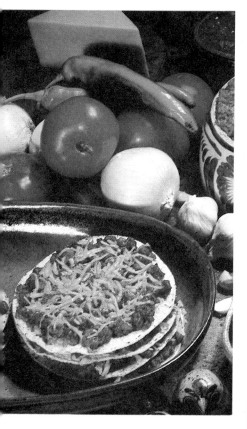

Above: Tortillas are a form of unleavened bread. *Right:* Leavening agents not only cause doughs to rise, they also produce differences in flavor, lightness, texture, and nutrients in baked products.

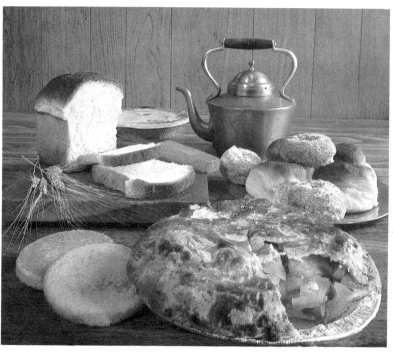

206

pancakes, waffles, doughnuts, coffee cakes, sweet rolls, and so on, all of which are varieties of leavened breads.

Different leavening agents produce great differences in flavor, lightness, texture, and nutrients. The most common types of leavening are yeast and baking powder, but bakers also use baking soda, egg white, or steam for leavening. Each of these leavening agents produces carbon dioxide gas. The gas may be held in the meshlike structure developed by the gluten or in the beaten egg whites or both.

Yeast. Unlike soda and baking powder, yeast is a microscopic plant and a good food in its own right. Yeast contains protein and it is rich in B vitamins and iron. Fifteen mL (1 T) of dry yeast yields 1.4 mg of iron. This is almost one-third more than one whole egg.

How does yeast leaven bread? The process begins when yeast is mixed with a warm liquid and sugar. An enzyme called zymase causes the mixture to ferment. The yeast plants then multiply in the bread dough. Carbon dioxide forms and the dough is thereby leavened.

Yeast grows and leavens best when warm. Therefore bread dough should be put in a warm place. It takes less time to make yeast bread if the amount of yeast in the recipe is doubled.

Sourdough yeast bread is made by a simple method that has been used for thousands of years. The method is still used in developing nations where many people lack refrigerators. To make sourdough, a portion of dough set aside from the last baking is added to a new batch of dough. The yeast plants in the saved dough, or starter, grow and leaven the new batch of bread. This process gives a special flavor to the bread.

Another bread with a special flavor is salt-rising bread. This was probably the first form of leavened bread. To prevent the formation of unwanted bacteria that give bread a bad flavor, large amounts of salt were added to the yeast. Today, bakers use bacteria cultures (*bacteria Clostridium*) rather than salt to produce fermentation.

Yeast must be stored carefully. Store dry yeast in a cool pantry. Store compressed or cake yeast in the refrigerator. Cake yeast works best at temperatures between 27 °C and 30 °C (80 °F and 86 °F). Dry yeast works best between 43 °C and 46 °C (110 °F and 115 °F).

Baking powder. Baking powder is the leavening agent used for most quick breads and cakes. All baking powders contain cornstarch and soda. Some baking powders also contain tartrate. In tartrate the leavening agent is tartaric acid, which reacts quickly when it comes in contact with liquid. Tartrate baking powders are not popular in the United States.

Baking powders containing phosphate (monocalcium phosphate or monosodium phosphate) produce about two-thirds of the total gas formed when they are mixed with the liquid. The other one-third is formed in the presence of heat in the oven. Too much phosphate gives food a bitter taste.

Yeast doughs are folded (*left*), kneaded (*right*), and allowed to rise (*covered bowl in both pictures*) one or more times before baking.

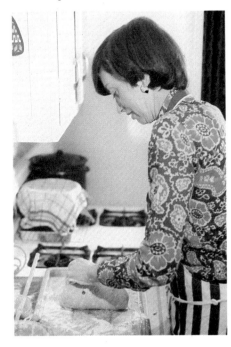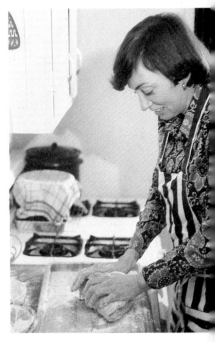

Baking powder containing SAS (sodium aluminum sulfate) are preferred by most bakers. As the SAS combines with liquid, some carbon dioxide is formed. But SAS is slower to act than other types of baking powder. It leavens in the presence of heat.

Baking soda. Before baking powder, soda was used for making quick breads that contained sour milk or molasses. The amount of carbon dioxide produced depends on the amount of acid in the liquid and the amount of soda used. Too much soda produces a bitter taste and turns white products a yellowish color. Baking soda darkens a chocolate cake. It destroys B vitamins and vitamin C.

Egg white. As egg whites are beaten, air becomes trapped in the fluffy foam. It is important to keep the air trapped when making angel food cake, spongecake, soufflé, and spoon bread. To do this, simply fold the flour or cereal mixture into the stiff foam gently with an under-and-over movement; do not stir or beat.

Steam. Steam leavens all baked flour products. Heat in baking changes water to vapor. This vapor expands about 1600 times in volume. Popovers, cream puffs, and poundcakes all depend on steam for leavening.

Other ingredients

Baked products made with flour use a variety of ingredients for flavor and texture.

Liquid. Liquid is essential for the starch to swell and the gluten to develop. The liquid may be plain water or the water from cooked macaroni, potatoes, and some vegetables or fruits. However, milk is better than water for producing a moist, tender, and nourishing bread.

Salt. Salt is used in making bread for two reasons. It enhances the flavor and it delays the growth of yeast plants in yeast bread.

Fat. Fat is added to flour mixtures to give tenderness in texture, to improve the flavor, and to encourage browning. It does this by shortening the strands of gluten in the flour. The fat coats the gluten strands and prevents them from holding together. Hence the term shortening is appropriate.

Eggs. Eggs improve the flavor, color, texture, lightness, and

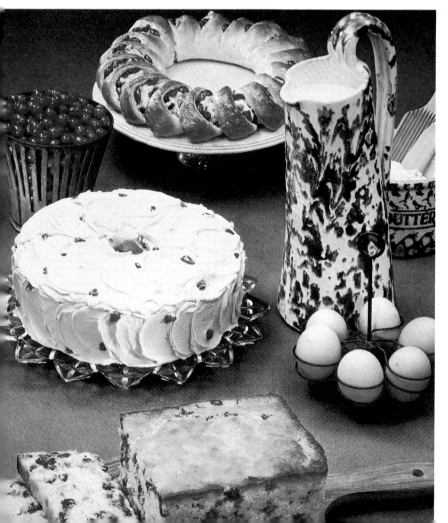

Sugar aids yeast in the leavening process and improves browning, as well as flavoring baked products.

browning or glaze of baked foods. They may be added to any bread or cereal dish to supplement the weaker protein in these foods.

Sugar. Sugar provides food for the yeast plants. It retards the development of gluten in flour. Sugar also improves browning and flavor.

The addition of a lot of sugar to doughs and batters has important effects. For one thing, sugary doughs do not rise as high as bread doughs. Secondly, sugar prevents the protein in eggs and flour from coagulating unless the baking temperature is increased. Cakes are baked in a moderate oven and quick breads in a hot one because the sugar and fat in cakes delay the development of gluten.

Other adjustments are needed when either molasses or honey is used in dough instead of white sugar. Less liquid and a lower oven temperature are required. Otherwise the food will burn.

A leavening agent, liquid, salt, fat, eggs, and sugar are the basic ingredients for breads and other products made from flour. For variety in flavor, flavoring extracts, spices, herbs, onions, garlic, or cheese may be added. Adding nuts and dried or fresh fruits increases the nutritive value but also adds to the cost and the calories.

COOKING CEREALS AND MACARONI PRODUCTS

Both cereals and macaroni products are ready to be boiled in water or other liquid. Select a pan that will hold about three times the volume of the food to be cooked. It should have a firm, heavy bottom and a lid.

How should you cook pasta and other cereal products? You can retain the maximum nutrients and produce a tasty, healthful, and attractive dish by following three steps.

1. Measure about twice as much water (or milk for cereal) as food to be cooked. Use more if you like a thin cereal or plan to use the macaroni water in a white sauce or a soup. Bring the water to a boil and add salt.

2. Add the cereal or macaroni. Stir slowly so that each piece is kept separate. This prevents sticking or lumping. When cereals boil vigorously for two to three minutes, the starch swells. The cereal will not settle to the bottom of the pot. When this happens, lower the heat, cover the pot, and just maintain boiling. Do not stir macaroni or rice while cooking.

Stirring may break the shape. If macaroni sticks together, lift the pan and use a circular motion to shake the mass apart.

3. Cook macaroni products and cereals until they are just tender. Do not overcook them. Serve while they are hot.

4. Cooking breakfast cereals in nonfat dry milk improves their health value. The milk also improves the flavor with only a slight increase in calories. Nonfat dry milk adds all the nutrients of whole milk to breakfast cereals except fat.

BUYING AND STORING GRAIN PRODUCTS

Buying guidelines

The place of breads and cereal foods in our meals is especially important when money is limited. Keep the following principles in mind.

1. Whole-grain breads and cereals yield more nourishment and more flavor for the money than any other kind. Gourmets who make an art of cooking prefer the flavor of whole grains. The whole grains are available in fine grind as whole-wheat flour and cereals for cooking. They are also available in flakes as raw oatmeal or as whole-wheat ready-to-eat cereal. They come in the form of cracked wheat as bulgur. They may be available precooked, as instant whole-wheat cereal. Unpolished brown rice and rolled oats are other kinds of whole grains.

2. Enriched, fortified, restored, and converted grain foods are next to whole grains in nutritional value. They are the best choice for those who prefer white breads and cereal foods.

3. Breads and baked foods made at home from basic ingredients cost less per serving than commercial ready-to-eat products. They cost less than partially

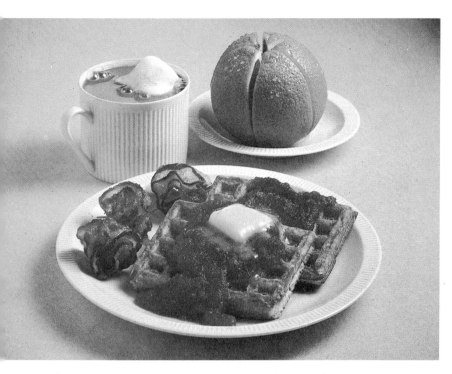

Some form of grain product is often the main dish in breakfast.

cooked, brown-and-serve, thaw-and-heat, separate-and-bake, and mix-and-bake products.

4. The cost per unit serving of ready-to-eat cereal is higher than the cost of any other type.

5. Sweet rolls, sweet breads, and breakfast cakes cost more than plain breads and rolls. They are higher in fat, sugar, and calories. Serve them as special-occasion foods and not as a regular alternative for plain bread.

6. Cereals with vitamins, minerals, and amino acids added may cost more. Remember that you can make up for the lack of certain amino acids in cereals and breads with milk, cheese, egg, or lean meat. You can balance the deficiency of vitamin C with fruits and vegetables. When money is limited, spend it for foods that bring nutrients to balance the whole meal.

7. Buy by net weight, not the size of the loaf or the package. The small loaf or package may be heavier than the large one. The weight of the box may be greater than the weight of the cereal in it.

8. Avoid sugar-coated cereals. You can add the sugar yourself for less money. You can also limit the amount used. It is important not to encourage a "sweet tooth."

9. Read carefully the nutritional and ingredient labels on all bread or cereals. The label tells the kind of cereal or bread. It tells whether the product is enriched, fortified, or whole grain. It describes the type of grind. It tells whether the product is raw, partially cooked, or ready-to-eat. It also tells whether chemicals or coloring are added and whether other ingredients are included, such as sugar, salt, malt flavoring, and vitamins. Labels help you select the cereal and bread that suit your taste, budget, and needs.

10. Plan bread and cereals to bring variety and nourishment to your meals at the lowest cost.

11. If storage space permits, shop for bread and cereals for an entire week. This saves time, fuel, energy, and money.

12. Buy "day-old" bread for lower cost. It can be eaten as toast or further dried and used as bread crumbs.

Storage guidelines

Adequate storage of breads and cereals is a part of good management. Commercial baked foods have chemicals added to retard mold. Ready-to-eat cereals contain chemicals to help retain freshness.

1. Store breads that are to be used immediately in a clean, fresh breadbox. In hot, humid weather, keep them in the refrigerator. This will keep your breads fresh and free of mold. Breads meant for long storage should be frozen.

2. Store ready-to-eat cereals and pasta products in the boxes in which they come. Once opened, tightly close the inner waxed paper container of cereal boxes to keep the product moisture-proof. Cereal loses crispness and becomes tough when it absorbs moisture from the atmosphere. The large bulk requires more storage space. This limits the amount that can be bought at one time. Storing cereals in a cabinet over the stove helps keep them crisp. If they become tough, heat them in a low oven to make them crisp before serving.

3. Store uncooked and partially cooked dry cereals and pasta in their original containers. Keep the lids on, or close the spouts securely when the product is to be stored. Once opened, cereal and pasta products may be stored in their boxes or transferred to glass jars with lids.

USING GRAIN PRODUCTS IN MEALS

You should have four servings of cereal or grain products in your daily diet. Any of the following is counted as a serving: 1 slice of bread; 1 roll, biscuit, or muffin; 3 average-size pancakes; 28 g (1 oz) of ready-to-eat cereal; 180 mL (¾ c) of cooked cereal, grits, or macaroni products.

Breakfast

At breakfast, we often eat toast or some other type of bread. Plain breads low in fat and sugar are the wisest choices for control of weight or of the fat content in the diet. Muffins, waffles, grits, griddle cakes, and biscuits are also good foods. You can make them at home with vegetable oil high in linoleic acid and fortified with nonfat dry milk. Cereal with milk is a better-balanced combination than bread eaten with butter and jam and no milk. When you choose bread instead of cereal, balance its nutrients with a glass of milk.

Use sweet rolls as a special treat, not as a habit. Remember that for the same amount of calories in one doughnut, you can eat 2½ slices of bread. Or you can have 180 mL (¾ c) of cooked oatmeal and a glass of skim milk.

Lunch

Consider the different ways you can make bread, rice, or macaroni an important part of your midday meal.

1. Sandwiches are popular lunch foods. You can use different kinds of bread to blend with meat, poultry, cheese, eggs, or fish.

2. Hot breads may accompany a salad. These may be in the form of hot rolls or corn, bran, wheat, or blueberry muffins. Popovers give an elegant, tasty touch when the main dish is a chef's salad or a fruit salad with cottage cheese.

Sandwiches are the focus of many lunches.

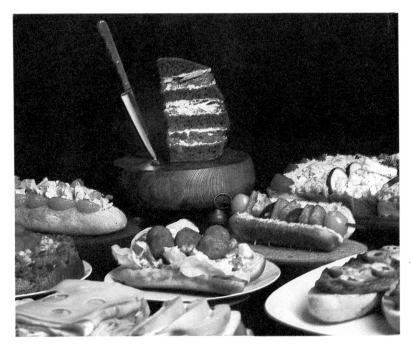

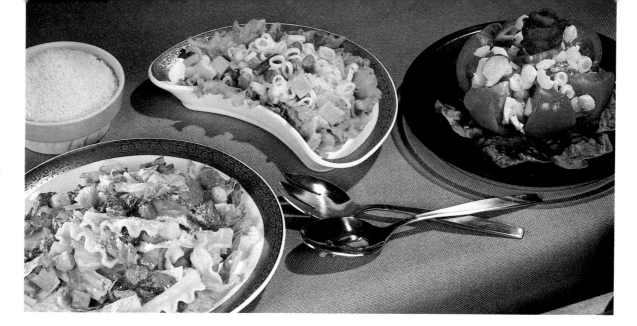

Macaroni in a salad is a way of using a grain product in lunch that is just as effective as bread in a sandwich.

3. As a main dish, bread may be in the form of pizza.

4. English muffins, hot biscuits, or corn bread may serve as a base for creamed chicken, turkey, or fish, or Welsh rabbit.

5. Crisp crackers or toast may serve as accompaniments to a soup or salad.

6. A main casserole dish or soup may include macaroni products, bread, or rice. All of these are excellent with tomato sauce, cheese, meat, fish, poultry, or vegetables.

Dinner

At dinner, grain products can be part of the main meal, as in a macaroni casserole, or they can accompany the meal in many different forms.

Spaghetti with a sauce that nutritionally balances the pasta is a sound dinner main dish.

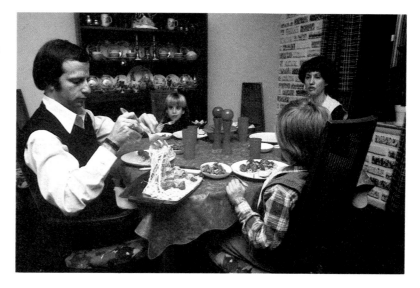

The proteins in the sausage balance the proteins in the rice in this casserole.

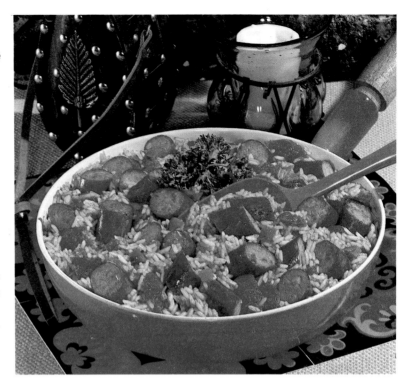

1. Hot biscuits, muffins, corn bread or sticks, or homemade yeast breads may be served with the main dish. With jam or syrup, they may serve as dessert.

2. Dumplings or hush puppies are delicious with poultry.

3. Stuffings are used in poultry, pork chops, fish, and breasts of veal or lamb. They are made of rice, bulgur, buckwheat groats (kasha), corn grits, corn bread, or stale wheat bread. Stuffings provide a good means of using left-over bread.

4. Grains are used in such desserts as rice or bread pudding and Indian pudding (made from cornmeal). They are used in fruit cobblers, pies, cakes, cookies, pastries, and sweet breads of all types.

Snacks and appetizers

Snack foods may be made of corn, wheat, soy, rye, or a mixture of grains with many types of seasonings. They are served plain, with beverages of various sorts, or as a base for canapés and dips. Many are quite high in fat and calories. For instance, only five small pretzel sticks yield 20 calories.

Popcorn, a whole grain, is one of the best snack foods. When you make it at home, you can control the amount and kind of fat added. A serving of 240 mL (1 c) of popcorn with no fat added has 25 calories.

Canapés use many different kinds of grain products as a base, especially breads and crackers.

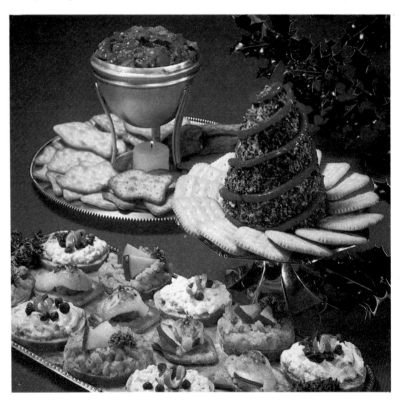

Popular grain products

Breakfast cereals   Macaroni products   Flour
*Whole-wheat flour   White flour   Cake flour   All-purpose flour
Self-rising flour*

Baking with flour

Leavening agents *Yeast   Baking powder   Baking soda
Egg white   Steam*   **Other ingredients** *Liquid   Salt   Fat ·
Eggs   Sugar*

Cooking cereals and macaroni products

Buying and storing grain products

Buying guidelines   Storage guidelines

Using grain products in meals

Breakfast   Lunch   Dinner   Snacks and appetizers

THINKING AND EVALUATING

VOCABULARY

aleurone
bran
endosperm
gluten
phosphate
salt-rising bread
SAS
self-rising flour
shortening
sourdough
tartrate

1. How is flour used in cooking?

2. Aside from wheat, what other grains are used to make flour?

3. How many different types of flour are you likely to find in the supermarket?

4. Which is the most nutritious flour? Why?

5. Which part of the wheat contains the protein? Which part contains the starch?

6. List the ingredients used as leaveners.

7. Why is salt added to baked products? Sugar?

8. Explain why it is so important to learn the right technique for cooking cereals and macaroni products. What is this technique?

APPLYING AND SHARING

1. With the information you have acquired about the grain foods group, make a trip to the market and, with notebook in hand, examine labels and compare cost per pound and cost per serving of

    a. the variety of whole-grain, enriched, and unenriched bread and cereal products in your market. Include flours, breads, plain yeast rolls, and those with added ingredients in different forms.

    b. quick breads

    c. raw cereals, quick-cooking cereals, cereals precooked and ready-to-mix with hot liquid, ready-to-eat cereals

2. From the preceding comparisons, what did you learn about

a. the price of flour per pound, as compared with the price of bread, rolls, and sweet breads made with yeast? Quick breads?

b. the cost of uncooked cereals? Quick-cooking cereals? Ready-to-eat cereals?

3. With the information from items 1 and 2, figure out the cost per serving of each type, allowing 28 g (1 oz) of flour or cereal, 1 slice of bread, or 1 roll per serving. Which is the most nourishing per serving? Do you see any relationship between the cost of bread and cereals and the health values they contribute to the diet? Explain.

4. Experiments in cooking and tasting:

a. Prepare yeast bread at school. With the class, mix and set the bread to rise the first day. Cooperate with other classes so that you may experience handling the dough, baking the bread, and test-tasting it. Discuss what mistakes, if any, were made and how they could be corrected.

b. Repeat this experience at home and make rolls with some of the dough. Which takes less time, bread or rolls? Which did your family enjoy more? How did your work at home compare with that at school? What was the cost per serving? If you can analyze your mistakes, try the bread again until you have a perfect result.

CAREER CAPSULES

Market researcher   Works for food company in product development; conducts studies and surveys to determine consumer needs and preferences, cost and pricing statistics. Required education varies; knowledge of statistical research essential.

Commercial baker   Works in a large or small bakery; supervises mixing, rising, and/or baking of the finished product. On-the-job training essential; vocational education helpful.

RELATED READING

Lappé, Frances M. *Diet for a Small Planet,* rev. ed. New York: Ballantine Books, 1975. Concentrates on combining different cereal grains, legumes, nuts, and milk to supply total protein needs.

Princess Pamela's Soul Food Cookbook. New York: The New American Library, 1969. Emphasizes nutritious ways of using corn, wheat, and rice that are characteristic of the South.

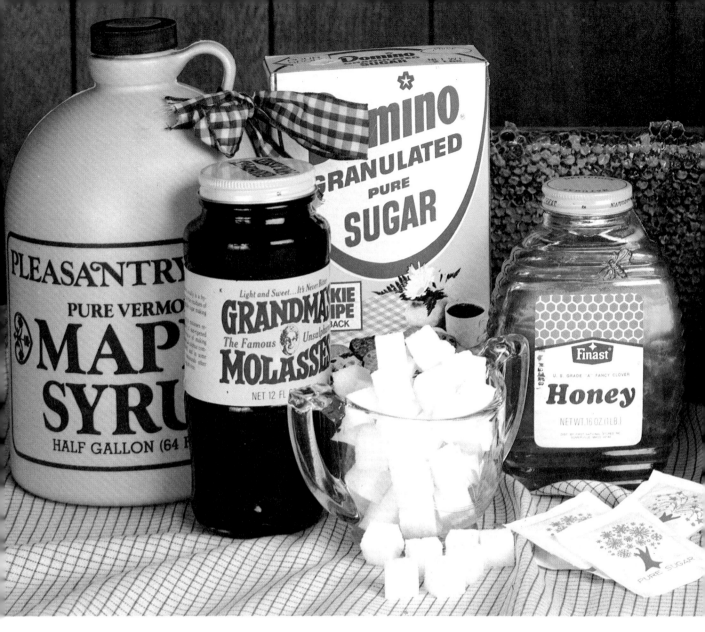

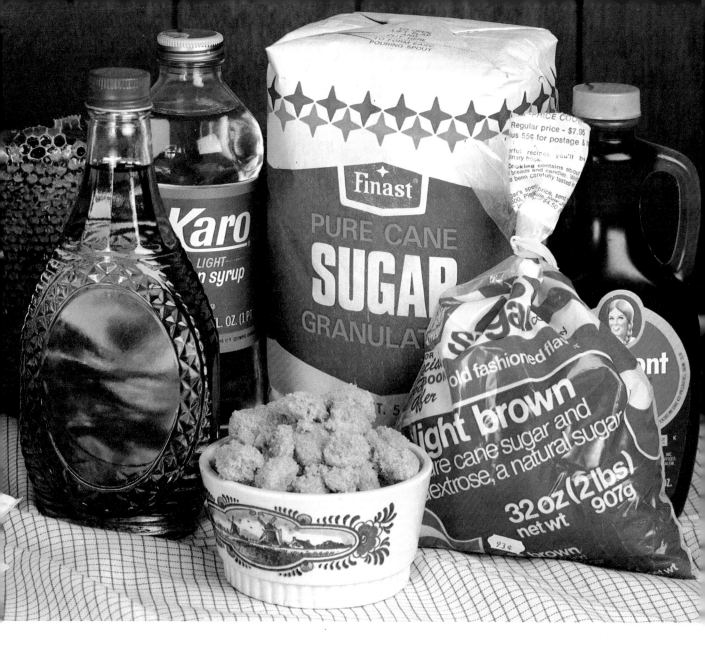

Sugar in your diet

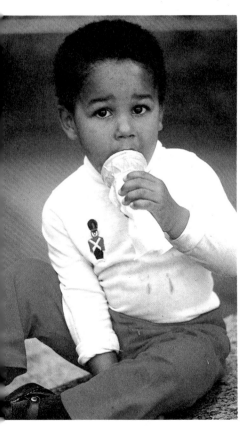

The main appeal of sugar is its taste.

Does the average American eat too much sugar? This question has been worrying a lot of people for a number of years. In 1968 an all-time high rate of sugar consumption was recorded in the United States. It amounted to 56 kg (125 lb) per person per year. There is evidence that some progress has been made toward reducing this figure. In 1975, according to the USDA, Americans ate 51 kg (114 lb) per person per year. Even so, the 1978 rate of consumption divides up into 504 calories a day. This is one-fourth the total calorie need for a person who requires 2000 calories daily.

Sugar, syrups, honey, and other sweeteners provided 16.2 percent of the total calories consumed by Americans in 1975. An additional 10 to 15 percent of our total calories came from sugar as it occurs naturally in fruits, vegetables, and milk. The amount of sugar we eat in an "invisible" form is staggering.

Value of sugar

Appeal. Sugar has been a popular food for thousands of years. Primitive people gained fiber and some nutrients from chewing sugar cane, even though they chewed it mainly for its sweet taste. Today, people sometimes eat sugar for the energy lift that it gives. But they, too, like it mainly because it makes foods and beverages tasty.

We associate sweet foods with festive occasions of all kinds—birthdays, weddings, holidays, and other happy occasions. So do people in other lands. The Turks, for example, enjoy sweets so much that they named their most sacred holiday *Seker Byram*, meaning Sugar Holiday. This holiday takes place at the end of Ramadan, the month of religious fasting. Children are given candy. Families and friends visiting one another are served cakes, candies, and other sweets, along with Turkish coffee or tea.

Energy source. Sugar is not only enjoyable to eat, it is also useful to the body as a source of energy. The body prefers sugar, in the form of glucose, to bring the energy from food to cell tissues.

In digestion, sugars and starch are changed into glucose, a simple sugar. Glucose is maintained at a nearly constant level in the blood. However, there is only a 10- to 15-minute supply in the bloodstream at any one time. There is about a 24-hour reserve stored in the body tissues as **glycogen.** When the blood sugar is lowered, the glycogen is changed back to glucose. The glucose is then burned to produce energy. But when we eat more sugar than the body requires for immediate use as energy and for glycogen reserves, the excess is stored in the body as surplus fat.

Classifications of sugar

Different kinds of sugars are found in different kinds of plants. They are classified chemically according to the three major subgroups of carbohydrates. Monosaccharides have one simple sugar per molecule. Disaccharides have two simple sugars per molecule. Polysaccharides are complex carbohydrate molecules. (See page 192.) Disaccharides and polysaccharides are converted by digestion to monosaccharides.

Monosaccharides. Glucose, fructose, and galactose are monosaccharides, or simple sugars. These sugars consist of one molecule each. After digestion, they are absorbed into the bloodstream; fructose and galactose are changed into glucose in the liver. All body cells use glucose for energy in performing all their functions. Fruits supply fructose. Galactose comes from the digestion of lactose, or milk sugar. About 50 percent of the solid matter in honey is fructose and glucose. The popularity of honey lies in its flavor; it is not a "magic" health food. Its 65 calories per 15 mL (1 T) compares with 40 calories in

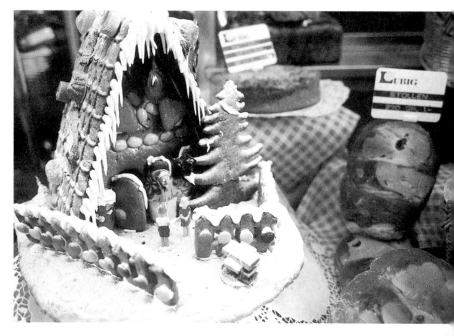

Much time and creative energy of cooks of all nations go into creating special sweets for special occasions.

Fruits are the best sources of monosaccharides, or simple sugars.

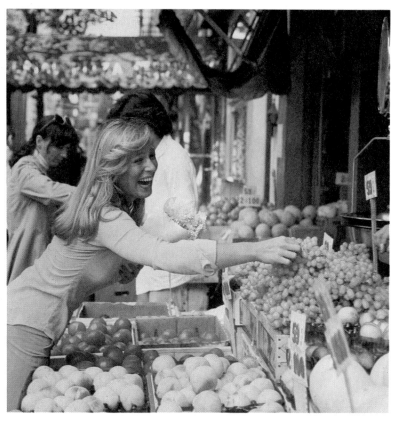

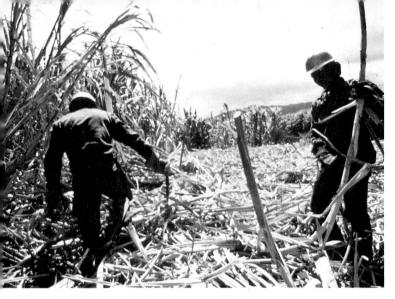

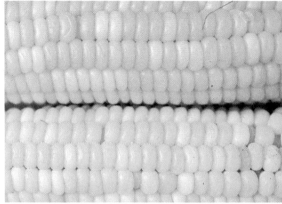

Left: Disaccharides occur in cane sugar, which is 99 percent sucrose. *Right:* The seeds of cereal grains are good sources of polysaccharides, or complex carbohydrates.

the same amount of granulated sugar.

Disaccharides. Sucrose (1 fructose molecule + 1 glucose molecule), maltose, and lactose are disaccharides, or double sugars. Cane and beet sugars are more than 99 percent sucrose. They contain hardly any nutrients at all, yielding only energy in the body. For this reason, we talk of the empty calories in sugar. Sucrose is also found in sorghum, maple syrup, pineapple, and many vegetables and fruits.

Polysaccharides. Polysaccharides are complex carbohydrates that include the starches and cellulose. Sugar changes to starch as some plants mature. It is stored as energy in tubers, roots, and seeds of vegetables and cereal grains. Many nutrients are derived in this way. For this reason, complex carbohydrates contain a variety of nutrients not found in simple sugars.

Forms of sugar

Sugar. When we use the word "sugar," we usually mean white table sugar. It can be cubed or granulated. Table sugar is 100 percent crystalline sucrose made from cane sugar or sugar beets.

Brown sugar. Table sugar that has been colored and flavored with molasses is called brown sugar.

The forms of sugar include liquids such as molasses, honey, and syrup as well as the dry products of sugar cane and sugar beets.

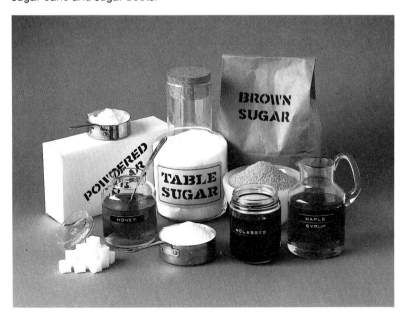

Powdered sugar. Powdered sugar is table sugar which has been ground to a powder. Confectioners' sugar is similar to powdered sugar, but it is even more finely ground.

Molasses. Molasses is the liquid that remains as a result of cane sugar processing. Molasses is 60 percent sugar. Dark molasses is also a good source of iron and some B vitamins.

Syrups. Syrups are available in many flavors and forms. Make your own syrups and save money. For instance, to 0.45 kg (1 lb) of brown sugar that has been boiled down with 240 mL (1 c) of water, add maple flavoring for a tasty substitute for much more expensive commercial maple syrup.

Read the labels on bottles marked "maple syrup." Avoid paying a high price for a small amount of maple syrup mixed with sugar, water, flavoring, and coloring. The shape of some bottles is deceptive. The net weights give the necessary information for determining the actual cost of the product.

Honey. Honey is popularly used as a syrup or as an ingredient in baking. Flavors vary according to the flower source of the nectar.

Artificial sweeteners. Many foods and beverages on the market are made for diabetics, dieters, and people who want sweets without calories. Americans consume millions of cases of low-cal-

orie soft drinks every year. At one time these drinks, and most of the other low-calorie foods, contained sodium cyclamate, an artificial sweetener. It seemed that sodium cyclamate was the perfect low-calorie sugar substitute.

A link with cancer became evident when experimental animals were fed large amounts of cyclamates. The FDA banned the use of cyclamates in 1970.

Saccharin, another sugar substitute, may also be unsafe. Fed to test animals, saccharin had undesirable effects. As a result, the use of saccharin was restricted in 1977. Research continues on the problem of sugar substitutes and their safety for human consumption.

SUGAR AND HEALTH

In 1973, Americans drank 23.56 billion L (6.2 billion gal) of soft drinks, amounting to about 114 L (30 gal) per person. This total was more than the combined total of all milk, tea, fruit juice, and vegetable juice consumed. For this $2 billion annual expenditure for soft drinks we got sugar, flavoring, color, and carbonated water. The calories contained in soft drinks are "empty" calories. They provide the body with an energy source but no nutrients.

Overweight

Too much sugar in the diet can create two major health problems. Excessive use of sugar can lead to overweight. You can add a pound of weight per week with 504 calories per day from sugar.

Too much sugar, particularly in snacks, may satisfy your appetite, but it also may keep you from eating other foods that carry the nutrients you require, thus undermining your good looks and

good health. Suppose you ate 504 calories of sugar a day. For the same calories you could eat a balanced breakfast consisting of a whole orange, a slice of toast, 5 mL (1 t) of margarine, one egg,

The concentrated sugar in sweet foods and snacks is usually an unnecessary supplement to the sugars provided by milk, grain foods, fruits, and vegetables.

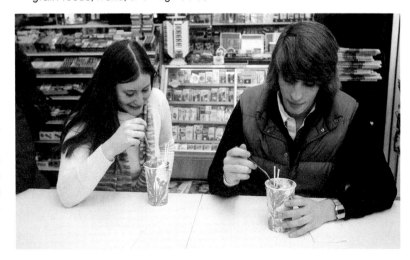

and a glass of whole milk. And you would still be about 100 calories short of the 504.

Diabetes

Some diseases develop because the body is unable to use sugar or starch normally. One such disease is diabetes. It ranks fifth among causes of death in the United States.

In the fifth to fourth century B.C., Hippocrates, a famous physician of ancient Greece, noted the "sweet urine" of the diabetic. Today we understand the meaning of what he observed. A person with diabetes has too much blood sugar and not enough insulin. The hormone insulin is secreted by the pancreas. It enables cells to oxidize glucose and release energy from food. When the bloodstream is deficient in insulin, glucose does not burn normally. The unburned sugar accumulates in the blood, and the kidneys excrete it into the urine. High blood sugar causes frequent urination, dehydration of body fluids and tissues, and extreme thirst.

Tooth decay

Many factors lead to tooth decay, or dental caries. One of the most important factors is poor choice of foods. Sugar contributes to tooth decay. Sucrose will ferment and cause acids that are harmful to teeth to form in the mouth. Thus, tooth decay is hastened when sweets stick to the teeth.

Studies show that about one-half of the 2-year-olds in our country have at least one decayed tooth. Ninety percent of the children up to 6 years of age have one or more decayed teeth. In 15-year-olds, the figure rises to 95 percent. It is unnecessary and undesirable that we "eat ourselves out of our teeth." Dr. J. H. Shaw of the Harvard School of Dental Medicine points out that the most successful way to give teeth a high resistance to decay is to have a good diet.

Gastric distress

Sugar eaten in large amounts at one time produces a feeling of overfullness in the stomach. The feeling comes from water being drawn into the stomach from our body tissues. This happens because of a scientific principle called osmotic pressure. A concentrated solution—in this case sugar—draws fluid into itself from outside. Water flows through a semipermeable membrane (the stomach wall) until the concentration is equal on both sides of the membrane.

USING SUGAR

Sugar in meals

The following points are guidelines for including sugar in your meals.

1. Get most dietary sugars from foods that carry other nutrients that you need, for example fruits, fruit juices, vegetables, cereals, grain foods, milk, and milk prod-

222

ucts. Eat dried fruits instead of candy for a quick energy lift. The glucose and fructose in dried fruit pass directly into the bloodstream. The sucrose in candy has to go through two steps in digestion.

2. Distribute the amount of sugar you eat in the day among the three meals. Try not to eat a large amount at one meal or as a snack. The time to eat a concentrated sweet is after a balanced meal, as dessert, and even then it should not be a large quantity. There is usually no need to give up eating sweets completely. Just remember to eat smaller amounts of them and to balance them with other foods in the day's diet.

3. Try to eat cereals and fresh fruits without adding sugar to them.

4. Learn to analyze the calories in the sweets you eat. For example, write down the ingredients in a recipe for sweet bread. Then make the bread and figure out the calories per serving by the method suggested in Chapter 4. Analyzing the amounts of sugar you eat each day will make you see how easy it is for the added calories of sugar to "sneak" into your diet (Table 13-1).

Breakfast. Sugar is often overused at breakfast. It is sprinkled liberally on cereal or fruit and put by the spoonful into coffee. Sweet spreads or syrup smother pancakes and waffles. Sugar is also present in coffee cakes, sweet breads, and doughnuts. Most of it is unnecessary to the diet, but even people with weight problems need not completely give up enjoying breakfast sweets if they use them sparingly. A teaspoon of marmalade spread

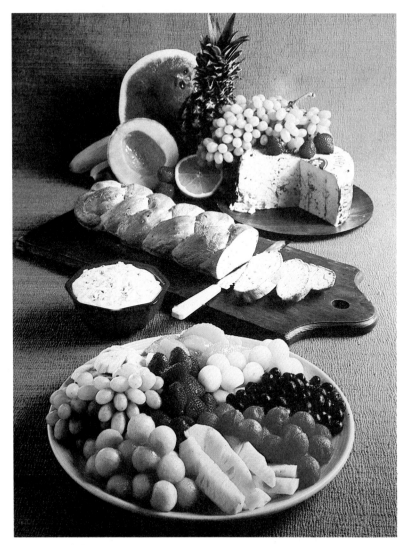

Fruit and cheese are a dessert that provides other nutrients as well as sugar.

thinly over bread is just as tasty as a larger quantity, and it adds only 18 calories to the basic meal. Dark molasses contains 45 calories per 15 mL (1 T) compared to 65 calories in the same amount of honey, and it has a few nutrients.

Lunch and dinner. Many nutritious lunch and dinner foods contain some sugar. Instead of a concentrated sugar dessert, eat a fresh apple or other fruit. Use canned fruit packed in light syrup or water rather than heavy syrup.

The calories from the sugar in the canned fruit will be cut down by 125 percent.

Custards and milk puddings are also good choices for dessert. They have a small amount of sugar and a lot of essential nutrients. Angel food cake, spongecake, plain cake, and gingerbread are all sweets with health values. So are deep-dish fruit pies.

Have your favorite pie or cake after a low-fat, low-sweet lunch or dinner, for example baked beans,

Table 13-1 Comparison of added sugar in two basic menus

MENU 1			MENU 2		
	ADDED SUGAR			ADDED SUGAR	
FOOD	mL	t	FOOD	mL	t
BREAKFAST			**BREAKFAST**		
Grapefruit, ½	10	2	Grapefruit, ½	0	0
Cereal, milk, sugar	15	3	Egg, soft boiled	0	0
Toast, spread, 15 mL			Toast, spread, 15 mL		
(1 T) jam	15	3	(1 T) jam	15	3
Coffee, milk, sugar	10	2	Milk, 240 mL (8 oz)	0	0
Total	50	10	Coffee, black	0	0
			Total	15	3
LUNCH			**LUNCH**		
Baked ham sandwich	0	0	Baked ham sandwich	0	0
Sweet pickle	5	1	2 leaves lettuce	0	0
2 leaves lettuce	0	0	Milk, plain, 240 mL		
Chocolate milk, 240 mL			(8 oz)	0	0
(8 oz)	15	3	1 banana	0	0
1 sliced banana, cream, sugar	10	2	Cookie, 1 med.	15	3
Cookies, 2 med.	27	5⅓	Total	15	3
Total	57	11⅓			
SNACK			**SNACK**		
Cola-type drink, 240 mL			Lemonade, 240 mL		
(8 oz)	30	6	(8 oz)	10	2
DINNER			**DINNER**		
Fried chicken	0	0	Fried chicken	0	0
Candied yams	15	3	Baked sweet potato	0	0
Frozen peas	1	⅓	Frozen peas	1	⅓
Green salad, dressing	1	⅓	Green salad, dressing	1	⅓
Apple pie	50	10	Raw apple	0	0
Coffee, sugar	10	2	Milk, 240 mL (8 oz)	0	0
Total	77	15⅔	Coffee, black	0	0
			Total	2	⅔
TV SNACK BEFORE BED			**TV SNACK BEFORE BED**		
Candy, 1 piece	35	7	Tangerine	0	0
DAY'S TOTAL (INCL. SNACKS)	249	50	**DAY'S TOTAL (INCL. SNACKS)**	42	8⅔
Total added sugar calories: 50 cal × 13 cal/t = 650			Total added sugar calories: 8⅔ cal × 13 cal/t = 112⅔		

Even fruit pies contain a great deal of added sugar and should be eaten as a dessert after a meal that is low in sugar.

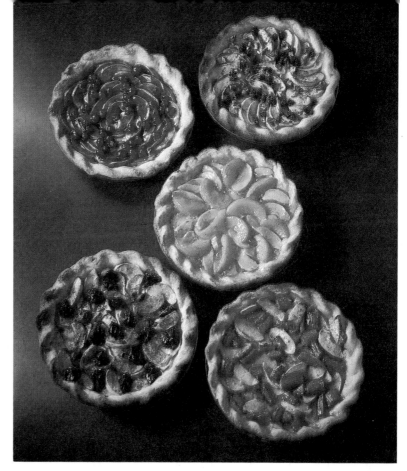

fish, liver, or a vegetable chowder of fish, meat, or poultry. If you have one food at a meal that is high in sugar, such as candied sweet potatoes, don't serve pie for dessert.

Sugar in candies and frostings

Crystalline candies and frostings. In crystalline candy and cooked cake frostings, the aim is a fine, smooth, creamy mixture produced by cooking liquid with sugar. Fudge frosting and fudge candy are cooked in similar ways. The only major difference is that the candy is cooked longer so that it will harden to a texture and thickness that will cut. The frosting must be creamy and soft enough to spread before it firms. Penuche, pralines, and fondants are other examples of crystalline candy.

Noncrystalline candies and frostings. Noncrystalline candies are brittle, sticky, or both. They include caramels, toffees, caramel popcorn, and all types of brittles. They are made by melting dry sugar until it is golden brown, but not burnt. Caramelizing changes the chemistry of the sugar, preventing the formation of crystals. Soda is added to increase the speed of caramelizing. Nuts or raisins may be added with the soda. Brittles should be spread quickly, for they harden quickly.

Buying and storing sugar

Granulated white sugar costs least per pound and maple sugar costs most, when compared with brown, lump, or confectioners' sugar. Granulated white sugar also costs less than molasses, syrups, and honey.

White sugar should be stored in a canister or jar with a tight lid.

Brown sugar becomes hard and dry when left in its box in a dry climate. Store it in the refrigerator in a closed metal or glass container. Add half a fresh apple to brown sugar to help retain moisture.

Once opened, natural maple syrup should be stored in the refrigerator. Molasses and honey keep well on a shelf in a cool place.

Sugar is the main ingredient in crystalline (*left*) and noncrystalline (*right*) candies and frostings.

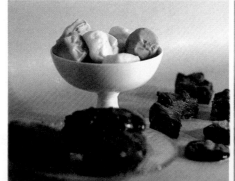
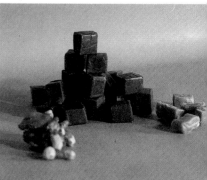

Facts about sugar

Value of sugar *Appeal* *Energy source*
Classifications of sugar *Monosaccharides* *Disaccharides*
Polysaccharides **Forms of sugar** *Sugar* *Brown sugar*
Powdered sugar *Molasses* *Syrups* *Honey* *Artificial sweeteners*

Sugar and health

Overweight Diabetes Tooth decay Gastric distress

Using sugar

Sugar in meals *Breakfast* *Lunch and dinner* **Sugar in candies and frostings** *Crystalline candies and frostings* *Noncrystalline candies and frostings* **Buying and storing sugar**

THINKING AND EVALUATING

1. How does the body use sugar for energy? How and where is sugar stored in the body?

2. Name the various classes of sugars and explain their nature.

3. In what forms would you find sugar on the supermarket shelf? Explain what these forms are.

4. How can too much sugar consumption interfere with health and a balanced diet?

5. List the guidelines for including sugar in meals.

6. Explain the difference between crystalline and noncrystalline candy. Give examples of each.

APPLYING AND SHARING

1. Record all the food and beverages you consumed yesterday. Using the table of nutritive values on pages 404-430, calculate

  a. the total number of calories; calories from complex carbohydrate foods and from sugars; protein in grams and calories; fat in grams and calories.

  b. the number of calories from concentrated sweets.

  c. the number of "hidden" calories from sugar.

2. How did this day's diet compare with your RDA? How would you improve this dietary record?

VOCABULARY

artificial sweeteners
crystalline
dental caries
diabetes
disaccharides
empty calories
glucose
glycogen
insulin
monosaccharides
noncrystalline
polysaccharides
saccharine
sodium cyclamate

226

3. Research the latest information on artificial sweeteners in the diet and sugar in the diet. Include information on nutrition, general health and well-being, disease, federal regulations monitoring use in processed foods, and cost. Report your findings to the class.

CAREER CAPSULES

Food stylist Usually works as free lance for publishers, food companies, advertising agencies, photographers; tests recipes and prepares foods for still or television photography. Required education varies; knowledge of home economics and photography helpful.

Dietetic assistant Works under a registered dietician in various settings; assists with diet planning, food service, or administration. Vocational education required.

RELATED READING

Cassela, Dolores. *A World of Baking.* Port Washington, N.Y.: David White, 1968. Discusses flavorful sweets—desserts, cakes, breads.

Field, Hazel E. *Foods in Health and Disease.* New York: Macmillan, 1964. Explains why certain foods are recommended or condemned by doctors.

Mikesh, Verna A., and Leona S. Nelson. "Sugar, Sweets Play Roles in Food Texture and Flavoring." *Food for Us All: Yearbook of Agriculture, 1969.* Washington, D.C.: USDA, 1969. Discusses nutrient values of sugar, emphasizing that no one sugar is more healthful than another.

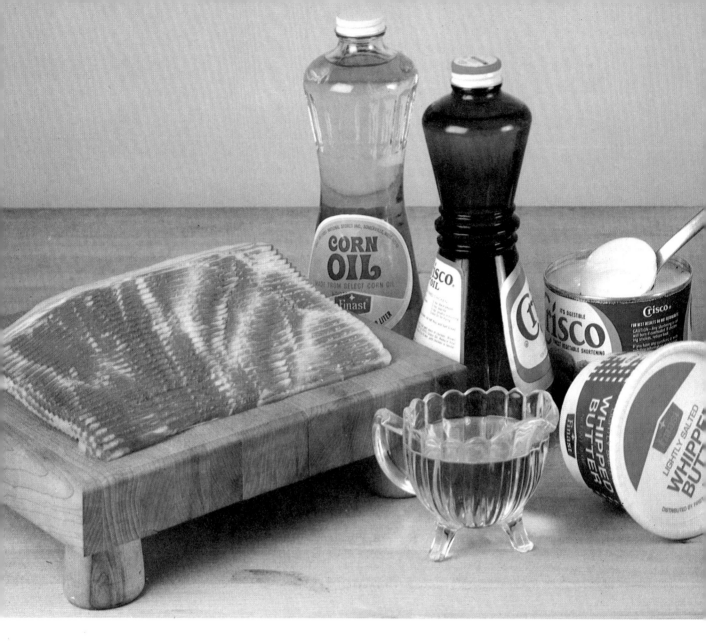

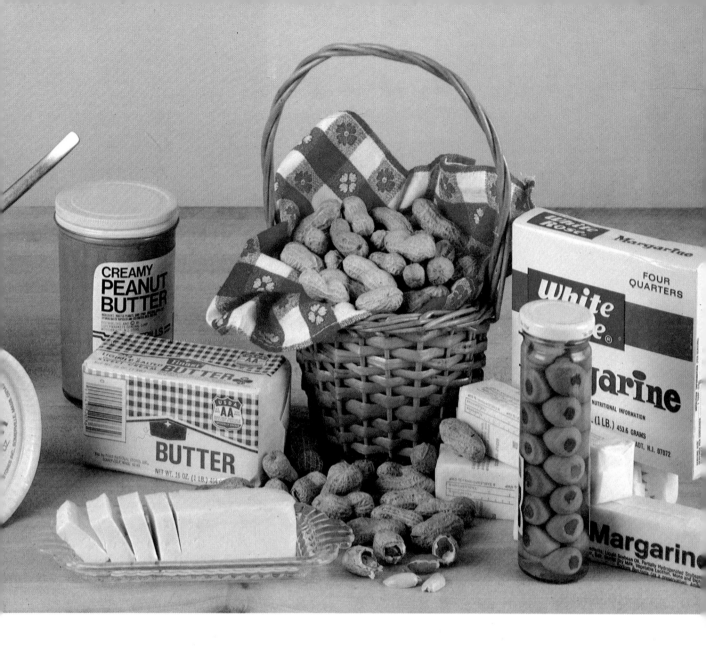

Fat in your diet

WHAT IS FAT?

Figure 14-1 Chemical differences distinguish the three different types of fat. In a saturated fatty acid molecule, all carbon bonds are filled with hydrogen. A mono-unsaturated molecule has one double carbon bond, reducing by 2 the number of hydrogen atoms in the molecule. Polyunsaturated molecules contain 2, 3, 4, or more double carbon bonds with a corresponding decrease of 4, 6, 8, or more hydrogen atoms.

Adapted from Callie M. Coons, "Fats and Fatty Acids," *Food: Yearbook of Agriculture, 1959* (Washington, D.C.: USDA, 1959), p. 77.

Fats used as foods come from two sources—animals and plants. Butter, cream, lard, and suet (from beef) are all animal fats. Olive and corn oil are examples of plant, or vegetable, oils.

The chemical name for fats and oils is lipids. Fats and oils are made up of fatty acid molecule chains of various lengths. Milk fat, or cream, and coconut oil contain fairly short chains of fatty acids. Fish oils have relatively long chains of fatty acids. The fatty acids themselves are composed of carbon, hydrogen, and oxygen. But the amount of oxygen in fatty acids is relatively small.

Fat is the most concentrated source of food energy. One gram of fat yields 9 calories, compared to 4 calories supplied by one gram of either carbohydrate or protein. Fat-soluble vitamins are mentioned throughout this book. Vitamins may be classified in two groups—fat-soluble and water-soluble. Fat-soluble vitamins include

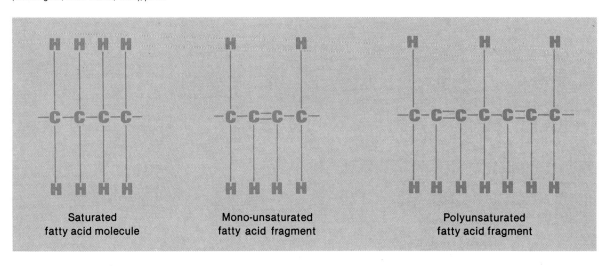

Saturated
fatty acid molecule

Mono-unsaturated
fatty acid fragment

Polyunsaturated
fatty acid fragment

vitamins A, D, E, and K. The rest are water-soluble. The names imply one of the chemical properties of each group: one dissolves in water, the other in fat. The differences in the two groups have implications for food preparation and meal-planning. There is little loss of fat-soluble vitamins in cooking water. But too little fat in the diet or interference with the body's fat absorption can result in a lack of these vitamins in the body, even if they are included in the diet.

Classifications of fats

Food advertisements speak about saturated and unsaturated fats, but few people understand what these words mean.

Saturated fats. Look at the formulas for fatty acids at the bottom of page 230. The formula at the left shows a segment of a saturated fatty acid. Notice that each of the carbons is attached to two hydrogens. Saturation means that the molecule can hold no more hydrogen. Butter is a food that is high in saturated fatty acids. In the other two groups at least two carbons are double-bonded to each other rather than to two hydrogens.

Mono-unsaturated fats. The center formula shows the structure of a section from a mono-unsaturated fatty acid chain. Oleic acid is a mono-unsaturated fatty acid. It makes up 50 percent of egg yolk, about 50 percent of peanut oil, about 75 percent of olive oil, and 43 percent of lard.

Polyunsaturated fats. Polyunsaturated refers to fats that contain molecules which have more than one double-bonded carbon. "Poly" is a Greek word meaning many. Look at the formula on the right on page 230, which shows the structure of a small segment of a polyunsaturated fatty acid. In this segment two pairs of carbons are double-bonded to each other rather than to other hydrogen atoms. A larger segment would show more such carbons. The fatty acid is polyunsaturated, or unsaturated many times.

Of common fats and oils, safflower oil has the highest proportion of polyunsaturated fatty acids. Peanut oil contains about one-third polyunsaturated fatty acids.

The length of chains, the amount of saturation, and the order in which fatty acids are joined in the chains determine the hardness or softness of a fat, the point at which it melts, and its flavor.

Polyunsaturated fats tend to be liquid at room temperature. Margarines and vegetable shortenings contain some fatty acids to which hydrogen has been added during processing so they will be firm at room temperature.

Saturated fats comprise 40 to 45 percent of the fat in the average American diet. The tastiest fats are saturated. We eat them in meats, whole milk, cream, butter, cheese, egg yolk, ice cream and lard. Saturated fats are hidden in many processed foods such as chocolate.

Polyunsaturated fats are the most desirable type of fats in the diet.

Linoleic acid is a polyunsaturated fatty acid essential for life. It contributes generally to the body's good appearance and health. It is essential for growth and normal reproduction, and it provides partial protection against radiation. Linoleic acid helps prevent excess

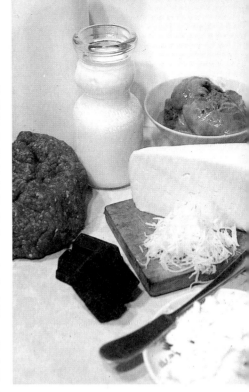

Saturated fats comprise 40 to 45 percent of the total fat in the average American diet.

Olive oil and pork contain high percentages of mono-unsaturated fat.

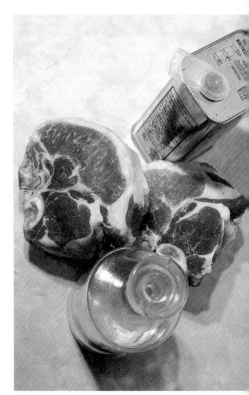

Table 14-1 Saturated and unsaturated fatty acids in oils and fats (percent of total fatty acids)[1]

FOOD	POLY-UNSATURATED FATTY ACID	MONO-UNSATURATED FATTY ACID	SATURATED FATTY ACID
Safflower oil	76	15	8
Sunflower oil	66	21	12
Corn oil	55	30	12
Soybean oil	55	21	18
Cottonseed oil	51	22	26
Peanut oil	31	50	19
Olive oil	8	80	12
Butter	3	35	59
Margarine[2]	9	60	27
Shortening, hydrogenated	8	68	24
Lard	11	48	40

Adapted from Callie M. Coons, "Fatty Acids in Some Animal and Plant Foods," *Food: Yearbook of Agriculture, 1959* (Washington, D.C.: USDA, 1959), pp. 84–85.
[1]The figures across the three columns add up to 99 percent. The remaining 1 percent is other unsaturated fatty acids.

[2]Margarine varies according to kind.

Turkey contains a high proportion of linoleic acid to saturated fatty acid.

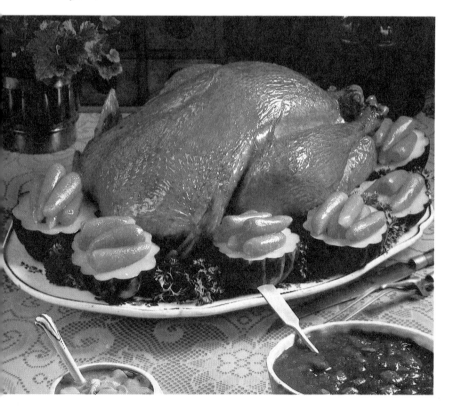

loss of water from the skin. It plays a key role in helping lower the cholesterol level of the blood.

Linoleic acid cannot be made in the body. It must be supplied through the food we eat. In the common foods we use, the best sources of linoleic acid are vegetable oils. Corn oil, soybean oil, and cottonseed oil contain from 51 to 55 percent linoleic acid. Safflower oil is the richest source, with 76 percent linoleic acid, and coconut oil is the lowest, with 0.5 percent.

Fat content of foods

Chicken, turkey, pork, and fish contain more linoleic acid and less saturated fat than lamb or beef (Table 14-2). Pork contains less saturated fats than other red meats. Scientific evidence has exploded the false belief held by many that pork is a "fattier" food than either beef or lamb. Vegetables contain practically no fat. Only two fruits—avocados and olives—contain enough fat to merit mention. The avocado is high in total unsaturated fat and low in saturated fat. Olives, on the other hand, contain less than half the linoleic acid of avocado. The whole grains are all high in linoleic acid and low in saturated fat.

Table 14-3 shows how meats and other foods compare in total amount and kinds of fat. A serving of 84 g (3 oz) of regular hamburger has 245 calories. Of the total weight, 23 g are protein. Multiplying these 23 g by the 4 calories that each gram of protein contains gives a total protein yield in the hamburger of 92 calories.

Of the total weight of the hamburger, 17 g are fat. Multiplying 17 g by 9 calories per gram of fat, we get 153 calories. Half of the fat in the hamburger is saturated fat. The other half is mono-unsaturated fat. A hamburger has only a trace of linoleic acid.

Fats for seasoning and cooking

Oils. Oils are fats that stay liquid at room temperature or when refrigerated. Most oils come from the plant seeds. Olive and coconut oils come from the fruit.

Oils are similar to other fats in many ways. They make food tender, crisp, and tasty. They provide a concentrated source of energy. They taste and feel greasy and become rancid when exposed to air. They also absorb strong odors and flavors from

Table 14-2 **Unsaturated and saturated fatty acids in some animal and plant foods (percent of total fatty acids)**

FOOD	UNSATURATED FATTY ACIDS			SATURATED FATTY ACIDS
	Polyunsaturated	Mono-unsaturated	Other	
MILK				
Whole cow's milk	3	35	3	59
Skim or nonfat milk	—	—	—	—
Buttermilk	—	—	—	—
Human milk	8	36	8	48
MEATS, FISH, POULTRY				
Beef	2	46	2	50
Pork	9	44	9	38
Lamb	2	37	2	59
Liver, pork	5	28	31	33
Salmon	—together, 27—		55	16
Tuna	—together, 26—		48	26
Chicken	21	40	5	34
Turkey	22	46	4	30
EGG, WHOLE	21	40	11	34
NUTS				
Almond	21	70	—	9
Coconut	1	7	1	91
Peanut	30	46	1	23
Pecan	21	70	1	8
Walnut, English	65	16	12	7
FRUITS AND VEGETABLES				
Avocado	15	50	13	22
Olive	7	80	1	12
WHOLE GRAINS				
Corn	47	37	4	12
Oats, rolled	43	33	1	23
Rice	38	42	1	19
Wheat	48	28	6	16

Adapted from Callie M. Coons, "Fatty Acids in Some Animal and Plant Foods," *Food: The Yearbook of Agriculture 1959* (Washington, D.C.: USDA, 1959), pp. 84–85.

Table 14-3 Fatty acids and calories in common foods

FOOD	MEASURE	SATURATED FATTY ACID g	cal	POLYUNSATURATED FATTY ACID g	cal	MONO-UNSATURATED FATTY ACID g	cal
FATS							
Margarine, soft	15 mL (1 T)	2	18	4	36	4	36
Butter	15 mL (1 T)	6	54	trace		4	36
Margarine, firm	15 mL (1 T)	2	18	3	27	6	54
Lard	15 mL (1 T)	5	45	1	9	6	54
Corn oil	15 mL (1 T)	1	9	7	63	4	36
Cottonseed oil	15 mL (1 T)	4	36	7	63	3	27
Soybean oil	15 mL (1 T)	2	18	7	63	3	27
Olive oil	15 mL (1 T)	2	18	1	9	11	99
Safflower oil	15 mL (1 T)	1	9	10	90	2	18
MEATS							
Pork							
·bacon	2 slices	3	27	1	9	4	36
roast, fresh	84 g (3 oz)	9	81	2	18	10	90
Roast beef	84 g (3 oz)	16	144	1	9	15	135
Hamburger							
regular	84 g (3 oz)	8	72	trace		8	72
lean	84 g (3 oz)	5	45	trace		4	36
Steak, broiled	84 g (3 oz)	13	117	1	9	12	108
Lamb roast, leg	84 g (3 oz)	9	81	trace		6	54
Chicken, boneless, broiled	84 g (3 oz)	1	9	1	9	1	9
Veal breast	84 g (3 oz)	7	63	trace		6	54
Salmon, pink, canned	84 g (3 oz)	1	9	trace		1	9
NUTS							
Almonds, shelled	80 mL (⅓ c)	2	18	5	45	17	153
Peanuts, halved	80 mL (⅓ c)	5	45	7	63	10	90
Peanut butter	15 mL (1 T)	2	18	2	18	4	36
Walnuts, shelled	80 mL (⅓ c)	1.3	12	12	108	9	81
OTHER							
Milk, whole	240 mL (1 c)	5	45	trace		3	27
Milk, nonfat or skim	240 mL (1 c)	0	0	0		0	0
Egg, large	1	2	18	trace		3	27
Avocado	1	7	63	5	45	17	153
Bread							
white, enriched	1 slice	trace		trace		trace	
whole-wheat	1 slice	trace		trace		trace	
Corn muffin	1	2	18	trace		2	18

Adapted from *Nutritive Value of Foods,* Bulletin No. 72 (Washington, D.C.: USDA, rev. 1977).

foods. All oils become undesirable for eating if heated to the point of burning. Oils differ from solid fats in flavor, melting point, smoking point, congealing point, the rate at which they become rancid, and ability to "shorten" or make a baked food tender.

Corn, soybean, and cottonseed oils have about two-fifths more linoleic acid than peanut oil. They have six-sevenths more linoleic acid than olive oil. Competitively priced safflower oil is highest in linoleic acid. Processors often blend low-cost coconut oil with other oils in order to bring expenses down. Because coconut oil is highly saturated, it is wise to buy a pure oil of corn, soybean, cottonseed, or safflower.

Butter. Butter is a highly saturated, firm fat made from both sour and sweet cream. It contains about 80 percent fat, of which 57 percent is saturated, 33 percent is mono-unsaturated, and 3 percent is polyunsaturated. It may or may not contain salt. The rest of the butter is milk solids and water. Usually color and flavoring are added to butter, even though the additions are not stated on the label. There are no federal restrictions against this practice as its contents are standardized (refer to Chapter 2).

Margarine. Margarine is a manufactured alternate for butter. It is made by heating vegetable oils under pressure. A metal catalyst is used to bring about a chemical reaction. As hydrogen bubbles through the vegetable oils, the double carbon bonds are forced open. Each carbon bond takes on hydrogen. Thus a polyunsaturated oil becomes partially or completely saturated. This

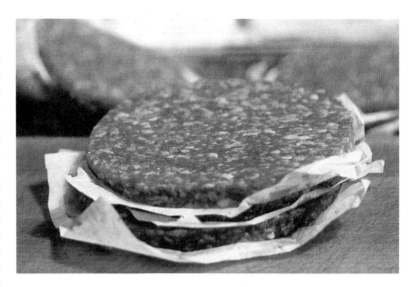

The fat in hamburger contains only a trace of linoleic acid.

process for making margarine is called **hydrogenation.**

Margarine must contain at least 80 percent fat. This is a standard set by the Federal Food and Drug Administration. Most margarines also contain whole or nonfat dry milk, salt, and the required 15,000 IU of vitamin A per pound.

Manufacturers produce four forms of margarine—regular, soft, whipped and diet. In general, the firmer the margarine, the higher the degree of saturated fat in it. The most desirable margarine is made only in part from hydrogenated oil. An oil high in linoleic acid is blended into the margarine. The linoleic acid reduces the risk of fat causing heart or circulatory diseases.

The amount of linoleic acid in margarines varies from 22 to 48 percent. Your clue to linoleic acid content is the list of ingredients on the package. The first ingredient listed on a margarine package is usually the chief ingredient. One soft margarine lists as its first ingredient "partially hydrogen-

ated vegetable oils." This means that the margarine contains more saturated fat than any other ingredient, even though the manufacturer also says on the label that the margarine is low in saturated fat. At least one margarine states on its label: "Made with liquid safflower oil, hardened safflower and cottonseed oils . . . polyunsaturated." For the informed shopper, this means that the chief ingredient is liquid safflower oil. Hence it is high in linoleic acid. The shopper can decide which to buy on the basis of facts not the advertiser's claims.

"Imitation" or diet margarines contain less than 80 percent fat and a high ratio of linoleic acid. Imitation margarines usually cost less than other margarines.

Butter and margarine look alike and have similar flavor. Their food value is similar except that the vitamin A content in a pound of margarine is always 15,000 IU. Butter costs more to produce and costs more per pound, but with increased cost of the oils used to produce margarine, the difference in cost to the consumer is decreasing.

Hydrogenated shortening. Shortening is also made by hydrogenating vegetable oils. It usually contains no color, vitamin A, or butter flavoring. Shortening is spoken of as a "plastic" fat. It is creamed by whipping air in during hydrogenation. It is easy to mix with flour and sugar for baking. Chemicals are added to prevent oxidation and rancidity, to give moistness, and to increase volume. These chemicals are monoglycerides and diglycerides, the same chemicals added to commercial bread as "softeners."

Lard. Lard is the fat from hogs. It is about 40 percent mono-unsaturated and has almost four times as much linoleic acid as butter. It is also high in arachidonic acid. Lard is the preferred fat among chefs for pastries. It is soft at room temperature and firm when refrigerated.

Lard and vegetable oils yield between 110 to 120 calories per 15 mL (1 T). Butter, margarine, and shortenings have 100 calories. About 210 mL (⅞ c) of lard or vegetable oil equals 240 mL (1 c) of butter or hydrogenated fats in baking —about 30 mL (2 T) less per 240 mL (1 c).

HOW THE BODY USES FATS

Digestion of fats

The fats that have the lowest melting point are easiest to digest. Milk fat, egg yolk, and vegetable oil are about 97 percent digestible, as compared with 93 percent for beef fat and 88 percent for lamb fat. This principle is significant in planning and preparing meals for people who need help in digesting fat.

Digestion of fat begins in the stomach, although most of it takes place in the small intestine through the action of bile and an enzyme called lipase. The mineral magnesium and vitamins B_6 and E are also needed for the body to use fat well. As the fat is digested, it is split into a fine emulsion of fatty acids and glycerol. Tiny fat globules absorb the fat-soluble vitamins. They then pass through the intestinal walls into the blood and lymph systems and circulate to all tissues. The tissues trap the

fat and vitamins they need.

For most young people, the fat level of the blood returns to normal before the next meal. The process takes from three to six hours. But in older, inactive people, especially people with some kinds of disease, the fat level does not return to normal as quickly.

Ideally, the calories from foods we eat should be the same as the total amount of calories used for energy. If the calorie intake is consistently higher than needed, we become overweight. If the supply of calories from the diet—whether from fat, protein or carbohydrate—exceeds the body's needs, the excess is changed into fat and stored in fatty tissues. These tissues are the body's storehouse for energy. They release the fat, as needed, into the bloodstream in a form that is usuable by the cells.

The reserves of fat in the body can be burned if the total daily calorie intake is reduced below that which is needed. Weight control is discussed in Chapter 16, pages 265–279, heart disease, Chapter 17, pages 281–291.

Functions of fats

Scientists say that the kind and amount of fat in our diet are clearly related to heart and circulatory diseases. Supported by nutritionists and the American Heart Association, they have repeatedly urged the U. S. public to eat less fat, particularly saturated fat.

The flavor of fatty foods tempts us to eat too much of them. Too much fat in the diet can cause us to gain excess weight, causing bodily processes to slow down and operate inefficiently. Too much fat increases the chances of illness. If fat piles up in the bloodstream, blood may clot more easily, causing heart attacks, strokes, and circulatory ailments.

Fats are an important component of the diet when properly used, however. They become harmful only when they are overused or misused. Following are the beneficial functions of fat in the diet.

Fat is our most concentrated source of energy, providing over twice as many calories as an equal amount of carbohydrate or protein. Fat gives "staying power" to a meal. Of all the nutrients, it takes longest to digest. Thus, it delays hunger. Our ancestors needed fat to sustain them as they worked long hours at hard physical labor. Today we are less active physically and therefore need less fat.

Unless fat is present in the diet, the body cannot absorb and use the fat-soluble vitamins A, D, E, and K. Instead, these vital nutrients are eliminated as waste.

Fat brings out flavor in food. It gives a crisp texture to fried foods and tenderness to baked products. It makes meat juicy and tender. Fat also seasons vegetables and other foods.

Fat also lubricates the digestive tract and aids in normal bowel action. Too much fat causes diarrhea. Mineral oil, often used as a supplementary laxative, cannot be absorbed or used by the body. It absorbs fat-soluble vitamins and eliminates them as waste. It thus deprives us of nutrients we need.

A thin fatty sheath under the skin helps control body temperature against excessive heat or cold. It pads the organs and joints to ensure greater comfort. It also rounds out the figure.

Fatty foods are beneficial if used intelligently in correct proportion to other foods.

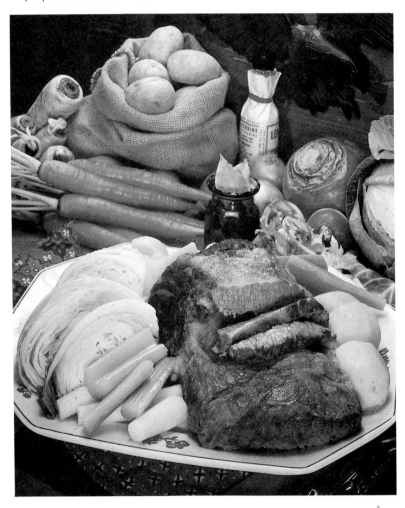

Cholesterol is a waxy, fat-like substance that is found in all animal tissue. The body needs some cholesterol just as it needs some fat. Cholesterol comprises 11 percent of the dry weight of the brain, where it is thought to form a protective sheath. It is also the major component in earwax. It works with a team of nutrients to form vitamin D when the sun shines directly on the skin. It also helps promote good vision.

Cholesterol forms part of the liver, spleen, sex glands, and hormones. It is also essential for the formation of bile salts needed for digestion of fat. Since fat is lighter than water, cholesterol is important in helping to transport fat through the bloodstream. It forms a part of white blood cells. It helps to prevent water evaporation from the skin. A nutrient that contributes so much to life needs to be understood.

Cholesterol in the body comes from two sources—from the food we eat and from the body itself. From our daily diet, we take in about 500 to 600 mg of cholesterol. The body manufactures 2000 to 3000 mg daily if it needs this amount of cholesterol for normal functioning. Most of the body-made cholesterol is manufactured in the liver. But it can also be made by the skin, intestinal mucosa, and other body tissues. Food alone is not responsible for raising the level of blood cholesterol. If we don't get cholesterol from the foods we eat, the body makes it.

Cholesterol and heart disease

Cholesterol was first suspected of contributing to heart and circulatory disease when large amounts of cholesterol were found in the blood serum of patients with certain types of heart disease. Cholesterol was also found in plaques that thickened the artery walls. Plaques are deposits of cholesterol and other forms of fats in the connective tissue of blood vessel walls. As a person grows older, the plaques harden and reduce the diameter of arteries. Blood cannot flow as well through the reduced openings.

Table 14-4 **Cholesterol content of common foods (mg per 100 g)**

FOOD	CHOLESTEROL CONTENT
Beef brains	2000
Eggs, fresh whole (2)	550
Liver, raw	300
Butter	250
Oysters and lobster (meat only)	200
Cheese, Cheddar	100
cottage, creamed	15
cream	120
American process	155
Lard and other animal fat	95
Shrimp and crab (flesh only)	125
Heart, beef, raw	150
Veal	90
Beef, round, medium-fat, raw	70
Chicken, raw, flesh only	60
Fish fillet or steak	70
Lamb and pork	70
Ice cream	45
Milk, whole	11
skim, liquid	3
Vegetable oils	0
Plant foods	0

Composition of Foods, Agriculture Handbook No. 8, (Washington, D.C.: USDA, 1963), Table 4, p. 146.

238

The development of plaques in arteries appear to occur for complex reasons. Some of these are heredity, the amount of exercise a person has, smoking, and diet.

In the past, people believed that heart disease occurred only in older people. But plaques have been found in the arteries of people in all age groups—even in infants.

Current research reveals that a diet low in cholesterol does not always solve the problem of heart disease. People with low cholesterol levels may still have heart ailments. People with high blood cholesterol levels may never suffer from heart disease. As a general preventive rule, however, it is wise to keep cholesterol intake low.

From a scientific technique allowing us to follow the cholesterol molecule through the body, we have learned that blood cholesterol may be higher than normal under many circumstances:

In women, during menstruation or during or after menopause

In men, after the age of 25

When a person's family has a history of coronary disease

When the thyroid gland is underactive

When a person is putting on weight

When the diet is too high in protein (a high-protein diet is often used by food faddists to reduce weight)

When too much sweet food is eaten at one time and quickly absorbed

When large amounts of foods rich in animal fat or other saturated fat are eaten

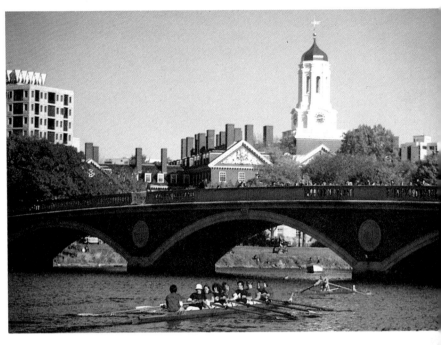

Exercise helps keep cholesterol under control.

When too much alcoholic beverage is consumed

When the diet is too high in cholesterol

When a person indulges in overeating in any form

When a person experiences emotional stress in any form

When a person does not exercise regularly

All these conditions may be guarded against by intelligent use of foods rich in cholesterol. Fruits, vegetables, and cereal grains contain no cholesterol. Familiarize yourself with the cholesterol content of other foods in planning your day's diet (Table 14-4).

Exercise also helps keep cholesterol under control. In a study at Harvard, medical students each ate 5000 calories of food a day—enough for a lumberjack. Yet they exercised enough to maintain steady weight and steady cholesterol levels. As soon as they stopped exercising, both their weight and their blood cholesterol rose.

Cholesterol and the diet

Long-term studies have shown that changes in the diet can lower the amount of cholesterol in the bloodstream. Although cholesterol is not the only factor in cardiovascular disease, there is evidence that consistently lower levels of blood cholesterol are related to declines in disability and death from heart disease.

The amount of fat in the diet of Americans is high—about 40 percent of calories from fat. In addition, a high proportion of this fat is saturated. Overall reduction of fat in the diet can help reduce blood cholesterol levels. Moreover, there should be a high ratio of unsaturated to saturated fats in the diet. In *Textbook of Medical Physiology,* Authur C. Guyton points out ways to reduce the concentration of cholesterol in the blood. He maintains that a diet low in saturated fat is more important than a diet low in cholesterol.

Guidelines

Both saturated and unsaturated fats are as nutritionally important as lean meats, nonfat milk, eggs, fruits, vegetables, and cereal grains in a balanced diet. In 1977, the Senate Select Committee on Nutrition and Human Needs recommended that 30 percent of our calories should come from fat, in equal proportions of polyunsaturated, monounsaturated, and saturated fat.

The following are suggestions for planning and preparing meals that contain more polyunsaturated and less saturated fat.

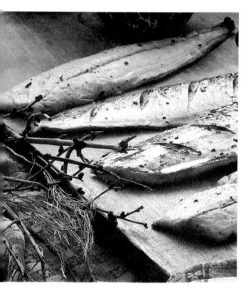

Most fish is low in animal fat.

When meat is broiled or roasted on a rack, much of its saturated fat runs off.

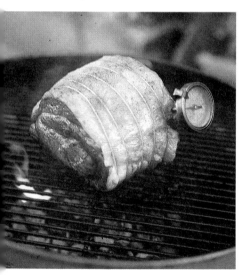

1. Use margarine as a spread. Be sure to read the label when you buy. See that the first ingredient listed is liquid safflower, corn, soybean, or cottonseed oil. These oils have a high percentage of linoleic acid.

2. Use vegetable oil high in linoleic acid for baking. To improve the taste of cakes and cookies, use more flavoring, spices, or lemon or orange peel. Oil brings out the flavors in herbs and spices. Most convenience baking mixes contain saturated fat.

3. Use vegetable oil to season vegetables, white sauce, casseroles, salads, and other foods. Use herbs, onions, garlic, and other seasonings with the oil.

4. Use vegetable oil to fry or sauté lean meat or to brush lean meat in broiling or baking.

5. Cook cereals in skim milk and add 5 mL (1 t) of oil per serving. Fry or scramble eggs in 5 mL (1 t) of oil.

6. Use low-fat animal sources of protein such as chicken, turkey, fish, shellfish, and veal in the diet. Cooked beans seasoned with vegetable oil and herbs, onions, and garlic make a flavorful meat alternative.

7. Trim all visible fat from red meat before cooking. This fat is saturated. Trim the marbling fat away as you eat red meat. Plenty of fat will remain in the fine marbling that you can't trim out. Skin poultry and remove all visible fat before cooking. Roast and/or broil meats on a rack so that the fat will run off.

8. Divide the amount of fat used among the three meals of the day. During the day you will probably be more active and burn up fat. Studies show that a high-fat meal in the evening followed by inactivity can cause the fat level in the bloodstream to be high for as long as twelve hours.

9. Keep a sharp eye out for "hidden" saturated fats in fried foods, snacks, and other foods (Table 14-5).

10. Study each recipe for the kind and amount of fat it contains before using it. You can prepare tasty foods that have the correct kind and amount of fat by using the implied guidelines in the tables and recipes in this book.

11. Read labels when shopping to find out the kind and amount of fat used in processed foods.

12. When eating out, analyze dishes for fat content. For example, you know that French fries are usually fried in oil. The oil most often used for deep-fat frying in public places is inexpensive coconut oil, which is almost completely saturated. Knowing this, you might want to order a baked potato instead of French fries.

13. Plan menus so that the kinds and amounts of fat in each meal are balanced. When you have a steak, use fresh fruit for dessert. Season the salad and vegetables with an oil high in linoleic acid. When fish, liver, broiled chicken, or beans are used as the main protein dish, then have your favorite dessert that is high in fat (preferably polyunsaturated).

14. Don't assume that ice milks are better for you than standard ice cream. It is true that ice milks contain less fat than ice cream. But the proportion of saturated to unsaturated fats is higher in ice milk and also in imitation coffee

cream and whipped cream. The oil used to make them is 85 percent saturated. Milk fat, in ice cream, is only 59 percent saturated.

Storing and cooking with fats

All animal fats should be stored in the refrigerator. Vegetable shortenings have chemical additives to prevent oxidation and rancidity. They may be kept at room temperature for short periods of time. However, it is well to store margarines in the refrigerator. Oils that are not promptly used should

Table 14-5 "Hidden" calories from fat in common foods

FOOD	MEASURE	CALORIES FROM FAT	TOTAL CALORIES
MEAT			
Sirloin steak, broiled	168 g (6 oz)	486	660
Bacon, fried	2 slices	72	90
Hamburger, regular	84 g (3 oz)	153	245
Lamb, roast	84 g (3 oz)	144	235
Pork, roast fresh (lean only)	67 g (2.4 oz)	90	175
Ham, cured, roast	84 g (3 oz)	171	245
Chicken, half breast, fried (with bone)	92 g (3.3 oz)	45	155
Drumstick, fried	58 g (2.1 oz)	36	90
Chicken, canned boneless	84 g (3 oz)	90	170
Crabmeat, canned	84 g (3 oz)	18	85
MILK AND MILK PRODUCTS			
Heavy cream	15 mL (1 T)	54	55
Cream cheese	84 g (3 oz)	288	320
Ice cream	84 g (3 oz)	45	95
Malted milk	240 mL (1 c)	90	245
NUTS			
Peanut butter	15 mL (1 T)	72	95
Peanut halves, roasted	120 mL (½ c)	324	420
Almonds, shelled	120 mL (½ c)	347	425
Pecan halves	120 mL (½ c)	347	370
Walnut halves	120 mL (½ c)	338	345

Table 14-5 cont. on next page

Table 14-5 (cont.)

FOOD	MEASURE	CALORIES FROM FAT	TOTAL CALORIES
LUNCHEON MEATS			
Bologna	2 slices	63	80
Frankfurter	1	94	170
DESSERTS			
Devil's food cake with chocolate icing	26 cm² (4 sq in)	81	235
Fruit cake, dark	10.5 cm² (1.7 sq in)	18	55
Plain cake			
no icing	46 cm² (7 sq in)	108	315
with boiled white icing	46 cm² (7 sq in)	108	400
Angel food cake, no icing	40 cm² (6 sq in)	trace	135
Brownie	32 cm³ (2.7 cu in)	54	95
Apple pie	59 cm² (9 sq in)	135	350
Mince pie	59 cm² (9 sq in)	144	365
Lemon meringue pie	59 cm² (9 sq in)	108	305
Pumpkin pie	59 cm² (9 sq in)	135	275
SALAD DRESSING			
Mayonnaise	15 mL (1 T)	99	100
French	15 mL (1 T)	54	65
Home-cooked	15 mL (1 T)	18	25
Thousand Island	15 mL (1 T)	72	80
SNACKS AND APPETIZERS			
Potato chips	10	72	115
Pizza	127 cm² (19 sq in)	54	185
Olives			
ripe black	2 large	trace	73
green	3 large	trace	78

Adapted from *Nutritive Value of Foods,* Bulletin No. 72 (Washington, D.C.: USDA, rev. 1977).

also be tightly capped and stored in the refrigerator.

When a fat smokes and turns brown during cooking, the fat molecule is breaking down. Such fat should be discarded. It is unpleasant to smell and taste. It is also an irritant to the digestive tract. Butter and margarine burn or smoke at the lowest temperature of any fat. They are not suited to frying, but they may be used for low-heat sautéing. Oils and shortenings are used for frying because they can reach a very hot temperature before starting to smoke or burn. Shortenings may be heated to 177 °C (350 °F). Lard may be heated to 182 °C (360 °F). Corn oil and other vegetable oils may be heated to 227 °C (440 °F). When frying in deep fat, use a thermometer to determine the heat of the fat.

RECAP

What is fat?

Classifications of fats   *Saturated fats*   *Mono-unsaturated fats*
Polyunsaturated fats   **Fat content of foods**   **Fats for seasoning and cooking**   *Oils*   *Butter*   *Margarine*
Hydrogenated shortening   *Lard*

How the body uses fats

Digestion of fats   Functions of fats

What is cholesterol?

Cholesterol and heart disease   Cholesterol and the diet

Using fats in meals

Guidelines   Storing and cooking with fats

THINKING AND EVALUATING

1. What contributions does fat make to a well-balanced diet? What are its disadvantages?

2. How are fatty acid chains held together?

3. Will a diet high in saturated fat affect your health differently from one high in polyunsaturated fat? Illustrate.

4. Name the different classes of fat. How do they differ chemically? In what foods can each be found?

5. What is linoleic acid? Why is it important?

6. How is fat digested? How is excess fat stored?

7. What is cholesterol? Where does it come from? How does it affect health?

8. Describe the guidelines for including fat in the diet.

APPLYING AND SHARING

1. List the fat-rich foods you like best. List the fat-rich foods you ate yesterday and today.

   a. From these lists, note the foods rich in saturated fats; the foods high in linoleic acid.

   b. Consult Table 14-5 and make a list of "hidden" calories from fat in the foods you ate yesterday and today.

   c. Multiplying the number of grams of fat in each food by 9, calculate the total calories from saturated fat and those from linoleic acid (polyunsaturated fat). What did you learn that can help you when planning meals?

VOCABULARY

cholesterol
fatty acid
hydrogenation
linoleic acid
lipase
lipid
mono-unsaturated fat
plaque
polyunsaturated fat
saturated fat

2. Visit the market where you shop and in a notebook list the different kinds of fat and the price per pound of oils, shortenings, firm margarines, soft or "special" margarines, and lard.

    a. Using Table 14-1, list the percentage of saturated fat and the percentage of linoleic acid in each one. Discuss with the class what you have learned.

    b. Do you need to change the kind of fat you use in cooking? The amount? Your table spread? Why? Is your family agreeable to a change? Why or why not? Discuss what you have learned.

3. Plan balanced menus for four days, lowering the total fat intake to 30 to 35 percent of the total calories and making about 50 percent of your fat calories foods high in linoleic acid.

4. Prepare for a debate. One-half of the class will prepare arguments for eating as much of the fat-rich foods as you wish. The other half will prepare arguments on controlling the amount of total fat to 35 percent of the calories, with a third to a half of the calories from linoleic fatty acids. Select three people on each side to debate the subjects. Draw conclusions from what you learned.

5. Explain how you can help your own life and the lives of your family by knowing how to prepare and serve balanced meals using the best knowledge of fat we have.

CAREER CAPSULES

Test kitchen home economist Works for a food company, larger newspaper, magazine, publisher, television station; develops recipes for consumer use. Four-year college education in home economics required.

Cookbook writer Works free lance or as food editor for newspaper, magazine, or book publisher, plans books, supervises development and testing of recipes, checks accuracy of final product. Two- or four-year college education in home economics and/or journalism helpful.

RELATED READING

Bond, Clara-Beth, et al. *The Low-fat, Low-cholesterol Diet.* New York: Doubleday, 1971. Discusses all aspects of controlled-fat cooking and contains summary on nutrition with special attention to the controlled-fat diet.

Brown, Helen B. *Low-fat and Vegetable Oil Recipes.* Cleveland, Ohio: Cleveland Clinic, n.d. Contains recipes for fat-controlled and fat-restricted diets with tips on low-fat cooking.

Kilgore, Lois T. "How to Avoid Confusion in Fats and Oils Buying or Use." *Food for Us All: Yearbook of Agriculture, 1966.* Washington, D.C.: USDA, 1966. Suggests ways of differentiating between the variety of oils and fats on the market.

CHAPTER 10

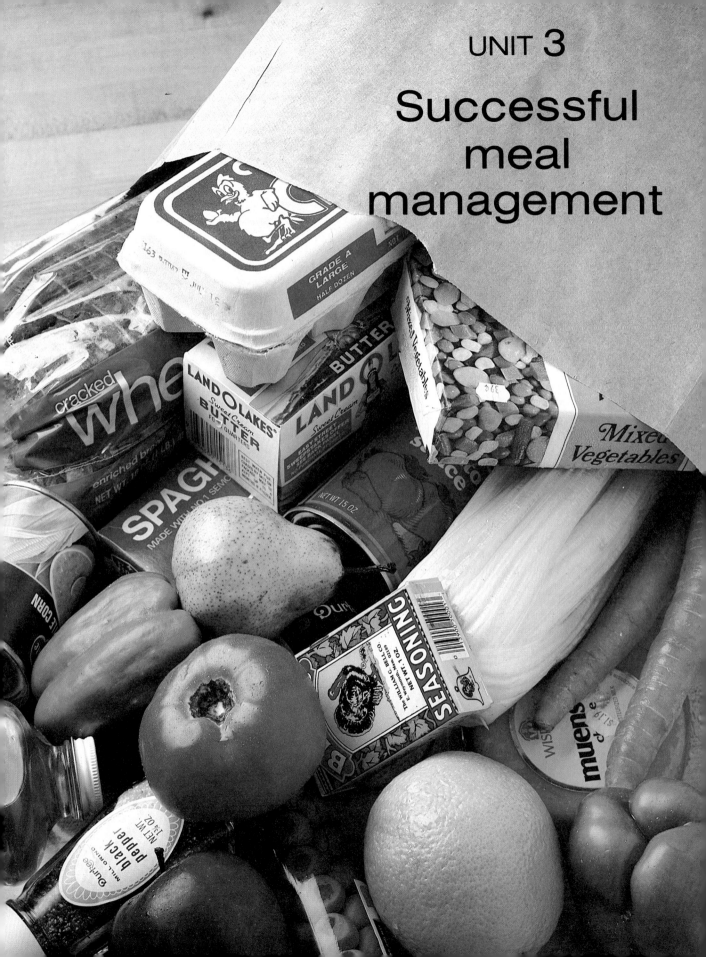

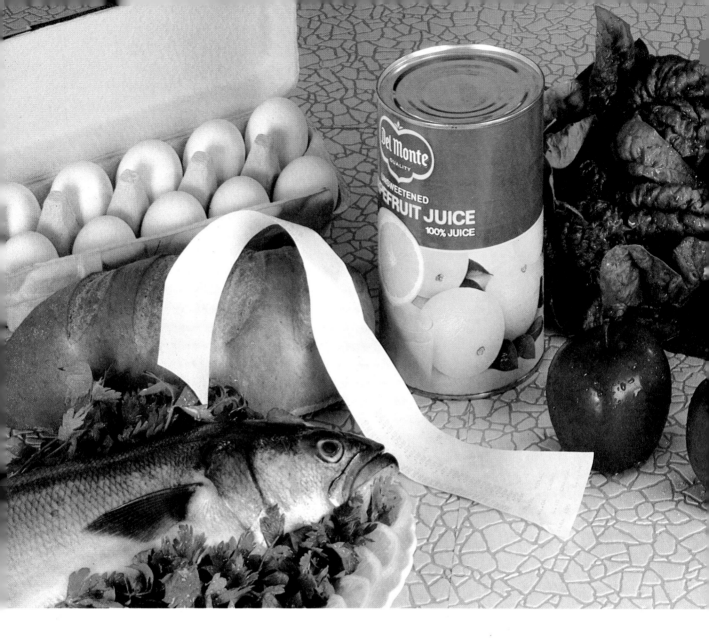

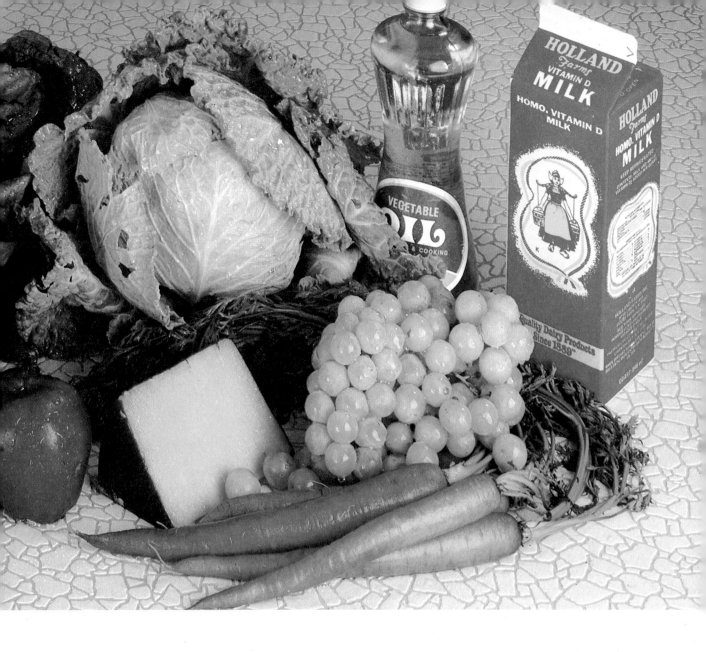

Managing your meals

MEAL PLANNING

Since men are increasingly sharing with women the responsibility for taking care of all aspects of home and family, everyone needs to learn the basic principles of menu planning, shopping for food, and cooking and serving meals. Managing meals is like managing a business. The following business principles can be applied to meal management.

1. Acquire accurate, up-to-date information about all aspects of the job. Know your equipment and resources.

2. Learn the best procedures to follow.

3. If you live with others, organize and assign the different jobs that must be done. Help family members feel that they are involved in the important business of providing nourishing meals. Set high standards in each phase of meal preparation.

4. Give clear, simple, and accurate directions to those who help you with shopping, food storage, meal preparation, and meal service.

5. Show enthusiasm about the task of serving nutritious meals. Successful executives communicate enthusiasm about their goals to people who work with them.

The ultimate in home meal management—budgeting, menu planning, preparation, timing, and appearance—is an elaborate holiday dinner.

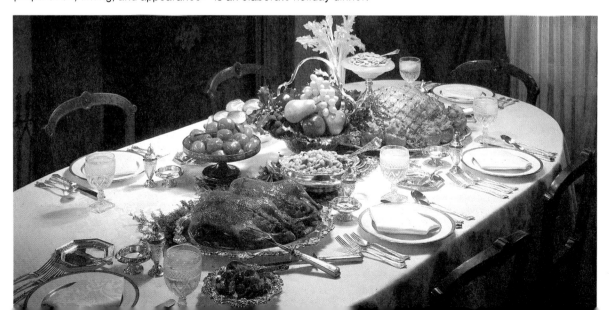

Place of food in the budget

Many of the decisions we make during our lifetime in some way involve money. As we try to decide how to divide income between necessities and luxuries, budgeting becomes a necessary skill. How we use our income depends on our personal tastes and values, but no household should sacrifice a balanced diet in favor of more expensive living quarters, furnishings, or clothing.

To prepare a budget, begin with total available income. Then set up a column for fixed expenses. These include food, housing, furnishings, and clothing. Make another column for flexible expenses—transportation, insurance, medical care, drugs, recreation, and education. Budget planning allows for a certain amount of flexibility. Experiment with various financial formulas until you find one that satisfies your needs and also allows for some pleasures.

After you have figured out what you *can* spend on food to meet your budget, figure out what you actually spend. You will probably realize that you need to economize on food in order to meet your budget. First ask yourself if you are spending too much on snack foods. Then ask yourself if you are getting a balanced supply of nutrients each day.

You can be as well-fed on a low income as on a high income. If you are well-informed about the nutritive values of different foods, you can plan balanced meals using the foods you can afford. The meals you eat daily should be varied enough to balance one another's nutritional strengths and

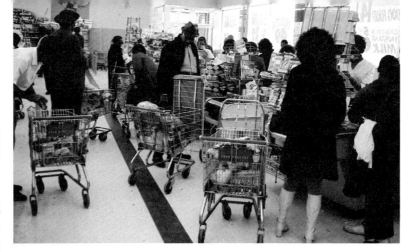

You can be as well-fed on a low budget as on a high one.

If you depend on fruits, vegetables, cereal foods, and milk products for most nutrients, a small amount of meat in the diet will suffice for the animal proteins required.

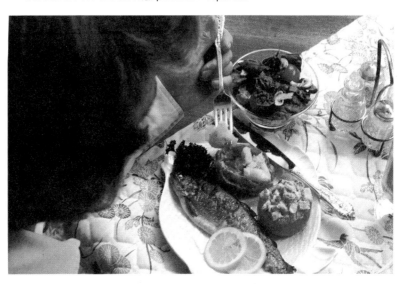

weaknesses. On the basis of three meals a day, each meal should provide enough nutrients to meet about one-third of the body's need for the day.

Economical sources of nutrients

Vitamin A. The most economical sources of vitamin A are dark-green and deep-yellow vegetables, fruit, egg yolk, margarine, and whole milk.

Riboflavin. The best sources of riboflavin are milk, cheese, and foods made with milk. Bread and cereal foods, eggs, and vegetables contain lesser amounts.

Thiamin. Potatoes rank first in amount of thiamin for money spent. Bread and cereal foods rank second. Dried beans, peas, and nuts rank third.

Niacin. Dried beans, peas, and nuts provide the most niacin for the money spent. Potatoes and bread and cereal foods follow.

Managing your meals **249**

Vitamin C. Citrus fruits in any form are the most economical source of vitamin C. Other good sources of vitamin C are tomatoes, potatoes, raw cabbage, and other vegetables and fruits.

Protein. Meat, poultry, and fish consume most of the food dollar, but they yield less protein and more fat for the money than nonfat milk, nonfat milk products, eggs, dry beans, peas, lentils, cereals, bread, and potatoes. Since the protein in animal foods contains all of the essential amino acids in generous amounts, the best policy is to combine animal proteins with vegetables, fruits and/or grain products in a ratio of 1 to 1 or less. You can then get the full benefit of the protein in the less costly plant foods, as well as the benefits of the animal foods.

Calcium. Milk and milk products are the most economical sources of calcium. No other foods compare.

Iron. Dried beans, peas, and nuts are the most economical sources of iron. Potatoes are second. Bread and cereal foods are third. Deep-green and yellow vegetables are fourth.

Planning a menu

An organized, businesslike approach to meal management, a knowledge of nutrient sources, and skill in budgeting simplify your menu planning. Use the following guidelines to help you plan your menus.

1. Reread the principles for planning balanced meals in Chapter 4.

2. Write down the amount of money you can spend for food in one week.

3. Encourage all family members to share their thoughts on the foods that will meet their nutritional needs and their favorite foods. If possible, include in a menu favorite foods that contribute to nutrition. If some favorite foods are "junk" foods, discuss the nutritional and economical reasons that nutritious foods must come first.

4. Plan your menus for each day of the week. Write them down in a notebook. Keep this notebook as a record for future reference. Allow space for comments on how the meal was accepted and how it might be improved.

5. Plan to use fresh foods in season. This helps you save money, and it makes the diet more varied and nutritious.

6. Evaluate the advertised food "specials" for the week. First, decide whether you need the product. Second, determine whether it is a genuine bargain.

7. Divide the money you can spend among the most essential foods—milk and milk products, bread and cereals, vegetables, fruits, meats, and eggs.

8. Select healthful recipes.

9. Carefully compare the cost and nutritional value of convenience foods with foods you can make yourself.

Shopping for food

Before doing the food shopping, you want to be sure that you and the people who live with you observe the highest sanitary standards in storing and using foods.

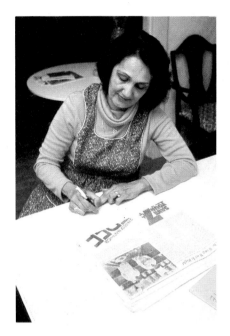
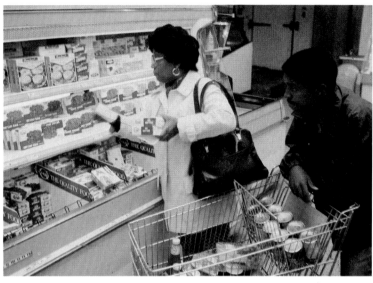

Left: A shopping list planned around the week's menus and the market's "specials" helps you to stay within your food budget. *Right:* Picking up frozen foods at the end of your shopping trip reduces the possibility of their thawing before you put them into the freezer at home.

High sanitary standards will ensure healthfully prepared meals and keep your food supply fresh for the maximum period of time. Clean the refrigerator with warm water and baking soda. Make sure storage cabinets, counter tops, and work areas are also clean.

1. Try to shop when the supermarket is not crowded.

2. Provide yourself with a shopping list. A carefully prepared list geared to your week's menus should help you shop quickly and more economically.

3. When shopping, select packaged foods first. Select fresh vegetables, fruits, meats, and dairy foods next, and frozen foods last. Reading the labels for nutrition information also help you make the best use of your food dollar.

4. Knowing about unit pricing will also help you. Unit pricing means the cost per unit of measure such as price per kilogram (pound), per gram (ounce), per liter (quart or pint). Look for the unit price on the shelf near the food.

5. Keep a record of the money you spend for food in each food group. Should you make any changes? Are you neglecting any important foods? Overusing any?

FACTORS AFFECTING MEAL PREPARATION

Every dish in a meal should be served at its peak of perfection. Getting everything to come out together requires a keen sense of timing that comes with experience. It you are a beginning cook, you may be frustrated at first by the problem of timing the preparation of a meal. But your timing will soon improve if you do each separate task well, one step at a time. The key is to plan ahead.

Decisions and timing

A meal plan requires decision making about the menu, meal management, and how the food will be served. Decisions must be made about the use of energy, time, money, equipment, space, your energy, as well as your experience and ability. This is the mental portion of meal management. (Preparing and serving the food is the physical part.) A plan is most important.

1. First, determine the number of

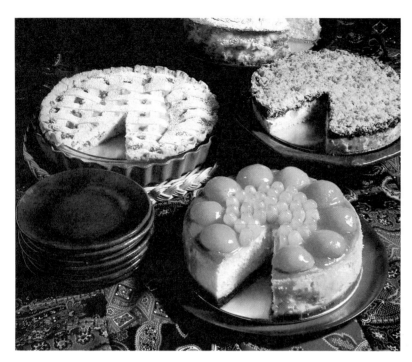

Many desserts can be made well in advance of a meal.

An attractively set table enhances the enjoyment of a meal.

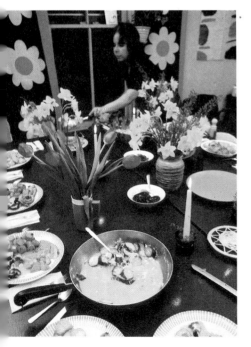

5. Remember to give time and attention to arranging the table for serving. Choose the setting, room, and table appointments for the meal.

6. Plan in terms of the entire day's foods. Take snacks into account during your meal planning. Make them a part of the total plan.

Table service

To decide how to serve your meal, consider the menu, the time of day, the occasion, the number of people, and where the meal will be eaten—outdoors or indoors.

1. A family service has all food on the table, and everyone serves themselves from the dishes.

2. A buffet service will permit you to easily serve large or small numbers of guests. People serve themselves from dishes placed on a separate, buffet table.

3. For more formal occasions, food may be served at the table or served on plates in the kitchen before they are brought to the table.

4. Use attractive trays or dishes when serving snacks, too.

The serving time for each meal should be agreed upon by the household. Every member should consider it an obligation to be at meals on time. Guests or family members who are late for a meal are being discourteous to the people who prepared it.

Taste, texture, temperature

Taste depends on our taste buds, which are located in the papillae

people you intend to serve. This number will influence the food you select, as well as how it can be easily served.

2. Select reliable, tested recipes that you understand and that will provide nutritious food.

3. Study the menu, or perhaps the entire day's food, to decide which foods will require more time to prepare. List these in order, according to preparation time. In the beginning, it may be necessary for you to write out a work plan so you can have everything ready at serving time.

4. Organize the work space and equipment to avoid clutter. Put ingredients away after you have used them. Put equipment you have used in or near the sink. Clean up as you work so the kitchen will be orderly by serving time.

on the tongue. A taste bud lives about seven days before a new one replaces it. As a person ages, the taste buds may become less acute. Alcohol, when taken in excess, diminishes the ability of the taste buds to distinguish subtle flavors. Hot peppers and heavy spices overpower subtle flavors in food.

There are only four basic flavors: sweet, sour, salty, and bitter. Yet we can distinguish hundreds of subtle flavors because the basic flavors mix together in different combinations. The range of taste has been compared to the color spectrum. A few primary colors blend into many new shades.

If the tastes of the individual foods in a meal both contrast with and complement each other, enjoyment of the meal is enhanced. The same principle applies to texture and temperature. A combination of foods of subtly contrasting crispness and softness is more enjoyable than a meal of all one texture. Hot foods should be hot and cold foods cold. Nothing is more unappealing than lukewarm mashed potatoes or a lukewarm green salad.

Looks

The first impression a meal makes on the diners is its appearance when served. If the serving dishes or plates are attractively arranged, appetites are increased.

The colors of the foods play the greatest role in the appearance of a meal. Consider the following menu: cream of celery soup, chicken à la king on mashed potatoes, creamed cauliflower, a wedge of iceberg lettuce with mayonnaise dressing, milk,

bread, margarine, and a vanilla pudding. Nutritionally, it is a good meal, but the colors are poorly planned. They are all variants of white! To improve this meal, add some bits of red pimento to the chicken à la king, and serve it on crisp whole-wheat toast. To the mashed potatoes, add some finely minced parsley or onion tops. Serve tomato juice instead of soup. Serve a mixed green lettuce salad with radish and pickled beets grated on top and a French dressing. Cook the cauliflower with soft margarine, then garnish it simply with strips of green pepper. Change the dessert to fresh cold watermelon in season or other fresh fruit. While you are improving the appearance of the meal, you are also improving the balance of its nutrients and textures.

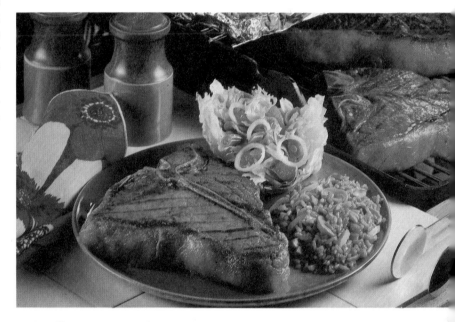

Top: The tastes, textures, and temperatures of a meal should complement each other. *Bottom:* The colors of foods play the greatest role in the appearance of a meal.

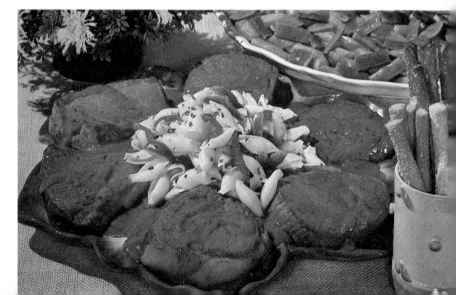

Tables 15-1, 15-2, and 15-3 give menus of meals that are economical, nutritionally well balanced, and attractive to look at. They combine flavors, textures, and temperatures. They are also relatively simple to prepare well and time efficiently. At any of these meals, bread, margarine, and coffee or tea may be served if desired.

Table 15-1 Easy breakfasts, low to liberal cost

CITRUS JUICE READY-TO-EAT WHOLE-GRAIN OR ENRICHED CEREAL BANANA GLASS OF MILK WITH 120 mL (½ C) NONFAT DRY MILK	HALF-GRAPEFRUIT SOFT-BOILED EGG WHOLE-GRAIN OR ENRICHED WHITE TOAST SOFT MARGARINE　MILK
CITRUS JUICE OR WHOLE ORANGE "INSTANT" HOT CEREAL BANANA MILK FORTIFIED WITH NONFAT DRY MILK	WHOLE ORANGE, SLICED SCRAMBLED EGG WITH 60 mL (¼ C) COTTAGE CHEESE TOAST　SOFT MARGARINE MILK
CITRUS FRUIT OR JUICE CHEESE SANDWICH MILK	HALF CANTALOUPE POACHED EGG 2 SLICES CRISP BACON TOAST　SOFT MARGARINE MILK
WHOLE PEELED ORANGE OR ½ GRAPEFRUIT READY-TO-EAT WHOLE-GRAIN OR ENRICHED CEREAL BANANA GLASS OF MILK WITH 120 mL (½ C) NONFAT DRY MILK	CITRUS JUICE QUICK-COOKING OATMEAL RAISINS　CINNAMON 5 mL (1 t) VEGETABLE OIL TOAST　SOFT MARGARINE MILK
CITRUS FRUIT OR JUICE PEANUT BUTTER AND JELLY SANDWICH MILK	FRESH BERRIES IN SEASON WITH 120 mL (4 oz) MILK PANCAKES (made from mix) SOFT MARGARINE　SYRUP MILK

Breakfasts

Breakfast is the most frequently skipped meal of the day. Our usual excuses are that we don't have the time or the energy to prepare breakfast, or that we are trying to lose weight. A good breakfast need not be time consuming to prepare, nor need it be "fattening." Table 15-1 gives examples of quickly prepared and economical balanced breakfasts.

Following are some principles to think about when planning breakfasts.

1. Eat foods you enjoy at breakfast, as long as they provide nutrients in the amounts you need. If you enjoy beans, corn bread, tomatoes, and milk, have them instead of the "usual" breakfast foods.
2. Skipping breakfast does not help you lose weight or control it. If you skip breakfast you may eat a snack later or be so hungry at lunch that you eat too much.
3. Skipping breakfast lowers the morning energy level and attention span. Fatigue sets in more quickly. An adequate breakfast helps you produce a normal morning work load better than either a coffee break or a midmorning breakfast.
4. A good breakfast provides one-fourth to one-third of the day's calories and total nutrients to meet individual needs.

Lunches or brunches

Lunch, too, should be nutritionally well balanced and provide roughly a third of the day's calories and total nutrients. Lunch need not be rich foods that cut down efficiency for afternoon work.

Lunch is a good time to use up nourishing leftovers in soups, casseroles, sandwiches, or salads. The following lunches can be eaten at home, carried to school or work, or bought in restaurants.

Soup: Bean; pea; lentil; potato; vegetable; vegetable and meat; chicken or turkey with vegetables, noodles, or rice; fish or shellfish with vegetables and milk. Add milk, a salad or finger salad, crackers or bread, and fresh fruit or another type of dessert.

Salads: Chef's salad with lettuce, fruit, and cheese; shellfish, poultry, meat, or hard-cooked eggs; mixed raw and cooked vegetables. Serve with hot bread or fruit-nut bread, milk, or caramel custard.

Sandwiches: Fat-trimmed roast lean beef, veal, lamb, ham, fresh pork, chicken, turkey, tuna, sardine, egg, tongue, corned beef, hamburger, liverwurst, frankfurter, cheese, baked bean, or peanut butter. Serve on whole-wheat, rye, pumpernickel, or enriched white bread. Add milk and fresh fruit. Or use a pizza as an open sandwich, a taco, or an enchilada.

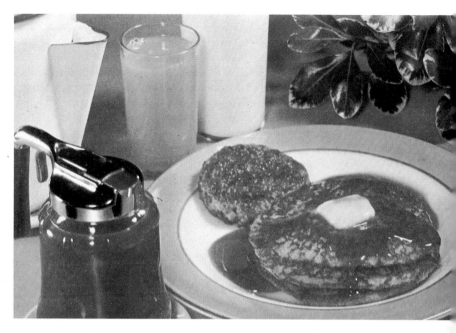

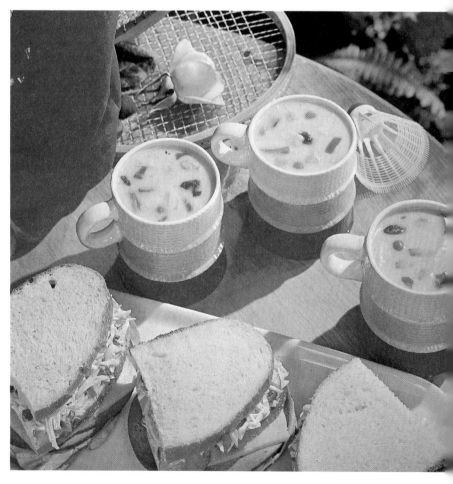

Top: A good breakfast is necessary to a balanced daily diet.

Bottom: Soups and sandwiches for lunch offer an opportunity to use up leftovers.

Table 15-2

Lunches or brunches

> FRESH STRAWBERRIES
> IN SEASON
> WAFFLES
> SOFT MARGARINE
> SYRUP OR MARMALADE
> MILK
>
> ---
>
> MELON IN SEASON
> CHICKEN LIVER OMELET
> BLUEBERRY MUFFINS   MILK
>
> ---
>
> FRESH SLICED PEACHES
> IN SEASON
> SPOON BREAD
> CANADIAN BACON
> CREAMED HONEY   MILK
>
> ---
>
> MIXED FRESH FRUIT COMPOTE
> HAM KABOB
> WITH CHERRY TOMATOES
> BROWN RICE   MILK
>
> ---
>
> WHOLE ORANGE,
> SLICED IN CIRCLES
> HAM   HOT POPOVERS
> HONEY OR PRESERVES
> MILK
>
> ---
>
> ORANGE-GRAPEFRUIT
> COMPOTE
> LEAN BROILED
> HAMBURGER ON TOASTED
> ENGLISH MUFFIN
> MILK
>
> ---
>
> MIXED DRIED FRUIT SOUP
> PANCAKES   HOT SYRUP
> MILK

Casseroles: Meat, fish, or poultry and vegetables with white sauce or cheese sauce and noodles, rice, bulgur, or macaroni products, if desired; macaroni and cheese; spaghetti and meatballs; baked beans. Add milk, bread and spread (if desired), and fresh fruit for dessert. These dishes may be prepared ahead with leftovers and used in the dinner menu.

Sauced dishes: Welsh rabbit; chicken à la king; creamed meat, poultry, or fish. Serve on toast, toasted English muffins, hot biscuits, or toasted corn bread. Add milk, a tossed or fruit salad, and either fruit or deep-dish fruit pie.

Any of the preceding combinations makes a good brunch. For a more elegant touch at brunch, serve a soufflé—cheese, chicken, or fish—or a spoon bread as the main dish. Table 15-2 gives examples of brunches that take more time to prepare than the quick breakfasts in Table 15-1. They are also more costly.

Dinners

The suggested dinner menus in Table 15-3 are moderate in cost. They may be scaled up or down to make lower-cost or higher-cost meals, if you wish. Include liver and fish in any week's dinner menus.

KITCHEN EFFICIENCY

Work centers

Whatever its shape, a kitchen should have good work centers. **Work centers** are needed around the sink, the range, and the refrigerator. Cabinets should be no higher than fingertip height at the base of the top shelf. Some base cabinets have drawers with fingertip control that slide out easily. They save time and energy by allowing you to select any pot or pan with a minimum of stooping.

The height of working surfaces has an effect on your posture, your energy, and even your appearance. Test the correct height for you by standing with your arms forward. Your hands should rest comfortably on the surface, and your back should be straight.

An allowance of a few inches of toe space beneath cabinets improves standing posture. Test your posture by imagining a line from your ear through your shoulder, hip, and ankle. If this line is straight, your posture is good. Your kitchen should have one place where you can sit comfortably with your lower back straight against a chair, and work with your feet and legs under a counter or table.

Large kitchen equipment

A stove, a refrigerator with a freezer, a sink, and cabinets are usually standard equipment in modern apartments, houses for rent, and often houses for purchase. A garbage disposal unit

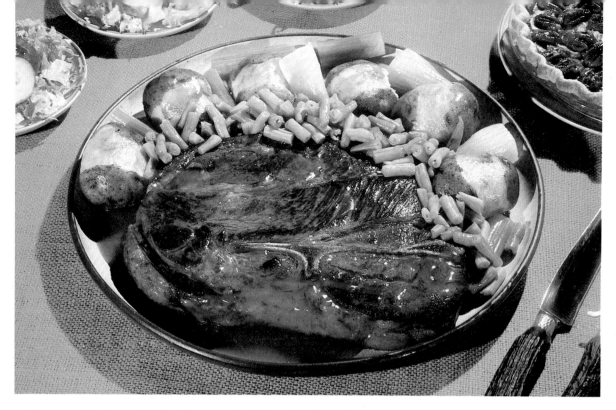

Because of our busy daytime lives—school, jobs, hobbies—dinner is usually the
most relaxed meal of the day.

Table 15-3 **Dinner menus**

ROLLED ROAST BEEF FRANCONIA POTATOES WHOLE BABY CARROTS MIXED GREEN SALAD ANGEL FOOD CAKE MILK	BAKED BEANS CORN MUFFINS OR STICKS BROCCOLI SLICED RED ONIONS ON LETTUCE CHERRY CHEESECAKE MILK	MEAT LOAF SCALLOPED POTATOES SPINACH CUCUMBER, TOMATO, AND LETTUCE SALAD PEACHES MILK
MACARONI AND CHEESE BLACK-EYED PEAS TOSSED GREEN SALAD FRESH FRUIT IN SEASON MILK	SAUTÉED LIVER WITH ONIONS ITALIAN SQUASH GREEN PEAS COLESLAW POTATO IN SKIN GINGERBREAD AND APPLESAUCE MILK	ROAST CHICKEN GIBLET GRAVY BAKED POTATO BRUSSELS SPROUTS GRATED CARROT AND RAISIN SALAD FRESH FRUIT COMPOTE MILK
BROILED FISH BROWN RICE CABBAGE-APPLE SALAD STEWED TOMATOES WITH ONION SUMMER SQUASH LIME PIE MILK	ROAST FRESH PORK BAKED SWEET POTATOES COLLARDS FINGER SALAD BAKED APPLE MILK	

Table 15-4 **Small kitchen utensils and appliances**

BASIC MEAL PREPARATION EQUIPMENT		TO BE ADDED LATER

1 set graduated mixing bowls
1 set graduated saucepans, with handles and tight-fitting lids
1 25.4-cm (10-in) frying pan
1 17.8-cm (7-in) frying pan
1 3.8-L (4-qt) pressure saucepan
1 0.95-L (1-qt) casserole, with lid
1 1.9-L (2-qt) casserole, with lid
2 layer cake pans, 20 × 3.8 cm (8 × 1½ in)
2 22.8-cm (9-in) pie pans
1 muffin pan (Teflon), 12 sections
1 cookie sheet
1 loaf pan (Teflon), 22.8 × 12.7 × 7.6 cm (9 × 5 × 3 in)
1 shallow roasting pan, with rack
1 teakettle
1 coffeepot
1 chopping block (small and light)
1 pastry blender
1 set graduated measuring spoons
1 set graduated measuring cups for dry ingredients
1 set graduated measuring cups for liquid ingredients
1 set: long-handled fork, slotted spoon, solid spoon

1 pancake turner with raised handle
2 spatulas (1 metal, 1 rubber)
1 eggbeater
1 colander
1 sifter
1 rolling pin
1 can opener–bottle opener
1 knife sharpener
1 grater–shredder
1 wide wooden spoon
1 wooden mixing spoon
1 potato masher
1 vegetable brush
1 fruit juicer
1 set of sharp knives: 12.7-cm (5-in) blade French type; 20-cm (8-in) blade for slicing bread and meat; paring knife
1 peeler
4 graduated refrigerator storage containers
1 toaster
1 timer
Pot holders
Dishtowels
Sponges

1 double boiler
1 5.7-L (6-qt) pot, with lid
1 30.5-cm (12-in) iron skillet
1 chicken fryer–Dutch oven
6 custard cups
Casseroles (additional)
1 angel food cake pan
Molds
2 muffin tins, 6 sections each
1 cookie sheet (additional)
1 loaf pan (additional)
1 pancake griddle
1 1.9-L (2-qt) pressure saucepan
1 pr. kitchen shears
1 kitchen stool, with steps
1 food grinder
1 garlic press
Electrical equipment as needed and allowed for in budget

Table 15-5 **Types of materials used in cooking equipment**

MATERIAL	ADVANTAGES	DISADVANTAGES
ALUMINUM	Attractive, strong, light in weight. Next to copper in spreading heat evenly. Cast aluminum better than stamped. Non-toxic and can be used for any kind of food. Moderate in cost. Stain does no harm. . Anodized surfaces provide better wear and heat spread than polished surfaces. Long life.	Thin, cheap grades dent easily and warp. Discolors and pits when alkaline foods are cooked in it or it is cleaned with alkaline compounds.
STAINLESS STEEL	Resists stains. Easy to clean. More useful if copper or other material is used in base to help spread heat. Holds heat well.	Expensive. Conducts heat slowly. Spot-burns, making cleaning hard. Shows water spots.

Table 15-5 (cont.)

MATERIAL	ADVANTAGES	DISADVANTAGES
GLASS	Holds heat well. Attractive. Permits watching food cook. Inexpensive to moderate in cost. Absorbs heat quickly.	Conducts heat slowly. Sensitive to sudden change of temperature. Breaks easily and must be replaced. More loss of riboflavin because of exposure of food to light.
EARTHENWARE	Conducts heat evenly and holds it well. May double to serve food on table. Does not discolor foods and is not discolored by them. Moderate cost.	Absorbs heat slowly. Needs to be glazed. Quick change in temperature may cause breakage. Lead in glaze may be hazardous to health, if not properly fired. Slow cooking destroys some vitamins.
IRON	Cast iron heats evenly, is thick and durable. Holds heat and shape well. Inexpensive. Sheet iron is thin, lightweight, and used as frying pans.	Cast iron heats slowly. Rusts easily when iron oxide coating wears off. Discolors acid foods. Heavy to handle. Sheet iron pans heat unevenly, warp, rust.
TIN	Conducts heat well. Light. Easy to clean. Inexpensive.	Not durable when tin coating is cut. Affected by acid foods. Turns dark, unattractive. Cuts easily. Bends.
NICKEL ALLOY	Strong, attractive. Doesn't scratch or dent easily. Doesn't rust. Affects color, flavor, and keeping properties of food very little, if at all. Extremely easy to keep clean and shining.	Doesn't conduct heat as well as copper. Costs more than aluminum. Will spot unless thoroughly dried.
TEFLON	Teflon is a finish that is coated on aluminum cookware usually, but might be applied to others. Its chief virtues are that foods don't stick in cooking and it requires no scouring. Some companies will replace the Teflon finish, if the guarantee covers it. Gives excellent browning.	Requires special care with hot temperatures or a quick change in temperature, such as pouring cold water in a hot pan. The finish is destructible.
ENAMELWARE	Made by fusing a glasslike material on iron. Best acid-resistant, has several coats of baked-on enamel. Absorbs and holds heat well. Colorful and decorative. Good grade expensive, others moderate in cost. Does not discolor food or affect its taste or keeping properties. Easy to clean.	Conducts heat slowly. Chips when dropped or exposed to sudden temperature change. Hard to clean if food burns. Marked by metal spoons and beaters. Food scorches easily. Some heavy, hard to handle.
COPPER	Quick, even heat. Sturdy. Attractive when kept highly polished.	Expensive. Must be lined with another metal. Tarnishes and discolors readily. Extremely difficult to keep clean.

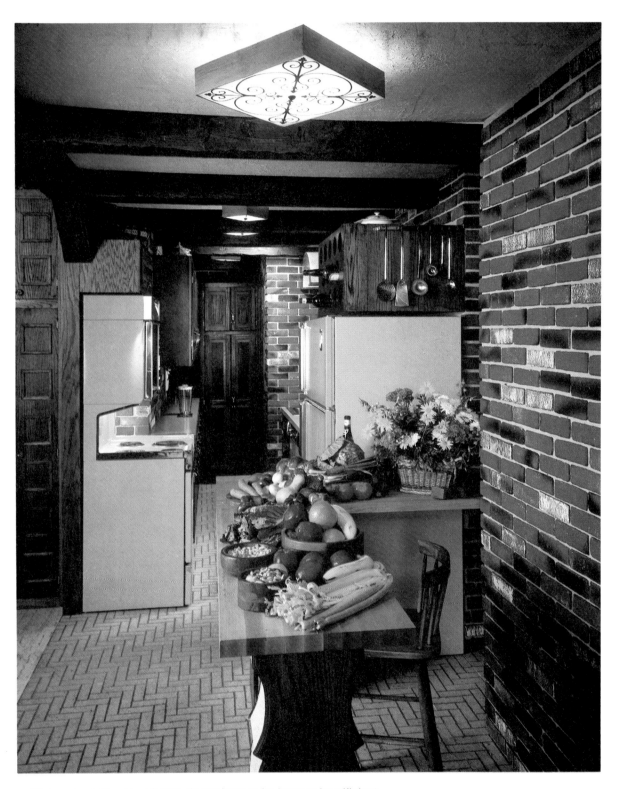

The work centers in a kitchen do not have to be large to be efficient.

and a dishwasher may also be included To keep informed about kitchen equipment, visit large department or specialty stores that sell a variety of brand names and models. Look at them and read the literature on each make and model. Compare and study the pamphlets to see what you are getting in each case for the price. Estimate how much of the price goes into nonessentials. Figure out how much it will cost to operate the equipment.

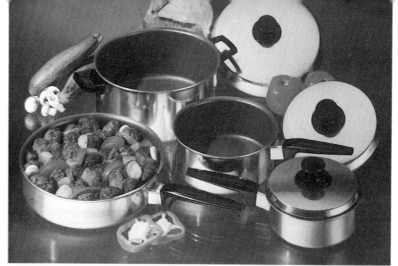

Small kitchen equipment

Various pieces of small equipment are needed to work efficiently in the kitchen (Table 15-4). Ask the following questions when buying small equipment. They will guide you in making wise choices.

1. Can you use this piece of equipment in more than one way?
2. Is the size right for your needs now? Can you continue to use it as your needs change?
3. Is the piece constructed well? Does it have a long life? What is the warranty?
4. Are the materials it is made of appropriate to your needs (Table 15-5)?
5. Is it safe and easy to use when directions are followed? Is it easy to clean?
6. Do you have adequate storage space for it? Will it fit in with what you have?
7. Does the cost justify the expenditure in relation to your total needs for meal preparation and service equipment?
8. Will you be happy to use it for many years, or prefer a newer model at regular intervals?

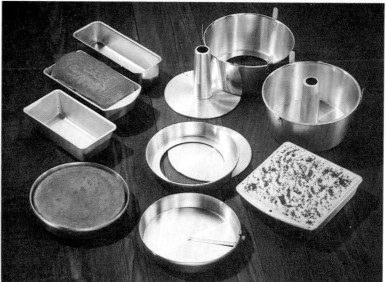

Sturdy, easy-to-clean pots and pans are a lifetime investment.

Pressure saucepans are available in a variety of sizes.

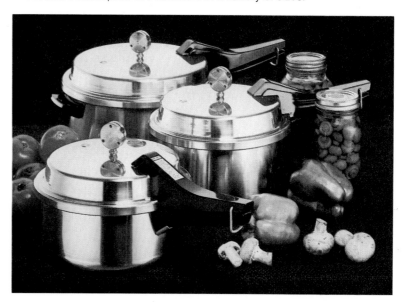

Meal planning

Place of food in the budget   Economical sources of nutrients *Vitamin A   Riboflavin   Thiamin   Niacin   Vitamin C   Protein   Calcium   Iron*   **Planning a menu**   Shopping for food

Factors affecting meal preparation

Decisions and timing   Table service   Taste, texture, temperature   Looks

Meal menus

Breakfast   Lunch or brunch   Dinner

Kitchen efficiency

Work centers   Large kitchen equipment   Small kitchen equipment

1. What are the principles of successful meal management?

2. How would you decide how much of your income could be spent on food?

3. Why is knowledge of nutrition important to meal planning?

4. What do you consider the key points to remember in effective shopping for food? What preliminary preparation do you need to do at home before you shop? What would influence you in selecting the place where you shop? The time? How would you organize your shopping list to be sure you buy all the foods you need for a week?

5. What factors affect meal enjoyment?

6. List the guidelines to meal preparation.

7. What are the types of table service? How can the type of table service affect enjoyment of the meal?

8. What elements add to the attractiveness of meals?

1. Analyze the work habits of someone you know and consider a good manager of family meals. A poor manager? How do these two people differ in their method of operation?

2. Given a gross income of $175.00 per week, plan a weekly food budget if your other fixed expenses include rent (appropriate for your area), a life insurance policy at $15.00 per month, and yearly car insurance payments of $200.00. Discuss the results in class.

VOCABULARY

budget

family service

fixed expenses

flexible expenses

papillae

unit pricing

work center

3. Discuss with your parents how they manage their food budget. Do they have a plan? If so, do you consider it as good as it might be? Could you find a tactful way to share with them what you have learned to help them manage family meals better?

4. Visit department or other stores that exhibit kitchen arrangements. Study the work centers and equipment. Do these kitchen layouts seem designed for efficiency? Explain.

5. Prepare and give a talk to a group or class of elementary school pupils that will help them choose snacks and meals wisely.

CAREER CAPSULES

Television or radio show personality Works in a television or radio studio and "in the field"; conducts informational programs on food and other areas of home economics, demonstrating techniques and products, interviewing guests, performing other duties as required by the format of the program. Required education varies; two- or four-year college education in home economics helpful.

Caterer Works out of own kitchen or company kitchen; provides food and sometimes service people and equipment for small and large, private and public functions, according to customer's request. Required education varies; knowledge of cooking and business administration helpful.

RELATED READING

Iowa Department of Health, Nutrition Service, in cooperation with the Iowa Dietetic Association. *Simplified Diet Manual with Meal Patterns,* 3d ed. Ames, Iowa: Iowa State University Press, 1969. Contains qualitative and quantitative guidelines for basic diets.

Nickell, Paulena, and Jean Muir Dorsey. *Management in Family Living.* New York: John Wiley & Sons, 1967. Covers meal planning, organized shopping, management in food preparation, use of time and energy; compares quality of convenience foods and home-prepared foods.

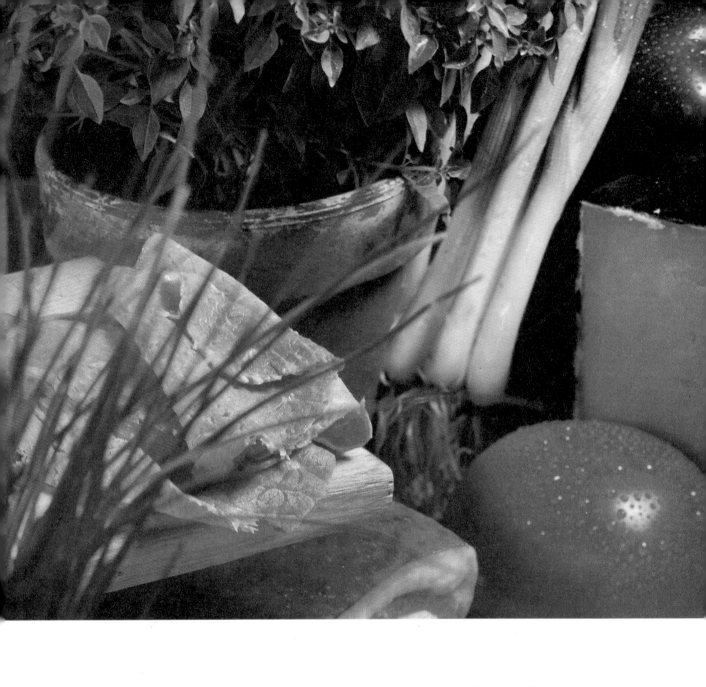

CHAPTER 16

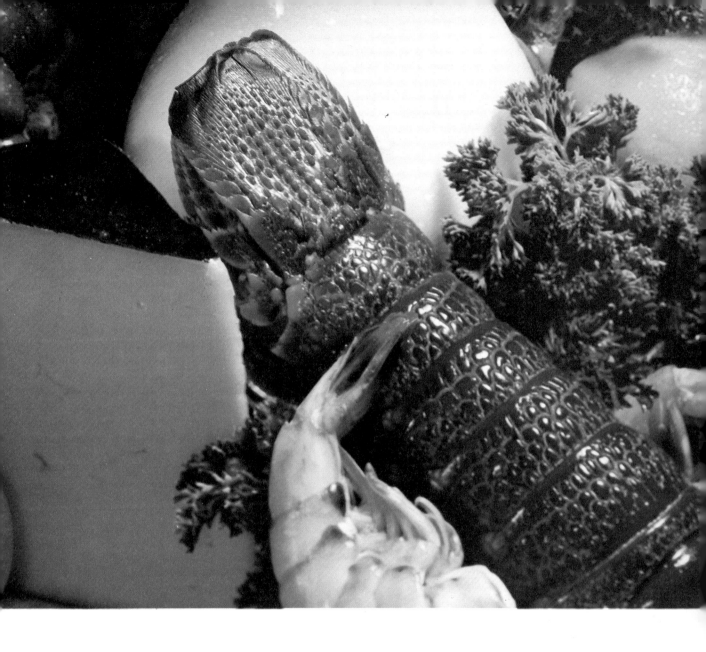

Weight control and diet

WHAT IS DESIRABLE WEIGHT?

The desirable weight for all of us is the weight at which we look and feel best. It varies for each of us, depending on height and bone structure.

Height—weight tables

Ever since we became nutritionally conscious, tables have been published that give recommended weights for people of various heights. The height–weight tables in use today are more realistic than those of the past. However, even they should not be followed slavishly. They should be used only as guidelines. In general, if you are above a recommended weight by 10 percent, you are considered to be overweight. If you are 15 to 20 percent above the recommended weight, you are considered to be obese.

The height-weight tables on page 401 are representative of those in use today. They consider whether a person's bone structure, based on the breadth of chest and hips, is small, medium, or large. The tables give weights and heights for fully clothed persons. Nude weights for women are 4 to 6 pounds less than those given in most tables. Those for men are 7 to 9 pounds less. Thus, if you use the guide and take off a light dress jacket, you are cheating.

The tables give a range of weights to allow for individual differences. Take, for example, a woman 5 feet 6 inches tall. If she has a small frame, her recommended weight ranges from 114 to 123 pounds. If she has a medium frame, the weight range is

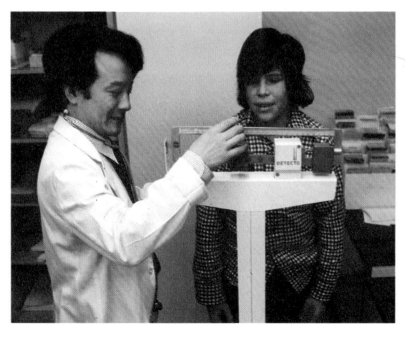

Weight control should be subject to the advice of a physician.

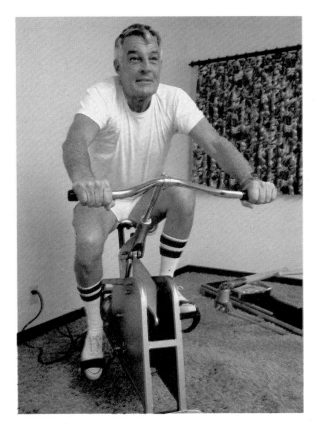
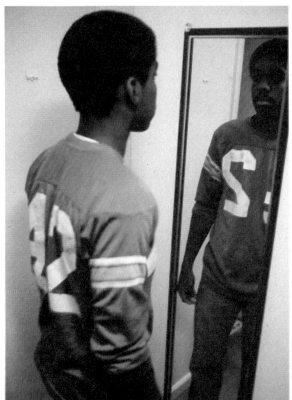

Left: The weight a man reaches at age 25 is usually the one he should maintain for the rest of his life. *Right:* Your appearance in the mirror tells you nearly as much about your weight as the scales tell you.

120 to 135 pounds. If she has a large frame, she should weigh between 129 and 146 pounds.

Notice that ages beyond 25 are not given. The modern concept is that the healthy weight for a woman at 22 years of age should be maintained for the rest of her life. For a man, the desirable weight is the one reached at age 25. Understanding this when we are young helps us gradually reduce the total calories we eat after we reach our full growth. As you grow older and become less active, you need to reduce your caloric intake. Begin watching this now. Notice when you gain the first 2 pounds. That is the signal to start reducing the amount you

eat. Reduce or omit the portions of the least important foods or beverages you are now eating.

Other tests of desirable weight

Dr. Jean Mayer suggests some other practical but "unscientific" tests that individuals can easily do themselves.[1]

Mirror test. According to Dr. Mayer, "looking at yourself naked in a mirror is often a more reliable

[1] Dr. Jean Mayer, *Overweight: Causes, Cost, and Control* (Englewood Cliffs, N.J.: Prentice-Hall, 1968), pp. 29–30. All quotations of Dr. Mayer cited in this chapter are from this work.

guide for estimating obesity than body weight. If you look fat, you probably are fat."

Pinch test. Dr. Mayer observes: "In persons under 50, at least half of the body fat is found directly under the skin." Body fat of this kind is found in the arms, back, calf of legs, abdomen, and below the shoulder blade. Try pinching together the skin and the tissue beneath it on the back of your arm. Is the layer of fold between your fingers more than 1 inch thick? If so, you have too much body fat. If your weight is normal, the pinched flesh should be between ½ to 1 inch thick. If it is well below ½ inch thick, you are abnormally thin.

Overweight is simply the condition of being too fat. Overweight is the number-one nutritional problem in the United States today. Approximately 45 million Americans are overweight. One adolescent in five is overweight. Another one in five is obese. Altogether, almost half the adolescent population weighs more than it should.

Table 16-1 **Relationship of overweight and life span**

	OVERWEIGHT (percent)	EXCESS IN MORTALITY OVER STANDARD RISKS (percent)
MEN	10	13
WOMEN	10	9
MEN	20	25
WOMEN	20	21
MEN	30	42
WOMEN	30	30

Metropolitan Life Insurance Company, "Overweight—Its Significance and Prevention," *The Build and Blood Pressure Study* (Society of Actuaries, 1959).

Table 16-2 **Relationship of disease and mortality in overweight people**

DISEASE	MORTALITY (PERCENT) Men	Women
Heart disease	43	51
Cerebral hemorrhage	53	29
Diabetes	133	83
Digestive system diseases	68	39
Malignant neoplasms (cancer)	16	13

Metropolitan Life Insurance Company, "Overweight—Its Significance and Prevention," *The Build and Blood Pressure Study* (Society of Actuaries, 1959).

Disadvantages of overweight

Physical drawbacks. People who are excessively overweight are more likely than others to suffer from poor health. Their expected life span is shorter (Table 16-1). They are also more likely to become ill and die from certain diseases, including heart disease and cerebral hemorrhage (Table 16-2). Diabetes is three times as common among the obese. Excess weight contributes to digestive and circulatory diseases, high blood pressure, gall stones, gout, some types of kidney disease, liver disease, and degenerative arthritis. It lowers resistance to many other diseases. There is a greater risk from anesthesia in surgery and also in pregnancy and childbirth.

Emotional and social disadvantages. The obese are likely to feel less at ease in social situations. They are likely to feel discriminated against in getting a job and holding it. They are more likely to feel unhappy with the way they look, with the difficulty and the cost of buying clothes, with being the victim of rude jokes.

Contributors to overweight

To understand the cause of a disease is the first step toward curing it. Overweight is not truly a disease, but it does relate indirectly to emotional pain and disease. Let us try to understand some of its major causes.

Obesity is a complex condition with no one cause. There are many causes that often have their roots in childhood. It is much more difficult to control obesity when the causes of it begin so early in a person's life. Knowing this, perhaps young people today will establish eating habits for themselves and their children that will prevent obesity.

The immediate cause of obesity is easy to explain. A person simply eats food with higher calorie content than the body needs or can use. The excess is laid down on the body as fat. However, saying that is like saying that alcoholics drink more liquor than they need or can handle. We must look at the interrelating causes of overweight.

Physiological factors. Dr. Jean Mayer and others have investigated the role that heredity may play in weight problems. They have found obesity genes in the dog, the mouse, and the chicken. The Aberdeen Angus cow will fatten more rapidly than will the Holstein. Because of its heredity, the razorback hog stays slim. The genetic factor in obesity has not been studied in human beings as extensively as in animals, but Mayer thinks it may contribute to obesity in people.

In a Boston study, it was found that about 40 percent of the children who had one obese parent were also obese. Among children who had two obese parents, 80 percent were obese. Only 8 to 9 percent of the children with parents of normal weight were obese. It is not clear that the problem of obesity is hereditary, however. People who are obese simply eat too much food. Eating habits are

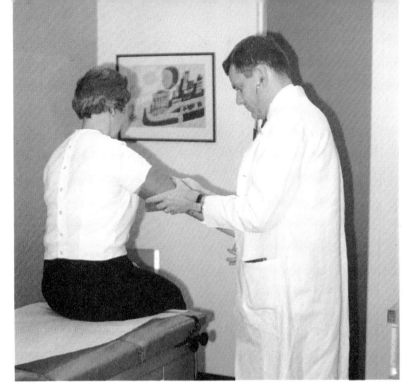

High blood pressure is one of the potential health hazards of overweight.

Overweight occurs when a person eats foods with a higher calorie content than the body needs or can use.

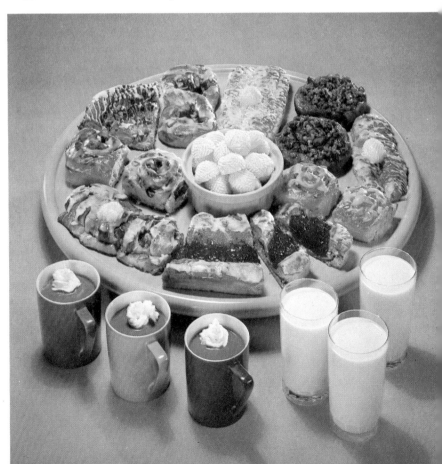

influenced by parents. Obviously obese parents set a bad example.

A favorite excuse given for overweight is improperly functioning endocrine glands or an underactive thyroid gland, but research shows that hormones are connected with overweight in less than 1 percent of the cases. It is interesting to note, however, that sex hormones—not endocrine or thyroxin—help make poultry and livestock fatten more quickly.

Women often gain a lot of weight during pregnancy and menopause. Their appetite increases and they eat more. At the same time, their physical activity often declines. The combination results in excessive weight gain. Puberty, pregnancy, and menopause are periods of glandular change. During each of these periods, therefore, it is wise to watch the diet and the scales and to increase your level of exercise.

We have all seen people who seem to have no signal to stop eating. They eat on and on and gain and gain weight. There may be a problem with a part of their brain called the hypothalamus, or appestat. The hypothalamus may control the switch that turns the appetite off.

Psychological factors. Some people overeat as a result of emotional disturbances. People may feel tense and anxious after a death in the family or of a loved one. They may feel worried or frustrated after a disappointment in love or a separation from home. They may overeat because of loneliness or depression.

Some children are excessively fed by their parents. They are not encouraged to engage in physical activity. The parents may be fulfilling their own emotional needs by making the children overdependent on them.

A recent study of obesity includes the following psychological reasons for obesity.

1. People overeat when they are tense but do not know what is wrong.
2. People overeat as a substitute joy in intolerable life situations.
3. People overeat as a symptom of a deeper emotional illness such as depression or hysteria.
4. People overeat because of an addiction to calorie-rich food.

POOR WEIGHT-CONTROL METHODS

How much you should eat depends partly on your age, sex, and level of activity. This is clearly shown in the RDA table on pages 402-403 The table recommends 2100 calories daily for girls aged 15 to 18 but only 1800 calories for women aged 51 or older. A young man of 15 to 18 should consume 3000 calories daily, but a man aged 51 or older should consume only 2400 calories.

Even these figures may be too high for physically inactive adults. The average woman weighing 121 pounds needs about 1400 calories daily. The average man weighing about 143 pounds needs about 1600 calories daily. As we get older, our metabolic rate slows down. We don't burn up as many calories. However, in many people the appetite remains the same. If older people eat as much as they did when they were young, they will of course gain weight.

Safe ways to control weight are discussed in the next section. However, many people try to deal with the age–activity–calorie triangle in unsafe ways. Because these methods are so common, it is worthwhile to dispel the false hopes the methods offer to the unwary.

Skipping meals

Meal skipping can contribute to overweight. The misinformed think they can lose weight by skipping breakfast or lunch or by eating a poor meal. It doesn't work. Instead of losing weight, they usually gain more. We know this to be true from many studies of both human beings and animals. Many people take multiple vitamin pills as a substitute for a meal. They deceive themselves into thinking that it doesn't matter what or when they eat. Vitamins do not provide the protein, fat, and carbohydrate that the body needs at regular intervals to help maintain normal body functions. Money and vitamins are wasted when they are not used in balance on a team of nutrients that come from food. That is the only role of vitamins in helping provide a good diet.

People who skip meals and eat one large meal become poorly nourished. The body regularly needs a variety of foods to keep it functioning properly. The skipped meals mean that for that period of time the body is operating without the nutrients it requires for normal functioning. Then the large meal overloads the system. This causes fat to store up and thus undermines health and appearance.

Snacking

Snacks and coffee breaks are important to us mainly for social reasons. They should never be regarded as meals. When they become a substitute for a missed breakfast or a poor lunch, they are a health hazard. Indeed, some people don't eat even one well-balanced meal a day. They eat only snacks from morning to bedtime. Both the affluent and the poor suffer nutritionally from this bad habit. Snacks are too often high in calories from sugar and fat and are low in needed nutrients.

On the other hand, the snack or coffee break can contribute to the total nutrients in a well-balanced diet for the day. Some schools, for example, do not allow candy bars or soft-drink machines. Instead, they provide vending machines with fresh fruit, fruit drinks, and milk.

Crash and fad diets

It is possible to lose weight on a crash reducing diet, but strong evidence proves that it is not possible to maintain the weight loss. Consider the constant parade of new reducing diets placed before us. This alone testifies to their failure and to our ignorance of the causes of excessive weight. The new diets usually offer only a new name for an old concept that has falsely attracted and disillusioned millions in the past.

Every once in awhile, a book or article is published describing a "miraculous" way to take off many pounds in a short amount of time. Fad diets often have catchy names and sometimes are endorsed by doctors. Most of them are nothing more than high-fat, low-carbohydrate diets. All have scientifically unsound and misleading suggestions. Any low-carbohydrate, high-fat diet causes weight loss because of water loss in the tissues. That is what makes it so dramatic (55 to 65 percent of body tissues is water). The weight lost on a dramatic shortcut diet has no long-term significance. People usually regain most of the pounds lost because they have not learned good eating habits. For example, Dr. Mayer suggests that "a diet high in fat, where calories . . . can be consumed at will . . . may increase serum cholesterol and precipitate atherosclerosis."

Fad reducing diets merely tempt overweight people to spend their money for a quick shortcut cure. Heavy dieters often talk about their temporary successes —and long-term defeat. Scientific research explains why their hopes are so often defeated.

Reducing drugs and pills

Drugs and pills for reducing are dangerous. Sometimes the consumer may purchase them over the counter. Sometimes an unscrupulous physician will prescribe them.

In June 1965, a federal court fined an advertising agency $50,000 for fraudulently promoting worthless regimen diet pills. The company manufacturing the pills was fined $53,000. The corporation's president was fined $50,000 and sentenced to 18 months in jail.

Many corporations cooperate with the Food and Drug Administration. Others, however, spend great sums of money to fight it. Consumers must always watch out for unscrupulous business practices. They must actively support the agencies working to protect consumer interests.

Another case involves the reprehensible use of the drug digi-talis. Drs. A. A. Kattus, Jr., B. W. Biscoe, A. M. Dashe, and N. H. Davis studied the effects of this drug on six patients who were suspected of having heart disease. The patients were of both sexes and ranged in age from 20 to 50 years. One of them—a healthy, vigorous, athletic 20-year-old girl—was denied a job as flight attendant because of an abnormal electrocardiogram. Her problem triggered the investigation. It was found that she and the five other patients had been taking various combinations of reducing pills containing digitalis, diuretics, thyroxin, amphetamine, and cathartics. Physicians had prescribed all these drugs for weight-reducing purposes.

The investigators point out that the use of such drugs can be ex-

To meet a lowered calorie need, increase the proportion of vegetables to other foods in your diet.

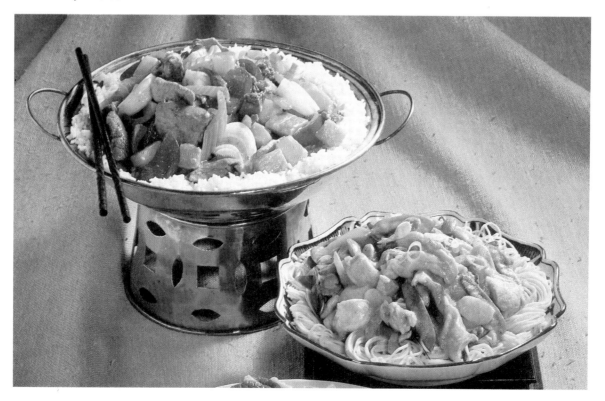

tremely dangerous. The scientists hope that the public will become aware of the dangers and that the doctors who prescribe such drugs will be exposed.

Fasting

Fasting is a popular though ill-advised way of losing weight. It is highly dangerous. It amounts to starvation and can cause death unless closely directed by an alert physician. Preferably, a patient who is losing weight by fasting should be hospitalized.

What happens when a person either goes on a starvation diet or stops eating foods containing protein? The body then breaks down about 30 grams of its own tissue protein a day to perform essential functions that preserve life. The body prefers glucose (carbohydrate) first and then fat as sources of energy. Because they are used first, it is said that carbohydrates and fats spare proteins. Remember that the reserve supply of carbohydrate (glycogen) is used up in 24 to 48 hours. Then fat is burned as energy.

When a person goes without protein or fat, the carbohydrate reserve is used up in 13 hours. If the person has 15 percent body fat at the beginning of a fast, all the fat is used up in five to six weeks. Then protein is broken down to use as energy. Soon after this the person usually dies, because body cells become depleted and cannot perform their duties. In effect, they are starved. The reserve of B vitamins and vitamin C is used up in about a week. This hastens deficiencies and destruction.

Formula diets

Formula diets (or liquid prepared diets) are advertised as having all the nutrients you need. They are also advertised as being a painless, permanent, perfectly safe way of losing and controlling weight. However, users of these diets have reported uncomfortable side effects such as diarrhea and constipation.

A formula diet may help achieve the goal of lost weight for a few weeks, but any diet of only 900 calories a day would do that. To be of permanent benefit, a reducing diet must help the user learn how to keep the desired weight by eating food, not by swallowing a formula like a pill. A formula diet is nothing more than a delaying tactic. It only postpones the day when you must learn to eat wisely.

ACHIEVING AND MAINTAINING DESIRABLE WEIGHT

Obesity and overweight can be cured, but it is much better if you prevent these problems before they start. A recent report about obesity emphasized that prevention is better than the cure.[2] Preventive care should be taken throughout childhood and particularly at any stage of growth when there is a physiological increase in body fat. There is an increase in body fat, for example, during the last growth spurt in adolescence.

If you decide you must go on a diet, have a physical examination by a competent physician. You can then find out the exact state of your health. If your weight is excessive, you may need medical guidance. You may also need to work with a nutritionist to whom the doctor may refer you.

Examine your reasons or motives for reducing. They must be strong if you are to succeed. When you decide the goal is worth the effort, stay with your decision and you will win. You might use the same approach as the Weight Watchers organization. It is similar to that of Alcoholics Anonymous. Eat what you need and no more, one day at a time, and don't worry about tomorrow. The tomorrows fall into place when you resolutely keep your routine today.

When you attain a normal weight, maintain it for at least two years without any relapses. Research shows that this is basic to maintaining a normal weight. It gives you confidence and assures you of future success.

Safe dieting

The safest and most permanently effective method of weight reduction is simply to eat a miniature

---

[2] E. M. Widdowson and M. J. Dauncy, *Nutrition Reviews, Present Knowledge in Nutrition*, 4th ed. (New York and Washington, D.C.: The Nutrition Foundation, 1976).

Table 16-3 Balanced weight-reducing and maintenance diets

	1200-CALORIE DIET			1800-CALORIE DIET
		Approximate calories		
BREAKFAST	½ grapefruit	50	65	1 whole orange
	28 g (1 oz) shredded wheat	90	197	1 egg scrambled with
	1 slice whole-wheat bread	60		60 mL (¼ c) low-fat cottage
	5 mL (1 t) safflower-oil soft			cheese and 5 mL (1 t)
	margarine	33		vegetable oil
	240 mL (8 oz) skim milk	90	90	240 mL (8 oz) skim milk
	Coffee or tea	0	60	1 slice whole-grain toast
			33	5 mL (1 t) soft special
				margarine
			18	5 mL (1 t) jam or marmalade
			0	Coffee or tea
	Total	323	463	Total
LUNCH	Tuna fish salad: 1 tomato,		165	Lean ham sandwich
	10 g (2 t) mayonnaise,			(fat-trimmed) on
	lettuce, diced celery,		60	1 slice whole wheat or
	parsley, 56 g (2 oz)			rye bread
	drained tuna	153	95	180 mL (¾ c) coleslaw with
	1 slice rye bread	60		10 mL (2 t) each safflower
	1 apple	70		oil and vinegar
	240 mL (8 oz) skim milk	90	90	240 mL (8 oz) skim milk or
	Coffee or tea	0		buttermilk
			60	½ cantaloupe
			0	Coffee or tea
	Total	373	470	Total
DINNER	½ broiled chicken breast	155	160	112 g (4 oz) baked fish fillet
	1 ear corn, 5 mL (1 t) soft		90	1 medium baked potato
	margarine	103	33	5 mL (1 t) soft margarine
	120 mL (½ c) broccoli,		40	120 mL (½ c) diced carrots with
	seasoned with 2.5 mL (½ t)			2.5 mL (½ t) margarine
	vegetable oil, onion		60	Tossed salad with 2.5 mL (½ t)
	flakes, celery salt, salt,			vegetable oil, 7.5 mL (1½ t)
	pepper	41		lemon juice, seasoning
	240 mL (8 oz) skim milk or			to taste
	buttermilk	90	178	180 mL (¾ c) low-fat yogurt,
	Coffee or tea	0		60 mL (¼ c) frozen
	1 orange	65		strawberries
			0	Coffee or tea
	Total	454	561	Total
	Total calories for day[1]	1150	1494	Total calories for day[1]

[1] The 1200-calorie and 1800-calorie totals may be made up as desired. Recommended snacks are raw vegetables and nonfat milk.

version of a well-balanced diet of three meals a day, skipping none. It takes 3500 calories to gain 0.45 kg (1 lb). Therefore, to lose a pound of weight a week, simply drop off 500 calories each day. This adds up to 4 pounds lost in a month and 13 pounds in three months. An enormous incentive! It is a safe way for growing young people to lose weight. An adult can safely lose 2 pounds per week by eating 1000 calories less per day.

Your diet should consist of those foods that contain all the essential nutrients. Look again at Table 14-5. It shows "hidden" calories from fat in common foods. Drop from your diet high-fat and high-sweet foods that contain unnecessary calories. To meet your lowered calorie need, increase the amount of vegetables and fresh fruits in your diet. Drink nonfat milk and eat low or nonfat cheese, poultry, fish, lean meat, and whole-grain breads or cereals.

This is a healthful diet plan that can work for you on a long-term basis. At the same time, the plan educates you in methods of sound eating. It helps you understand how a variety of foods can help you maintain the weight you desire throughout life.

There are two excellent diet patterns you could follow, according to your needs (Table 16-3). The 1200-calorie diet offers a total of 89 grams of protein for the day. The 1800-calorie diet offers 80 grams of protein. Each diet generously meets your needs, and the loss of weight on either diet is so gradual that it does not result in looseness of skin, wrinkles, or undue risk to health and appearance. It is very important to take a long-term view. Do not allow yourself to be in a hurry and seek a crash short cut.

Following are some hints for safe dieting.

1. Depend on raw and cooked vegetables and fruits in each meal for bulk. They help you feel full

When you are on a reducing diet, have fruit for dessert.

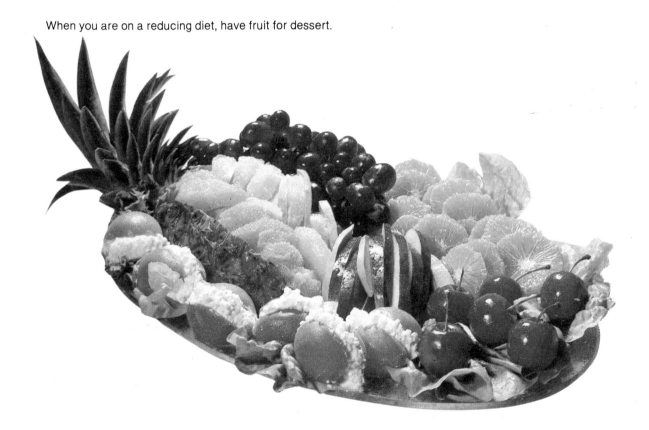

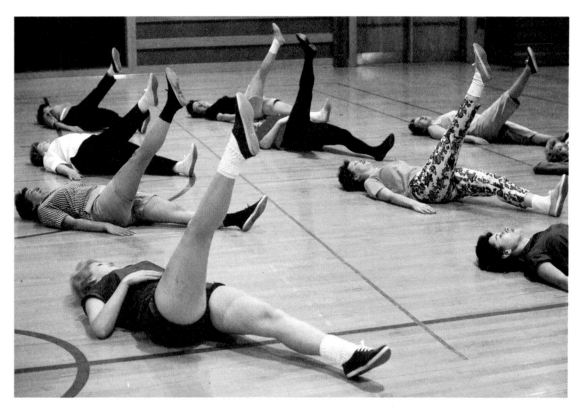

Exercise helps to control weight.

and satisfied without adding many calories to your diet.

2. For dessert, use fruit with no added sugar.

3. In seasoning vegetables, use such fat as vegetable oil or safflower margarine.

4. In each meal, use a nonfat milk or milk product in some form.

5. Select a snack—if you have one—that fits into your calorie allowance and nutrient need.

6. Eat an egg a day for its wide variety of nutrients, unless your physician disapproves.

7. Follow the suggestions for preparing food in Unit 2 and Chapter 17. These will help you in diet control and also in prevention of heart disease.

8. Stop eating before you feel full. If you plan to have dessert, allow yourself to feel a little hungry by eating less in the main meal.

When you have reached normal weight and can maintain it, allow yourself small servings of your favorite foods at intervals. You need not give up favorite foods completely. Simply eat only small amounts of them if they are rich and fattening.

Weigh yourself before breakfast every four days. Keep a record of your weight. If you have gained, take the excess weight off at once. Your aim is success and you can achieve it. Watch your diet. Watch your scales. Watch your mirror. Decide on exercise you can maintain each day or varied physical activities you enjoy.

Value of exercise

A key factor in the prevention and control of obesity is exercise. It is not enough to be concerned with caloric intake. We must be equally concerned with energy output. Some people doubt whether exercise expends much energy. They think that exercise only increases your appetite and your food intake. Dr. Jean Mayer points out that both of these ideas are harmful myths. Anyone who exercises every day knows how exercise helps to take off weight. This has been demonstrated with both animals and people, of all ages.

Regular exercise adds up collectively to wide benefits. For example, speeding up the circulation through exercise achieves the following.

1. Fat that has piled up in the bloodstream is burned up, thus possibly helping prevent heart or circulatory disease.
2. Waste products are eliminated from cell tissues and the body.
3. Nutrients and oxygen are carried to cell tissues more vigorously.
4. Muscle tissue is strengthened and built up.
5. Fatigue is lessened, and physical endurance is increased
6. Emotional well-being is promoted.
7. Appearance is improved or maintained.

Roughly, we burn about 1 calorie per hour per pound of body weight for ordinary activities. Swimming requires more energy and burns more calories than most other activities. Sleeping, of course, requires the least energy. A person who weighs 120 pounds and walks 3 miles in an hour burns 180 calories for the walk. If the person swam the crawl for only 15 minutes, that person would burn about 133 calories.

RECAP

What is desirable weight?
Height-weight tables   Other tests of desirable weight
Mirror test   Pinch test

What is overweight?
Disadvantages of overweight   *Physical drawbacks*
Emotional and social disadvantages   Contributors to overweight   *Physiological factors   Psychological factors*

Poor weight-control methods
Skipping meals   Snacking   Crash and fad diets
Reducing drugs and pills   Fasting   Formula diets

Achieving and maintaining desirable weight
Safe dieting   Value of exercise

VOCABULARY

appestat
crash diet
endocrine glands
fad diets
fasting
formula diets
hypothalamus
obesity
overweight

1. Analyze your weight. Do you consider yourself to be overweight? Obese? If so, list the different things you have tried to do about it. Are they sound? Do you think you need a new plan for improvement?

2. Explain why excessive overweight is undesirable.

3. What are the causes of overweight and obesity? Do any of them affect you?

4. Why is it so necessary to be concerned about exercise as well as calorie intake? Do you think you get enough exercise every day? If not, make a plan to improve.

5. Give your evaluation of meal skipping, snacks, and coffee breaks on the basis of the latest medical findings and also your own experience and observation. How would you advise a person who is overweight to manage these eating habits?

6. List the pitfalls of crash reducing diets. Which crash diets have you tried, if any? Did you get the permanent results you sought? Why do most crash diets fail? Why are most of them dangerous? Evaluate a diet scheme that you read about in a popular magazine or newspaper or heard described.

7. Prepare a plan to attain desirable weight and a diet for maintaining that weight the rest of your life. What are the advantages of this plan?

APPLYING AND SHARING

1. Research the latest literature on reducing and weight control. Be prepared to report to the class on your findings. Evaluate your findings. List any fad diet plans for weight control that you find.

2. Describe in your notebook for a two-week period all advertising of products for weight reduction you come across on television and radio and in newspapers and magazines. What are the products advertised? The prices? The psychology used to persuade you to use the product? How has this study helped you evaluate such advertising? How would you help a friend understand the waste of money and danger to health in what is presented? Discuss this problem. Draw conclusions.

3. Plan a week's menus that would meet your nutritional needs and at the same time enable you to reduce 1 to 2 lb (0.45 to 0.90 kg) of weight per week.

4. Plan well-balanced meals for a week for two adults and a three-year-old child that would be enjoyable to eat and would help each maintain normal weight.

5. Cooking:

    a. Prepare and serve at school and again to your family one breakfast, one lunch, and one dinner, using menus you planned for item 3.

    b. Prepare snacks for a child and an adult that fit in with what you have learned about weight control for yourself.

CAREER CAPSULES

Classroom home economics teacher Works in a school, university, vocational school; teaches one or more of the various courses in home economics. Four-year college education in home economics required as well as other certification demanded by the employing institution.

Food service worker Works in a restaurant, school cafeteria, hospital kitchen, catering establishment; may prepare, serve, or clean up after meals. High school or vocational education helpful; on-the-job training essential.

RELATED READING

Mayer, Jean. *Overweight: Causes, Costs, and Control.* Englewood Cliffs, N.J.: Prentice-Hall, 1968. Presents problems that relate to obesity for all age groups and offers suggestions for treatment.

Pillsbury's Family Weight Control Cookbook. Pillsbury Publications, 1970. Contains useful information on weight reduction, nutrition, and food purchasing and preparation.

Present Knowledge in Nutrition, 4th ed. New York: The Nutrition Foundation, 1976. Chapter 3 describes the physiological nature of fat cells in relation to obesity throughout the life cycle.

Siegel, Murray J., and Dolores Van Keuren. *Think Thin Manual and Cookbook.* Middlebury, Vt.: Paul S. Eriksson, 1971. Discusses altering and improving eating habits while losing weight on three nutritionally balanced meals a day.

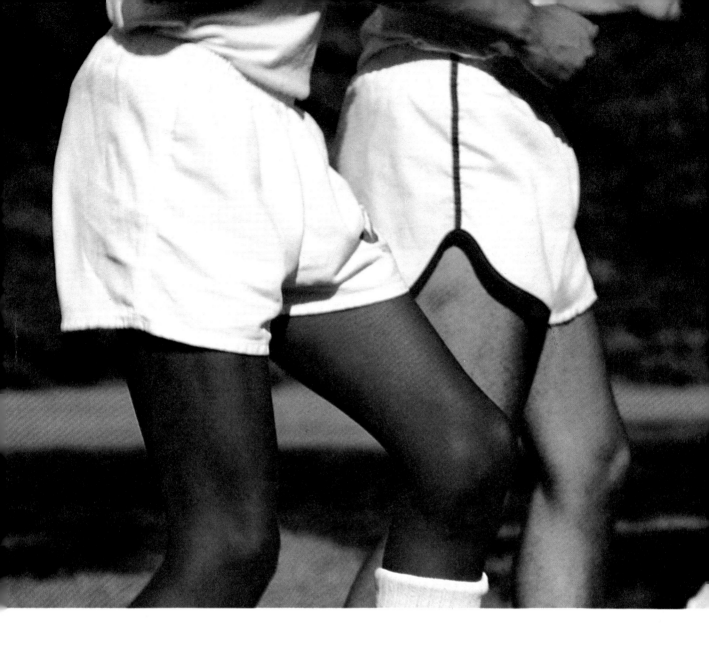

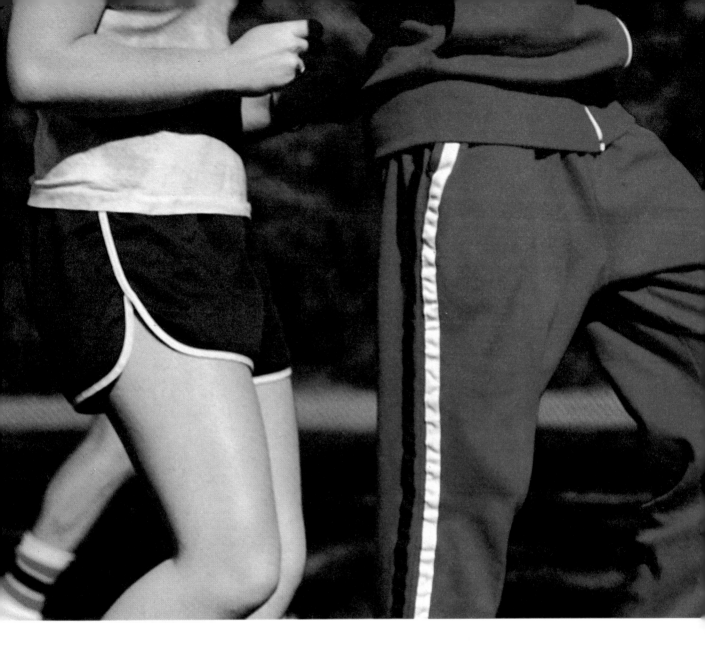

CHAPTER 17

Heart-circulatory disease and diet

After studying this chapter, you will be able to

- identify the factors that contribute to cardiovascular disease.
- explain how your eating habits can contribute to the prevention and control of heart and circulatory disease.
- determine how people involved in planning and preparing meals can contribute to the protection of people's health.
- plan and prepare low-fat meals containing polyunsaturated fat for yourself and members of your family.

Heart and circulatory diseases are the number-one cause of death in the United States (Table 17-1). They are not limited to the aged. They occur in all age groups. Autopsies performed on young soldiers killed in the Korean and Vietnam wars showed that a shocking number of these young men had advanced arterioscle-rosis. In other words, the inside walls of their arteries were abnormally thick.

Over a half-million persons per year in our country lose their lives to arteriosclerosis and almost that many to cerebral hemorrhage (stroke). Many of those struck down are still in the most vigorous and productive years of life. Recovering from an attack takes a person weeks, months—even years. Physicians tell us that the working hours lost because of this disease make working hours lost by strikes and work stoppage seem insignificant.

Why? And what can be done about it? Threads of the answers run through the chapters on food groups in Unit 2. In this chapter we will study the contributing causes and focus on the role that the diet plays in preventing and controlling cardiovascular (heart and circulatory) diseases.

What is coronary atherosclerosis?

First, let us take a look at the heart itself. The heart is a small muscle about the size of your fist.

The expense, waste, and tragedy of heart and circulatory diseases may be decreased by good nutrition.

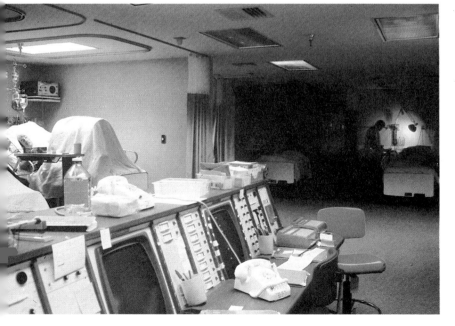

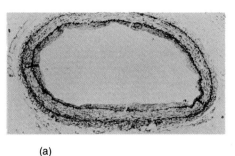
(a)

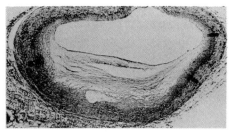
(b)

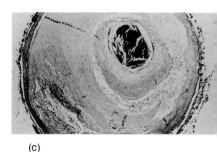
(c)

Figure 17-1   Plaques are fatty deposits in an artery. (a) Normal artery. (b) Plaques developing in the artery. (c) Blood clot has formed in the artery.

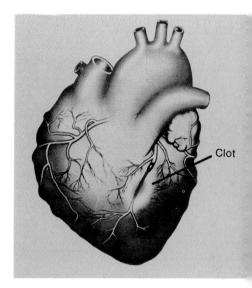

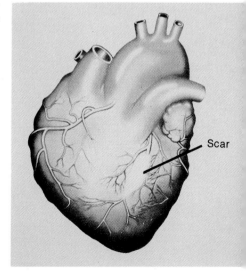

Figure 17-2   If a person survives a heart attack, a scar is formed on the heart muscle. *Top:* The clot causes the heart attack. *Bottom:* Scar tissue is formed.

Clot

Scar

It is only 1/200 of the body weight. But look at the work it does! Every 24 hours, the heart pumps blood through circuits equal in length to three times the circumference of the earth. The tissue along the entire route has to be kept in good condition. Therefore, to stay in good working order, the heart muscle consumes ten times the nourishment of other tissue.

Coronary atherosclerosis underlies most heart attacks. The arteries that supply the heart with blood become hardened. Arteries in the heart and in other parts of the body build up fatty plaques, which can gradually plug up the arteries, interfering with circulation.

Role of plaques in heart attacks

A team of San Francisco scientists has studied the coronary arteries of persons autopsied after heart attacks. The studies were conducted by Meyer Friedman, a cardiologist, and G. J. Vanden Bokenkamp, a physiologist, of the Harold Brunn Institute at Mount Zion Medical Center. Their work has given us clues about the way plaques are formed.

Figure 17-1a shows a healthy artery. Artery walls are normally smooth. They consist of an inner layer of tissue, a layer of muscle, and an outer covering. Figure 17-1b shows fatty plaques formed inside the artery. In Figure 17-1c the situation is more advanced. The artery has been blocked by a clot that blocks the passage of the blood. A coronary occlusion, or heart attack, occurs.

The San Francisco researchers discovered that plaques are composed mainly of fat, cholesterol, and calcium. They found that 39 of the 40 cases examined had ruptured. The debris was not pus, as in an abcess, but chalky fat.

When the artery is plugged by a clot, the heart is deprived of oxygen and nutrients. This condition can often be relieved if a competent heart specialist sees the patient immediately. If the patient survives the attack, a scar is formed (Figure 17-2). If the heart is strong, the person can resume a normal life, within limits.

Medically, there are several other names for heart attacks. Coronary thrombosis is caused by a blood clot within a blood vessel. Myocardial infarction results from death of localized tissue in the heart, caused by

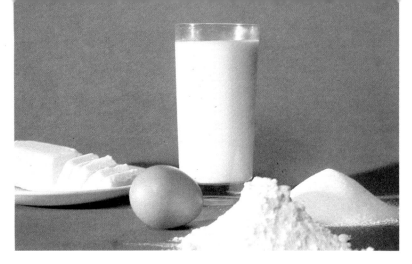

Many doctors restrict the amounts of eggs and butter, and substitute skim milk for whole milk in diets of heart and circulatory disease patients.

blockage of blood vessels by a blood clot. If the clot forms in the brain, the attack is called a stroke. If it forms in a limb (usually a leg), phlebitis is the name given the disease.

A. C. Guyton, a physiologist, notes that almost half of all human beings die of arteriosclerosis. Two-thirds of the deaths are caused by thrombosis or hemor-

Regular physical examination and attention to medical advice can help prevent and control heart and circulatory diseases.

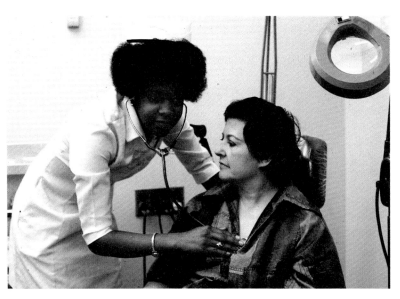

rhage of vessels in the brain, kidneys, liver, gastrointestinal tract, and limbs.

Contributors to heart and circulatory diseases

Cholesterol. Cholesterol may be one factor in the diet that causes heart attacks, although heart attacks occur in some people with low serum cholesterol and do not occur in some people with high serum cholesterol (reread the section on cholesterol in Chapter 14). Research shows that severe diabetes or a poorly functioning thyroid gland each can cause great quantities of cholesterol to be deposited on artery walls. Studies show that large amounts of cholesterol are made in the artery walls of animals. Thus serum cholesterol is not necessarily related to the amount of cholesterol in a person's diet.

Studies of fat have led to a real breakthrough in solving the riddle of the effect of cholesterol in the diet. In Oslo, Norway, for example, a cardiologist made a five-year study of 412 persons who had suffered a myocardial infarction. The group was divided equally. One unit served as a control and ate as usual. The other experimental unit of 206 people ate a strictly supervised diet. Their total fat intake was slightly over 40 percent of their total calories, which is considered high by professional nutritionists and the American Heart Association. However, their intake of saturated fat was quite low and of linoleic acid quite high.

People in the experimental unit were given only a little red meat, from which all visible fat had been removed. Instead of red meat, they ate poultry, fish, shellfish, and whale. They had one egg a week. They were not allowed any whole milk, cream, butter, margarine, lard, hydrogenized shortening, or olive oil. The fat they used was chiefly soybean oil. The experimental diet added up to 92 grams of protein a day (368 calories), 104 grams of fat (936 calories), and 269 grams of carbohydrate (1076 calories). The diet, eaten at home, was supervised by dietitians. What was the result? The experimental group had only 80 relapses, or sudden deaths, as compared with 120 in the group who ate as they pleased. In other words, there was a 30 percent survival rate among those who ate the controlled diet. Dr. Jean Mayer and others believe that controlled diets may be as valuable in preventing heart attacks as in treating them.

Heredity. Studies reveal that heredity is a factor in heart disease. Some people seem to have an inborn tendency to high blood serum cholesterol, despite low amounts of cholesterol in their diet. A. C. Guyton points out that this trait is sometimes carried in the dominant gene. Therefore, once the trait enters the family, the disease can be expected to occur frequently in the family's descendants.

Overweight. It is clear that overweight contributes to cardiovascular disease. Overweight persons are twice as likely to die from coronary disease as those with normal weight (review Chapter 16).

Age. Age is a factor in heart disease (Table 17-1). Although no age group is immune to heart disease, the mortality rate is higher with age, especially at middle age and later.

Table 17-1 Death rate from arteriosclerosis (per 100,000 population)

AGE		MALE	FEMALE
	Birth–1 yr.	0.3	0.2
	1–4	0.1	0.0[1]
	5–9	0.1	0.0[2]
	10–14	0.1	0.1
	15–19	0.4	0.2
	20–24	1.4	0.6
	25–29	4.7	2.0
	30–34	17.3	4.8
	35–39	53.6	11.1
	40–44	126.0	25.8
	45–49	257.1	50.8
	50–54	449.4	104.4
	55–59	725.5	202.3
	60–64	1099.2	399.8
	65–69	1702.8	714.5
	70–74	2322.2	1218.5
	75–79	3237.1	2018.7
	80–84	4729.1	3458.1
	85 and over	7754.0	6736.1

Facts on the Major Killing and Crippling Diseases in the United States Today (New York: National Health Education Committee, Inc., 1966). Figures are 1963 statistics.
[1]Less than .0.05 percent per 100,000 population.
[2]Zero rate: that is, no deaths.

Sex. Statistics show that men are affected by heart disease earlier in life, more severely, and in greater numbers than women. During and after menopause, however, women are vulnerable. The decrease in female hormones is considered the cause. The male hormones in women may accelerate the deposit of plaques inside the arteries, but the female hormone may protect against the formation of plaques.

Inactivity. Not enough regular exercise is a factor in the abnormal clotting of blood. Fat can pile up in the bloodstream following a fat-rich meal. Exercise helps burn up the fat, thus helping prevent the formation of plaques.

After a heart attack, scar tissue—sometimes called dead tissue—is formed. Exercise helps the heart muscle build corollary arteries to take over a part of the work once done by the healthy artery and its tinier branches. Exercise helps strengthen the whole heart muscle and all other body tissues. It improves a person's ability to relax and sleep normally. It also adds to the person's sense of well-being.

Stress and tension. Stress and tension seem to be factors leading to heart disease in some people. We live in a swiftly moving world filled with competition, pressures, changes in life styles, and anxiety. Each person must learn to cope with the stresses and strains in our society and in the family. The blood vessels constrict under emotional stress. This condition seems to be favorable to the formation of plaques.

On the other hand, soothing the emotions enables the blood vessels to relax. They become more elastic instead of tight. The effects of smoking, however, are puzzling. Smokers claim to derive from smoking emotional satisfaction that is relaxing. Yet physiologists find that smoking makes the blood vessels constrict, which favors the formation of plaques in arteries.

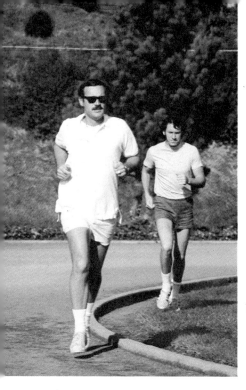

Regular exercise strengthens the heart and burns up fat.

DIET AND THE HEART

One of the most important goals in meal planning should be the control of diet to help prevent heart and circulatory diseases. A good diet for controlling heart disease varies only slightly from a good diet for regular nutritional purposes (Table 17-2).

As a young person, you can prevent or deter the dietary conditions that contribute to heart disease.

1. Establish a meal pattern and develop eating habits that provide the amount and balance of nutrients you need daily.
2. Establish a calorie level that includes the nutrients you need but at the same time maintains your desired weight.
3. Lower your total intake of fat to about 30 percent of the total calories.

Food selections

Fats. The correct proportions of different kinds of fat are still undecided. The American Heart Association recommends about twice as much polyunsaturated fat as saturated fat. Dr. Frederick Stare, a professor of nutrition at Harvard University, suggests a ratio of 1 to 1. The 1977 national dietary goals recommended that the calories from fat be divided equally among saturated, mono-unsaturated, and polyunsaturated fats. Each would comprise 10 percent of the total calorie intake for a total of 30 percent of the intake.

If you wish to increase the amount of polyunsaturated fat in

Everyone, not only heart patients, should eat recommended proportions of saturated, mono-unsaturated, and polyunsaturated fats.

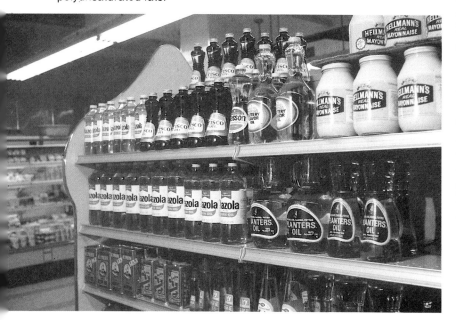

Table 17-2 Daily meal plans for fat-controlled diets

FOODS FOR THE DAY	1200 CALORIES	1800 CALORIES	2000–2200 CALORIES	2400–2600 CALORIES
SKIM MILK	480 mL (2 c)	480 mL (2 c)	480 mL (2 c)	720 mL (3 c)
VEGETABLES (at least one serving of yellow or leafy green vegetables)	3 or more servings	4 or more servings	ad lib (4 or more servings)[1]	ad lib (4 or more servings)[1]
FRUITS (at least one serving of citrus fruit or juice)	3 servings	3 servings	ad lib (5–6 servings)[1]	ad lib (6 servings)[1]
BREADS AND CEREALS	4 servings	7 servings[2]	ad lib (8–10 servings)[1]	ad lib (10–12 servings)[1]
MEAT, FISH, OR POULTRY	168 g (6 oz)	168 g (6 oz)	168–224 g (6–8 oz)	168–224 g (6–8 oz)
EGGS	3 or less per week	3 or less per week	3 or less per week	3 or less per week
FATS AND OILS	25 mL (1⅔ T)	45 mL (3 T)	45 mL (3 T) or more[3]	60 mL (4 T) or more[3]
SOFT MARGARINE	5 mL (1 t)	15 mL (1 T)	15 mL (1 T) or more	15 mL (1 T) or more
SUGARS AND SWEETS	none	30 mL (2 T)[4]	ad lib 60 mL (4 T)[4]	ad lib 75 mL (5 T)[4]

American Heart Association, *Note to the Physician* (New York: American Heart Association, 1968).

[1] Number of servings following *ad lib* were used to calculate diet plans.

[2] Some nutritionists prefer extra servings of vegetables, fruits, and skim milk, rather than so much bread-cereal.

[3] One additional tablespoon of oil will yield a diet containing 35% calories from fat and 13% calories from linoleic fatty acids.

[4] If simple sugars are to be restricted, substitute breads and cereals.

the daily diet, allow 15 to 30 mL (2 to 3 T) of fat per person, depending on the age and needs of each person. Safflower oil is about 38 percent higher in linoleic acid than corn, cottonseed, and soybean oil. This means that 30 mL (2 T) of safflower oil provide the same amount of linoleic acid as 45 mL (3 T) of the other oils mentioned and 120 fewer calories from fat.

Use spreads that are high in linoleic acid. The highest amount is in margarine made with liquid safflower oil added after hydrogenation (review Table 14-1). The first ingredient listed on the label should be liquid safflower oil, corn oil, or another oil high in linoleic acid. The ingredient listed first is more plentiful than other ingredients. For practical suggestions on how to achieve a balance

of fat in the diet, reread Chapter 14.

Meat. Protein foods should be included in each meal (also see Eggs, Legumes). Chicken, turkey, fish, and veal are the meats lowest in saturated fat and total fat. When using red meats in the diet you must be selective. Beef, lamb, pork, and processed foods made from them are quite high in saturated fat. For beef, choose rump

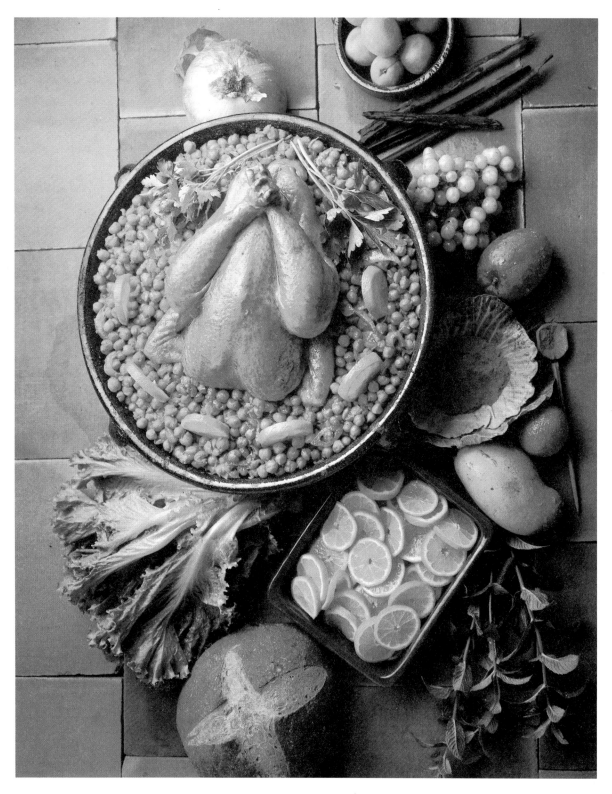

Legumes and meats low in saturated fats are advised for people concerned about heart disease.

or round roasts, or use these cuts as steaks or as ground meat. Use almost any cut of veal. For pork, use sirloin roast, chops, fresh center cut of steak, or ham. Trim the fat off the meat before cooking. Remove visible fat as you eat it. Roast, broil, or cook with moist heat. Skim off all fat and use the brown drippings. A serving of meat cooked is 84 g (3 oz).

Eggs. Some heart patients may eat all the egg whites desired because they contain no cholesterol or fat. But patients on restricted sodium diets may not eat egg whites because they have a high sodium content. The American Heart Association recommends two eggs a week. Few foods give such a variety of nourishment for so few calories. Remember that the cholesterol in one egg yolk is about one-fourth to one-eighth of the amount the body needs daily. The body will make cholesterol if it is not provided in the diet.

Legumes. Eaten in meals with milk, cheese or eggs, legumes like peas provide complete protein. The individual can determine the kind and amount of legumes that he or she can tolerate. Among the nuts, the plain dry-roasted kind (without oil) is best. The walnut is highest in linoleic acid.

Fruits and vegetables. Most vegetables and fruits help prevent and control heart and circulatory disease. They contain no cholesterol and little or no fat. A rich source of vitamin C in every meal helps to maintain the tensile strength of blood vessels and to hold cells together. Heart patients especially need the benefit of generous amounts of vitamins C and A. These vitamins are found

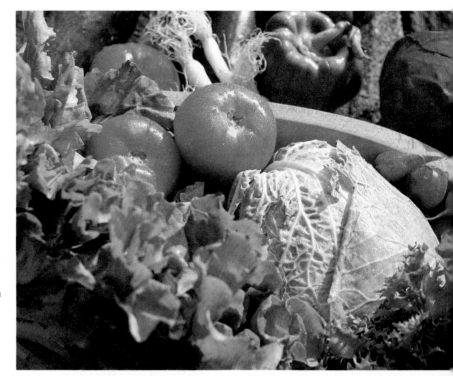

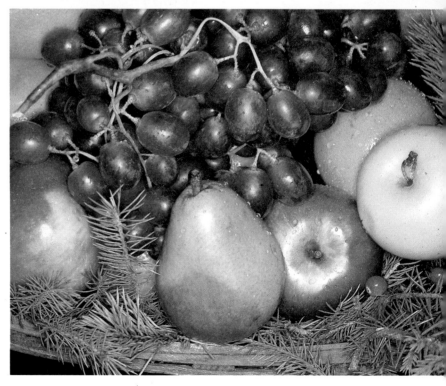

Vegetables and fruits contain no cholesterol and little or no fat.

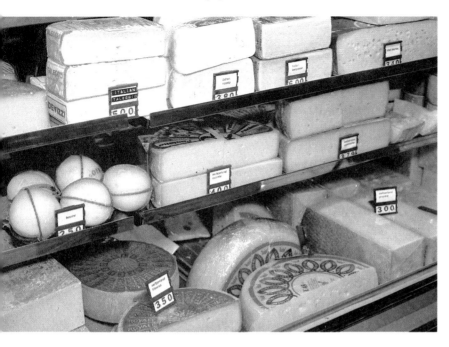

Cheeses made from low-fat or nonfat milk may be eaten by heart patients.

Make your own baked foods so that you can control the quantities of fats and sugar that go into them.

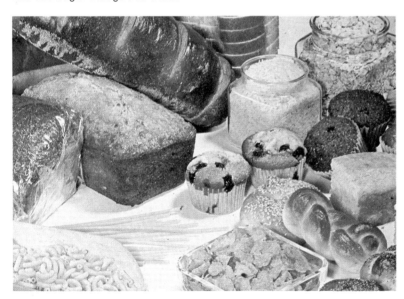

ing the body maintain its acid–alkaline balance.

Milk and milk products. Use nonfat milk and milk products. They give you the benefits of milk without the saturated fat. Read the label and buy the kind that is fortified with vitamins A and D.

Use the cheeses made from nonfat milk or low-fat milk. These include dry cottage cheese, mozzarella, farmer's cheese, ricotta, baker's cheese, sapsago, and Count Down (a 99-percent fat-free Cheddar-type brick cheese). When you make your own ice cream for a heart patient, you can put in it exactly what the patient needs. You might also use ice milk and low-fat yogurt, which is becoming a popular ice cream alternate. Low in fat and calories, yogurt supplies the other benefits of milk. You can make your own nonfat yogurt by using nonfat dry milk.

Grain products. Grain products in their natural state contain no cholesterol. The cereal grains are high in linoleic acid. However, many convenience grain products may be quite high in saturated fats. It is best to make your own bread and baked sweets or pastries. That way you can control all ingredients that go into them. Most mixes and ready-to-eat products are not for the heart patient. If you buy commercial bread, buy the nonfat type. Add your favorite spread, preferably one high in polyunsaturated fats.

When you eat dry cereal for breakfast, mix 120 mL (½ c) of nonfat dry milk with about 160 mL (⅔ c) of water. This mixture yields 12 g of protein. Add 5

in deep green, leafy vegetables, the yellow vegetables, fruits, and citrus fruits.

Heart patients also benefit from the undigested soft fiber of plant foods that help eliminate wastes. Along with milk, fruits and vegetables are key foods in help-to 10 mL (1 to 2 t) of vegetable oil high in linoleic acid. Remember that breads, cereals, and starchy vegetables are a much healthier form of carbohydrate than are sugars and sweets.

Small meals, snacks, other foods

Heart patients may need to eat four or five small meals a day or three small meals and a snack or two to get the good nourishment they need. The aim is never to overeat at one meal or in one day. This is not difficult for one who understands good nutrition.

Most commercially prepared snacks and tidbits are "off limits." They are usually loaded with saturated fat and calories. The same snacks suggested for overweight people are good for helping prevent and control heart and circulatory diseases (refer to Table 16-3). Fresh fruits, unsweetened canned fruits, and raw vegetables are especially good.

Except on rare occasions, avoid snacks and desserts that are made with saturated fat. Avoid those that are high in cholesterol. For example, avoid cream, whole milk, high-fat cheese, regular ice cream, butter, fish roe, caviar, and canned meats. Avoid frankfurters, sausages, cold cuts, high-fat meat (highly marbled), bacon, and goose, duck, chicken or turkey skin. Avoid commercially made quick breads, pastries, cakes (except angel food), pies, sweet rolls, whipped cream desserts, and imitation whipped cream. Avoid chocolate, coconut, commercial popcorn, whipped cream and coffee cream substitutes, commercially fried foods, and frozen and packaged dinners. Finally, unless the fat is skimmed off, avoid creamed soups, cream and other sauces, and gravy.

Alcohol causes a rise in blood cholesterol, and it yields high cal-

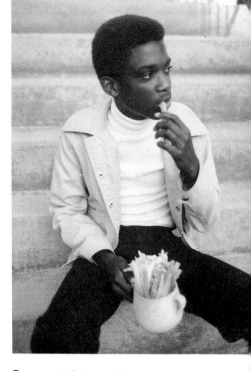

Raw vegetables and fruits are the best snack foods we can eat.

ories that may contribute to overweight or poor nutrition or both. The American Heart Association recommends moderation in the use of alcohol, sweets, ice cream, sherbet, and soft drinks.

RECAP

Heart disease

What is coronary atherosclerosis? **Role of plaques in heart attacks** **Contributors to heart and circulatory diseases** *Cholesterol Heredity Overweight Age Sex Inactivity Stress and tension*

Diet and the heart

Food selections *Fats Meat Eggs Legumes Fruits and vegetables Milk and milk products Grain products* **Small meals, snacks, other foods**

VOCABULARY

arteriosclerosis
cardiovascular disease
cerebral hemorrhage
coronary
    atherosclerosis
coronary occlusion
coronary thrombosis
myocardial infarction
phlebitis
plaques
stroke

THINKING AND EVALUATING

1. State why it is worth a young person's time and effort to develop eating habits that can help prevent and control cardiovascular disease. Do you think you have these habits? List the ways you would change.

2. Discuss why it is important for each member of the family to know how to plan and prepare balanced meals that can help protect each one from heart and circulatory diseases. What age groups are affected by such diseases?

3. Name the factors that contribute to cardiovascular disease. What can you and your family do about these factors, other than eating well-balanced meals?

4. Using what you learned in Unit 2, explain the different ways in which foods help prevent or control heart and circulatory diseases.

5. How would you prepare a low-fat diet, high in linoleic acid, to help prevent or control heart and circulatory diseases? What foods would you avoid?

APPLYING AND SHARING

1. List the ways in which the study of the preceding chapters of this book helped you understand this chapter better.

2. How do your own eating and exercise habits compare with the suggestions offered in this chapter? How could you improve these habits?

3. Write down the food you ate at meals and between meals yesterday. Was it a good, fair, or poor example of a diet for prevention of heart-circulatory disease?

4. Suppose you know someone whose physician advises certain precautionary measures to prevent the development of heart disease. The person must lose 20 pounds and maintain that loss. Make a plan of menus for one week showing a balanced diet that contains 1200 calories per day, is low in saturated fat and high in linoleic acid, and provides only 25 to 30 percent of the total calories from fat. In what other ways could you participate with this person in developing good habits to prevent heart disease?

CAREER CAPSULES

Research nutritionist Works in a hospital, higher educational institution, community health program, government health agency; researches the effects of diet on health. R.D. certification and advanced degree in nutrition required.

Processing plant quality controller Works in a cannery or other packing plant; checks end products and reports on accuracy of processing, ingredients, sizes. High school education and on-the-job training required.

RELATED READING

Eshleman, Ruthe, and Mary Winston. *The American Heart Association Cookbook.* New York: David McKay, 1973. Gives shopping advice, cooking hints, memos, and other features geared to a controlled-fat diet.

The Healthy Life. New York: Time, 1966. Illustrated text covers general fitness, emphasizing effects of diet and exercise on the heart.

Liebowitz, Daniel, M.D., W. James Brown, M.D., and Marlene Olness. *Cook to Your Heart's Content.* Menlo Park, Calif.: Pacific Coast Publishers, 1969. Discusses food preparation for a fat-controlled, sodium-restricted diet.

Zane, Polly. *The Jack Sprat Cookbook.* New York: Harper & Row, 1973. Emphasizes good eating with low-fat and low-cholesterol recipes; Appendix I discusses diet and heart disease.

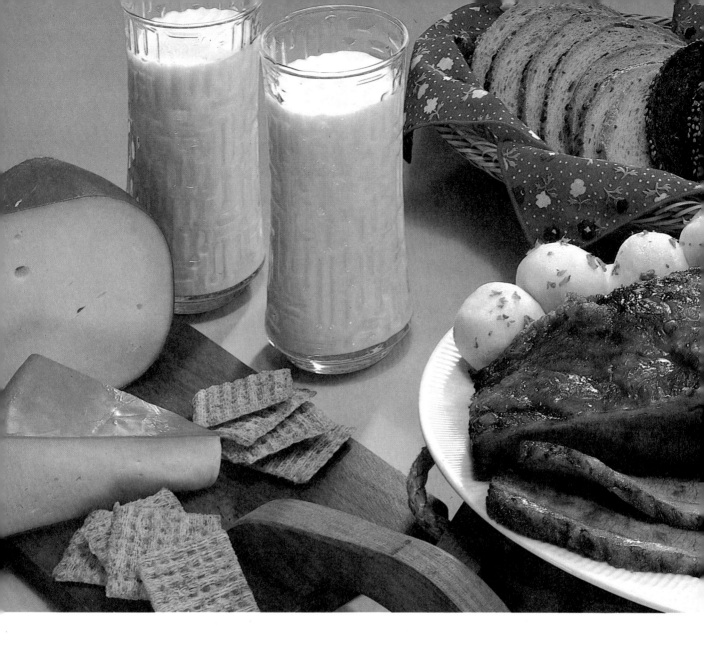

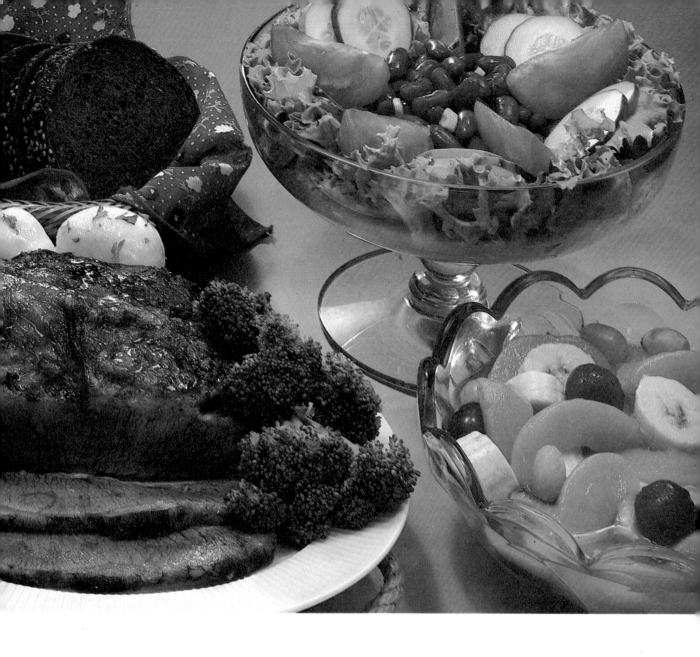

CHAPTER 18

Aging and nutrition

After studying this chapter, you will be able to

- list the ways in which good eating habits established now will delay the aging process.
- compare the nutrients and calories you need with those of an elderly person.
- plan and prepare balanced menus for yourself now that will continue to be a good pattern when you are older.
- draw conclusions on how this study can enrich your life now and in the future.

An older person looking in the mirror sees the effects of a lifetime of aging—and a lifetime of eating. How young this person looks will depend partly on how well he or she has eaten.

No one can escape aging. It starts when life begins and ends when life ends. However, each of us can influence the degree of premature aging by the foods we choose to eat each day. This is one good reason for learning the values of a balanced diet and establishing sound eating habits when we are young. We can thus help to extend the "prime of life" and delay the characteristics of aging.

Aging shows itself in many ways. Physical appearance deteriorates. Stamina and mental agility decline. Research shows that these changes are not only partly a matter of chronological age. More important, they result from impairment of tissues in the different parts of our bodies. How quickly or slowly our tissues deteriorate is closely related to nutrition, for it is food that makes us from the hair on our heads to the soles of our feet.

Of course, other factors affect aging and longevity besides diet. They include heredity, illness, alcoholism, inadequate rest and medical care, and physical and emotional stress. However, no one factor outranks the importance of the food we eat in building and maintaining the body.

Good eating habits can help to delay the characteristics of aging. Would you have guessed that this woman is 91 years old?

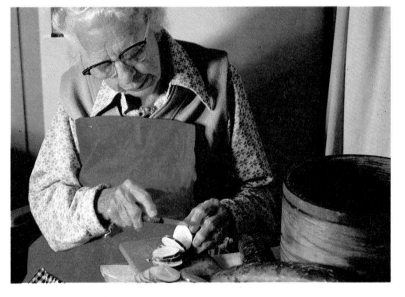

Fortunately, good eating habits work for you from the moment you establish them. You can easily judge whether a person is 16 or 26 years old, but some people at age 65 are as active and appear as young as others at age 55. Many people in their seventies seem younger, more creative, and more active than people in their sixties. How was the aging process slowed down in these cases? No doubt nutrition was partly responsible.

It takes time and effort to learn the essentials of nutrition and apply that knowledge, but this is a small price to pay for delaying the aging process. Aging accelerates at any period of life when the body does not have the proper balance of nutrients.

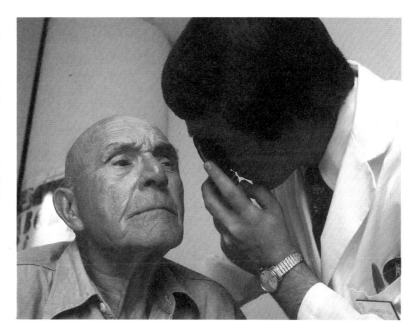

The health problems older people have are often related to poor lifelong eating habits.

LIFE EXPECTANCY

We are living longer today than ever before. In 1975, according to government reports, there were approximately 23.75 million persons in the United States who were 65 years old or more. This was an increase of nearly 4.25 million since 1960.

By comparison, at the height of the Roman empire, the average life expectancy of a citizen of Rome was only 23 years. In New England in 1850 life expectancy was 40 years. In 1900, it had increased to only 50 years. The most dramatic change came between the years 1920 and 1965. Life expectancy jumped in this short time from 50 to 70. By 1976, the Bureau of the Census reported that the life expectancy for the average male in the United States was 68.9 years and for the average female 76.6 years.

The Ten-State Nutrition Survey of the Department of Health, Education and Welfare found in 1973 that persons over 60 years of age showed evidence of general malnutrition, not restricted to the very poor or to any ethnic group. Like teen-agers, the elderly eat diets that are often too low in calcium, vitamins A and C, thiamin, and iron. The diets of the elderly in our country stand just one notch above those of teenagers, which are at the bottom of the totem pole.

NUTRITION EDUCATION FOR THE ELDERLY

Many older people do not understand what constitutes a nutritious balanced meal. In Rochester, New York, a study was made of 238 people 71 to 75 years of age who lived at home. Many of these people were woefully ignorant of facts about food and nutrition. Many were victims of food fadism. Others were on reducing diets.

Some of the older persons studied in Rochester had false ideas about food. One person thought milk is constipating. Another believed that bananas give

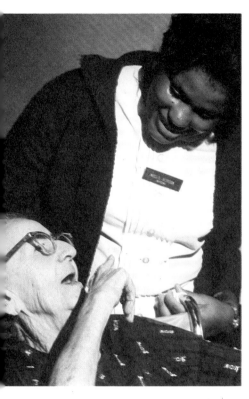

Older people often need guidance in planning and preparing balanced meals.

gas pains, a third that fat causes sour stomach. More than a third of the people did take vitamins, but often they did not choose the vitamins they needed most. Some people on a liberal food budget had poor diets, whereas about 10 percent of those on a low food budget chose adequate diets. Clearly, many older people need help in selecting a balanced diet, buying food, and properly preparing it.

Community involvement

In 1965, Congress passed the Older Americans Act. Nutrition research has been conducted under this act. It has helped open our eyes and our hearts to the nutritional needs of the elderly in our country, especially those with low incomes. Communities in many parts of the nation are devoting their time and energies to providing our older citizens with the nutrition they need. The following are examples of such programs.

1. Meals on Wheels regularly delivers good meals to homebound couples or single persons. How the program works in La Jolla, California, is fairly typical. Here volunteers use their own cars and deliver a well-balanced meal at noon with a bag lunch for the evening meal. The supper usually consists of a soup to be heated, a sandwich, fresh fruit, and milk. The recipient paid $2.75 in 1977 for a hot meal and the supper. In some cities Meals on Wheels delivers six days a week and leaves a frozen main meal for Sunday. Some communities also deliver breakfast, consisting of a can of fruit juice, individual packages of cereal, and milk. The maximum charge for three meals in Kalamazoo, Michigan, in 1975 was $3.50. In some communities, meals are prepared at a hospital, and a doctor's prescription is needed for the service.

2. The Older Americans Act of 1965 enables communities to receive funds for better nutrition from the federal government. Under this act, older Americans eat meals outside the home in some sort of community setting. For example, the meal may be served in a school cafeteria or a church hall. It is a nutritious midday main meal that meets one third of the daily recommended food allowances. It is also a boon to the morale of older people because it enables them to enjoy the company of friends.

3. Federal funds also sponsor the Golden Diners Clubs. Participants in this program may have

Many retirement communities serve three balanced meals a day.

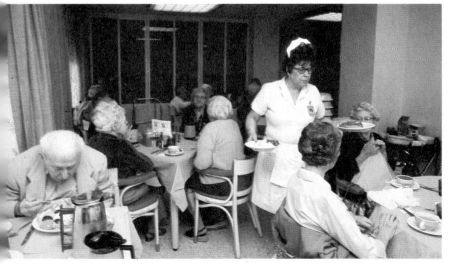

meals at one of several sites in a city or community at least five days a week. They are required to make a reservation on the day before. Usually they pay a sum they can afford.

4. There is a growing number of retirement communities that cater to the needs of people over 60 years of age. Such communities are planned for those who wish to maintain their independence and who can support themselves with the care that the facility may offer. The expense and care vary. Often one to three meals a day are planned by a dietitian. In many places, medical, recreational and other services are also provided.

How you can get involved

We are just now learning how to provide better nutrition for the elderly in the low-income group. We are learning how important it is for the elderly to have company at meals. Research shows that those living and eating alone are less interested in food. They become lonely and lose their self-respect when their health is poor, income low, and mobility reduced. We who can help improve their lives need to do so.

Studies show that about 80 percent of older people live independently. They often cook and eat alone or with one other person. Perhaps you have an older relative living in your home. Perhaps you know of older people living alone in your neighborhood. You might visit with them from time to time and even have a meal with them.

The following guidelines are designed to help older people enjoy nutritious, easy-to-prepare meals. You can help by passing these suggestions on to your older friends or relatives.

1. A person's attitude toward eating is important. Few people enjoy eating alone, but some cannot avoid it without special planning. Older people should plan to share meals together at one anothers' homes. They can also dine together occasionally in public places.

2. Advise your older friends to plan balanced meals for each day in the week. They can adjust plans to save money on seasonal foods. Stress the need for variety in the menus each day, so that meals include foods from each group. A person can try new combinations of meats and vegetables, or beans, peas, nuts, and low-fat cheese or yogurt. If on a special diet, an elderly person

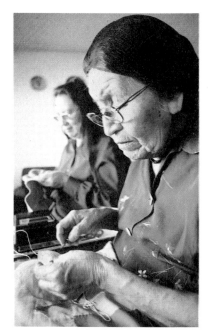

Sharing the company of others helps to keep up interest in eating.

Gardening and shopping are ways older people can sustain their interests in food, activity, and other people.

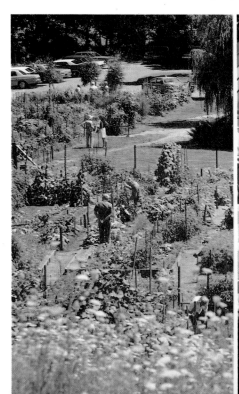

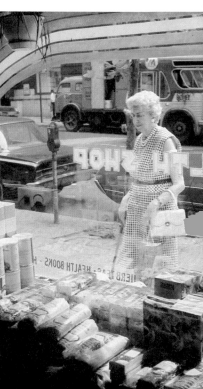

should take time to make the diet tasty with herbs and spices. Fruits should be served for dessert—especially fresh fruits.

3. Older people should use only those recipes that have been tested and found to be nutritionally sound. If there is adequate refrigeration, they should make larger quantities of the standard recipe. They should then freeze one or two serving portions and serve them on alternate days. The food should be reheated but not overcooked.

4. One-dish meals may be tastily prepared in small servings. For example, two or more vegetables may be added to cooked meat.

5. When shopping, older people should buy only what is needed immediately. If they buy more than this, the surplus should be stored properly.

6. Meals should be served attractively, whether they are on a

Poultry and cooked fruits are nutritious and easy to chew. Some people may have difficulty chewing raw foods such as radishes or cucumbers.

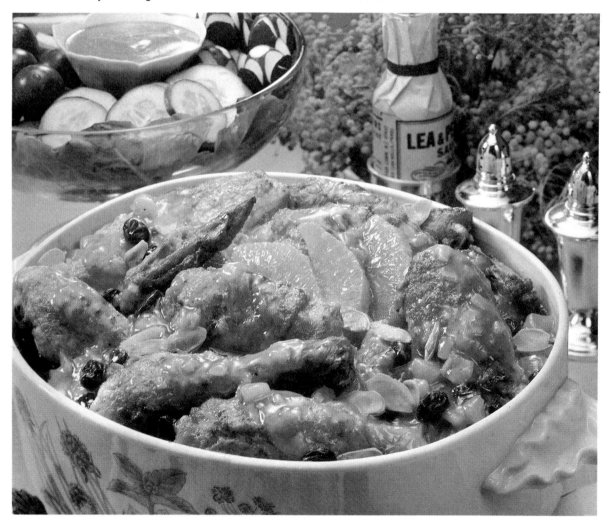

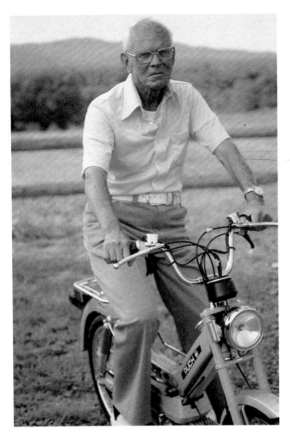
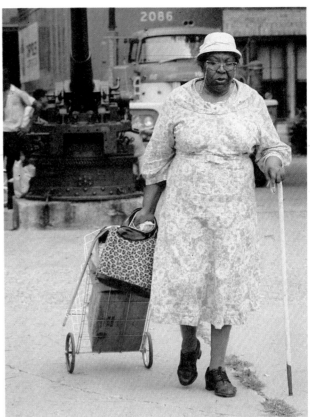

Moderate exercise improves morale, physical strength, and appetite.

tray or at the table. For example, pretty mats may be used in table settings, and a colorful garnish may be added to salad or fruit.

7. Older people should set a convenient time for the meal. They should allow enough time to prepare meals without rushing. They should eat small meals without skipping any.

8. An older person may have trouble chewing less expensive cuts and grades of meat. To correct this problem, meat can be braised in a pressure saucepan, sprinkled with a commercial meat tenderizer, marinated or ground. A roast that is thinly sliced is easy to eat. If it is impossible to chew pieces of meat, it can be broiled or pan broiled and ground through the food chopper. Fish and poultry should be eaten often. They are easy to chew, low in saturated fat, and have excellent protein.

9. Older people should neither overeat nor undereat. Their diet should be just enough to maintain normal weight. Their food should be cut in small bite sizes. If swallowing is difficult for them, they should chew food well and swallow before taking another bite.

10. Essential foods should be eaten first. Calorie intake is low for older people. They should know, therefore, that every calorie must contribute toward real needs. The best sweets that they can eat are fruits.

11. Foods that may make some older people uncomfortable are eaten with ease by others. Foods that sometimes cause problems are dried beans and peas, cooked cabbage, cauliflower, radishes, brussels sprouts, raw onions, and cucumbers. Raw and cooked vegetables, whole grains, and fruits provide the fiber that older people need.

12. Small living quarters make some people feel tired and lacking in appetite. Older people should take a brisk walk before they eat. Walking stimulates the appetite, keeps the figure trim, better utilizes nutrients, and improves the circulation. It often lifts the morale and enhances physical strength at any age.

Aging and nutrition   **301**

Process of aging

Life expectancy

Nutrition education for the elderly
Community involvement   How you can get involved

THINKING AND EVALUATING

1. List the ways this chapter has helped you understand how good eating habits established now can help you delay your own aging process.

2. Compare the nutrient needs of young people with those of the elderly.

3. Prepare a talk to your class on the major causes of poor nutrition among elderly people.

APPLYING AND SHARING

1. Name and describe five elderly men and five elderly women in the United States who continue to make outstanding contributions to our society. Discuss your findings in class. Do you like or dislike elderly people? Why?

2. Under what circumstances would you be willing to help an elderly person shop for food once a week and prepare a meal? Can you think of a person to whom you would offer such help? Discuss this and other ways the class could help in nutrition education for the elderly in your community.

3. You may know an older person who is a food faddist, a follower of a quack diet, or a reader of fad diet books or magazines. Make a plan to help that person correct false ideas about food.

4. Plan for an older person a balanced day's diet—three meals and one snack—that you would enjoy eating. The diet should provide good nutrition for each of you when the portions of food are properly adjusted.

5. Research a retirement community in your area. What emphasis does it place on nutrition for its residents? Interview some of the residents. Do they enjoy their meals? Why or why not? Do they have suggestions for improvement? Discuss in class.

CAREER CAPSULES

Administrative dietician Usually works in a hospital; supervises planning, operations, and budget of the entire food

VOCABULARY

aging
Golden Diners Clubs
life expectancy
Meals on Wheels
Older Americans Act
retirement communities

service department. Four-year college education in dietetics and R.D. certification required.

Consumer consultant Works in retail outlets; helps customers plan meals and parties, choose foods; advises store on latest nutritional, product, and equipment information. Four-year college education in home economics required.

RELATED READING

Present Knowledge in Nutrition, 4th ed. New York: The Nutrition Foundation, 1976. Pages 341–342 discuss the relationship between aging and the decrease of the trace mineral silicon in tissues such as the skin, aorta, and arterial walls.

Rockman, M., and M. L. Sussman, Eds. *Nutrition, Longevity, and Aging.* New York: Academic Press, 1977. Reports a 1976 symposium on the relationship between aging and lifelong nutrition; reviews both animal and human research.

Winick, M., Ed. *Nutrition and Aging,* Volume IV: *Current Concepts in Nutrition.* New York: John Wiley & Sons, 1976. Reports a 1974 symposium on nutrition and aging; focuses on the relationship of the aging processes and the diseases of aging.

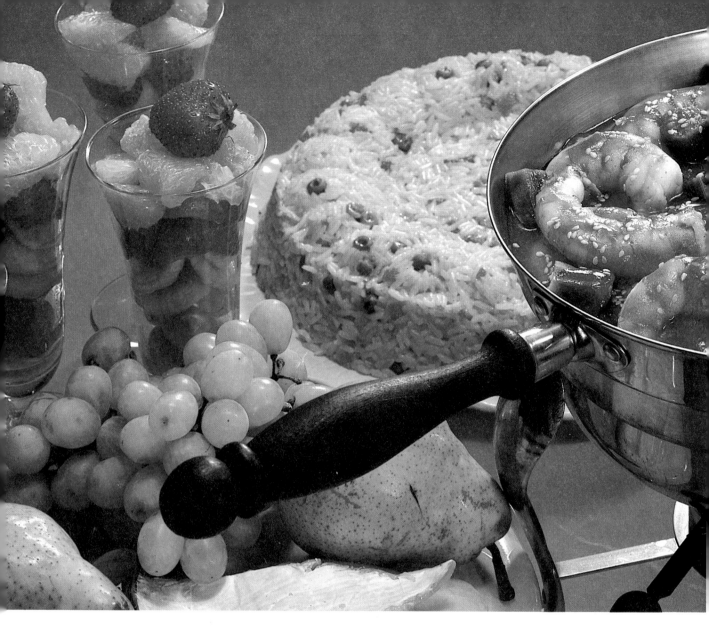

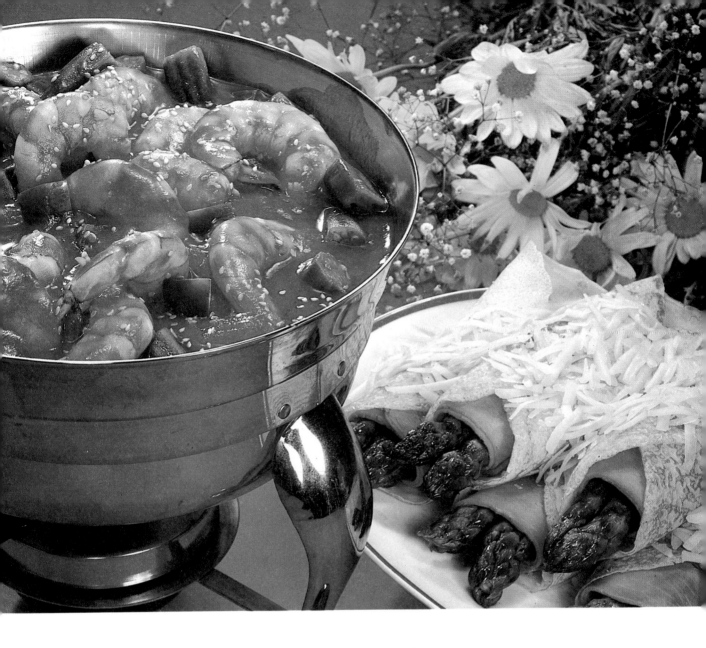

Gourmet meals

After studying this chapter, you will be able to

- define the modern meaning of "gourmet."
- explain why the French are identified with gourmet cooking.
- prepare a menu and a meal that are typical of another culture, and also a traditional American holiday meal.
- achieve the goal of preparing well-balanced meals that are beautiful, delicately flavored, and enjoyable.

THE MODERN GOURMET

A French writer once defined a gourmet as a person who can make a delectable dish out of amazingly little. Defined another way, a gourmet is anyone who enjoys foods that are prepared with taste and imagination.

Some people think gourmets are snobs who wish to impress others with exotic, rare, and ex- pensive foods. Others think of gourmets as being gluttons who overstuff themselves. Both notions are completely wrong. Gourmets are good managers who know how to create excellent meals without spending much money. They are imaginative, creative, and flexible. They select and prepare food artistically so

Swedish smorgasbord and Spanish paella are representative foods that have been brought to the United States from other countries by immigrants or travelers.

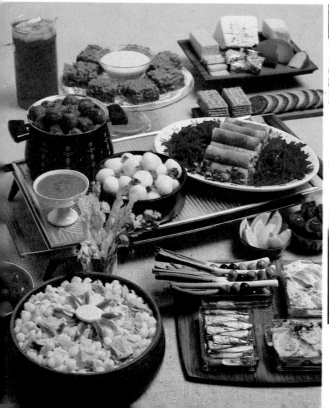
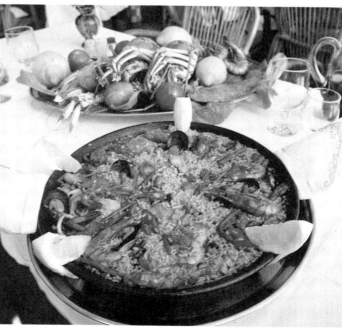

that the whole meal blends in flavor and each dish is a harmonious part of the whole. Gourmets are experimental. When they taste a new dish, they enjoy analyzing its flavor in the discriminating way that one might admire a poem or a piece of fine music. They are artists with food.

Young Americans are awakening to the possibilities of preparing gourmet meals. Our heritage is one reason for this interest. We are a nation made up of people who came from other lands. Each ethnic group brought its food traditions and favorite recipes and adapted them in the new homeland. Because of our mixed ancestry, we have a wide range of food tastes.

Twentieth-century Americans are developing gourmet tastes for another reason. Many of us have traveled and lived abroad. We have eaten and enjoyed the foods of other lands. We have learned how to prepare or adapt these foods for our own use.

A person once asked the founder of the first hotel school at Cornell University: "Where do you get your standard for the best cooking and style of serving meals—at the Waldorf?" "No," he replied, "the Waldorf and all other fine hotels get their high standards from the best of dining in the homes of this country and abroad." It is the home cook, then, who sets the standard for the best cooking and finest style of dining.

Gourmets of the past judged a meal only by its taste and appearance. Today's gourmets also consider whether the meal is low in calories and nutritionally balanced. Modern gourmets want to keep their figures and their health while they enjoy delicately flavored and beautiful meals.

Today, both men and women enjoy preparing gourmet meals. As members of gourmet clubs, people in all age groups dine in one anothers' homes on foods prepared by the members.

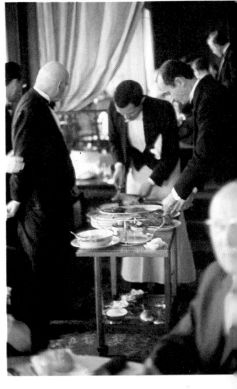

The gourmet tradition in France has culminated in famous restaurants believed by many to be the finest in the world. Here, the *Tour d'argent* in Paris.

THE ART OF GOURMET COOKING

When Napoleon invaded Russia in 1812, food supplies for the French army were meager and monotonous. The skills of Napoleon's French cook were tested to the utmost. Even so, the cook somehow managed to prepare meals for the general that were flavorful and varied. Napoleon was so pleased he awarded the cook a citation.

The story illustrates the ability of the French with food. They take pride in making ordinary foods taste extraordinary. The word gourmet (pronounced *goor-may*) comes from the

French language. Eating, to the French, means more than satisfying hunger. It is an aesthetic and intellectual part of life.

The gourmet style can be learned. You simply need to be awakened to the exciting flavors that can be created with simple foods. You can develop your own style with practice. You need a desire to experiment and improve. You can begin by studying the list of herbs and spices in Table 10-7. Learn to use herbs and spices imaginatively to help produce gourmet dishes and gourmet meals.

American gourmet cooking

Throughout our history as a nation, American gourmets have built up a rich heritage of delightful and savory dishes. Mark Twain was one of our most dramatic gourmets. He often wrote enthusiastically about even the simplest foods. Writing of the watermelon, for instance, Twain said, "It is the chief of this world's luxuries. . . . When one has tasted it, he knows what angels eat. . . ." He was right. Delicacies can be as simple as a good juicy watermelon. Ex-

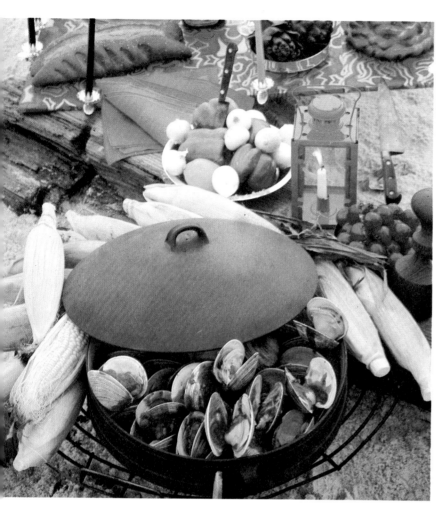

A beautiful American beach picnic is an example of the gourmet style of making a delectable meal out of simple native foods.

Seasoning is important in any French dish. *A bouquet garni* of several herbs—bay leaf, thyme, rosemary, parsley, or others—tied in cheesecloth is added to soups, meats cooked with moisture, and some vegetable dishes. The French use all members of the onion family—leeks, shallots, chives, and garlic—as well as regular yellow onions. Other common seasonings are celery seed, thyme, fennel, chervil, mustard, tarragon, pepper, orange and lemon peel, orange and lemon juices, nutmeg, cloves, vinegar, wine, butter, cream, bacon, olive oil, cheese, white sauces, brown sauces, watercress, and other vegetables.

Hors d'oeuvres. As appetizers or first courses, the French may serve thin slices of smoked salmon on pumpernickel bread. They also enjoy cucumbers, asparagus, deviled eggs, eggplant, artichokes, caviar, and canapés. They serve *pâté de foie gras* (goose liver *pâté*) with warm crusty French bread. Other favorites are radishes, mushrooms, peppers, celery, cheeses, and chicken in tiny stuffed rolls. Except for the vegetables, most of these foods are expensive. If you wish to use hors d'oeuvres wisely, select one or two rather than a wide variety of the expensive items. Use the less expensive vegetable hors d'oeuvres with them.

Soups. Several French soups are used internationally, including onion soup, *vichyssoise* (potato soup) served hot or ice cold, *consommé Madrilène,* and lobster bisque. The *pot-au-feu* (literally, "pot on the fire") is a mainstay for soup stock in most

citing food does not have to be laboriously prepared.

Each section of the United States can boast of its special culinary adventures. Table 19-1 lists a few examples of dishes that American home cooks have invented or discovered. Many of these dishes have become popular in other countries as well as in the United States.

French gourmet cooking

The French specialize in many kinds of dishes—hors d'oeuvres, soups, meats, vegetables, salads, cheeses, and desserts.

Table 19-1 **Some American food specialties**

SOUPS	MEATS AND FISH	FRUITS
Manhattan clam chowder	Barbecued spareribs	Cranberry sauce
New England clam chowder	Chicken a la king	Fruit cup
New Orleans chicken gumbo	Chicken and dumplings	Fruit juice cocktail
	Deviled crabs	Watermelon
BREADS	Hamburgers	Watermelon pickle
Biscuits	Lobster Newburg	
Blueberry muffins	Planked shad	**SWEET DESSERTS**
Corn bread	Roast turkey	Angel food cake
Hot cakes	Southern fried chicken	Apple pie à la mode
Spoon bread	Virginia baked ham	Baked Alaska
Yeast bread		Blueberry pie
	VEGETABLES	Cantaloupe à la mode
SALADS	Boston baked beans	Chiffon pie
Avocado salad	Corn on the cob	Coconut custard pie
Chef's salad	Corn pudding	Ice cream sundae
Chicken salad	Green vegetable with bacon	Molasses cake
Coleslaw	Harvard beets	Parfait
Crabmeat salad	Hominy	Pecan pie
Shrimp salad	Stuffed baked potatoes	Pumpkin pie
Stuffed tomato salad	Succotash	Strawberry shortcake
Waldorf salad	Sweet potatoes	Upside-down cake

French homes. Traditionally, the French toss every scrap of unused food into this kettle and simmer it. They toss bones of meat, fish, and fowl into the pot. They may add the outside leaves of lettuce and cabbage and all imperfect leafy vegetables. They throw in the peelings of all root vegetables and the hulls and pods of peas and beans. The soft remains, pushed through a strainer, go into the soup or another mixture. Many of the vitamins are lost in this process, but minerals and other nutrients remain. Accompaniments to the meal should provide the lost nutrients.

The French make a fish soup called *bouillabaisse.* People in Spain, Italy, San Francisco, and New Orleans make a similar fish soup. To make *bouillabaisse,* shellfish and fish fillets are cut in

Bouillabaisse or mixed seafood soup originated in Provence, an area of France that borders the Mediterranean Sea.

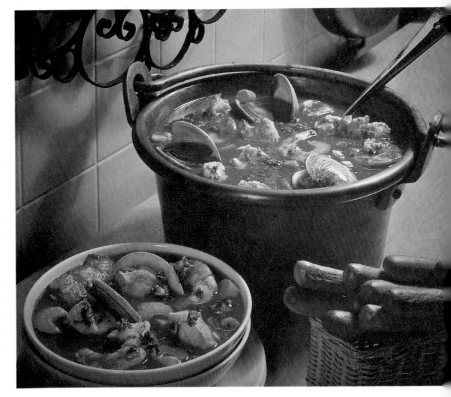

bite sizes. An assortment of vegetables, herbs, and seasonings is added. *Bouillabaisse* is the main dish of the meal. For nutritional balance, it is served with a tossed green salad, warm crisp French bread, and fresh fruit and cheese for dessert.

Soup is extremely important to the French. French children who take their lunch to school traditionally carry a jar of soup. French laborers carry soup to their work places.

Vegetables. In French villages, vegetables are usually garden fresh. In Paris and other French cities, vegetables are brought into the city fresh every day. There is also an increasing number of canned and frozen foods in the markets of European cities.

The French usually cook vegetables quickly, season them simply with salt, pepper, and a fat, and serve them at once. They split green beans "French-style" for artistic effect. They cook tiny onions and new peas together. Mushrooms, a favorite vegetable, may be served alone or with another vegetable, meat, or poultry. Artichokes and asparagus are widely grown and considered a delicacy in many homes throughout Europe. Dried beans, which all Europeans use in many ways, provide a fair share of their protein. The French people at first refused to eat potatoes when the first explorers to America introduced them, but now "French fries" are eaten around the world. Potatoes are also used in potato salad, soups, and many other

Some people consider a perfectly roasted and garnished chicken or duck to be the true test of a gourmet cook.

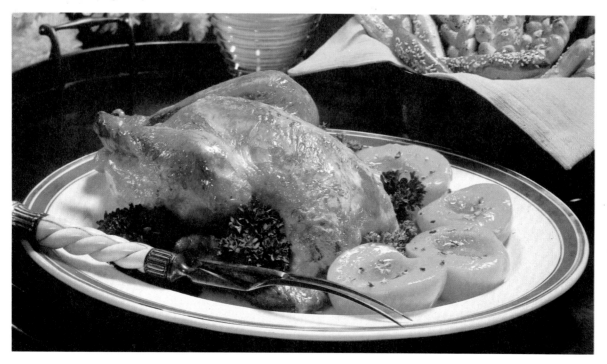

dishes. Europeans eat more turnips and rutabagas than we do. They include these vegetables in many types of soup.

Salads. The French respect salads so much that they usually serve them as a separate course, after the main dish. Their salads consist chiefly of green leaves of lettuce and simple French dressing.

Poultry. Cooking chicken is another French specialty. Among their most famous dishes are chicken Marengo, *coq au vin, poulet au vin blanc,* chicken à la Bourgogne, breast of chicken with grapes, chicken legs with mustard, and *poulet à la Valencienne.* The French cook each of these dishes in moist heat, using chicken stock, wine, or both as the liquid. They add different seasonings to vary the chicken's flavor. After the chicken is done, the cooking liquid is reduced and made into a rich sauce or saved for use in soups.

Meats. The French do not eat as much red meat as Americans do, but they are masters at preparing tough and low-grade cuts, for example a pot roast called *boeuf à la mode.* They brown the roast first on all sides in hot butter. Then they add vegetables

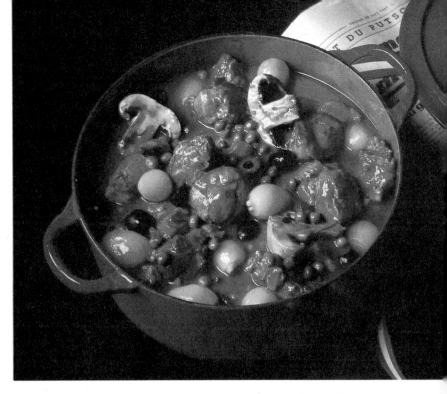

A stew of *boeuf bourguignon* (beef, mushrooms, and onions) is a hearty French provincial dish that can be varied in many ways—here, with the addition of peas and sliced olives.

and wine and simmer the meat until it is tender. Another kind of French pot roast is *boeuf bourguignon.* The French enjoy *steak au poivre* or steak with pepper. For lunch, they may eat a cold cut called *langue de boeuf froide* (cold beef tongue). *Pâté* made with pork liver and truffles has a superb flavor and superior nutritional value. *Porc au Maréchal* is a favorite pork chop dish served

with a sauce made of orange and wine. To make lamb stew, the French mix pieces from the neck or shoulder of lamb with vegetables, wine, and seasonings. Veal, a favorite meat, is served as stew, soup, or cutlets.

Fish. Fish is another food that the French prepare particularly well. They are famous for lobster thermidor. They cook sole in many different and delicious

French cooking has perfected the practice of using the seasoned liquid in which fish is poached as the base for a sauce

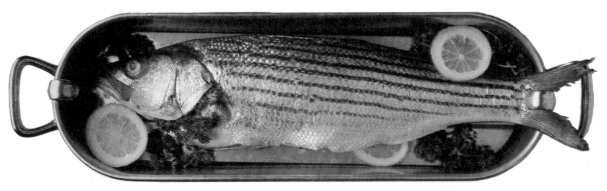

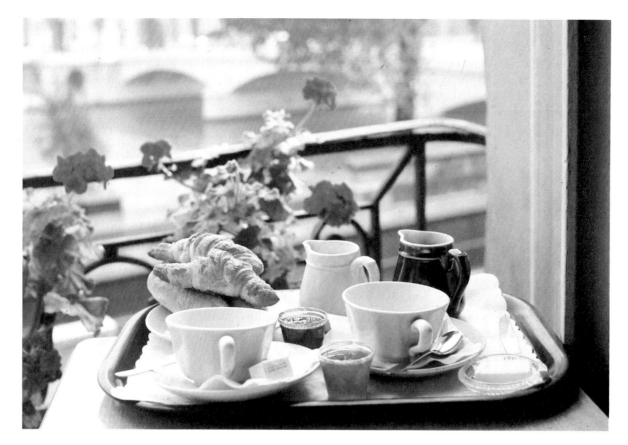

A French breakfast typically consists of *café au lait,* croissants, butter, and preserves.

Omelets may be filled or garnished with herbs, cheese, preserves, chopped meat, creamed vegetables, or cottage cheese and sour cream. Or they may be served with a tomato or cheese sauce.

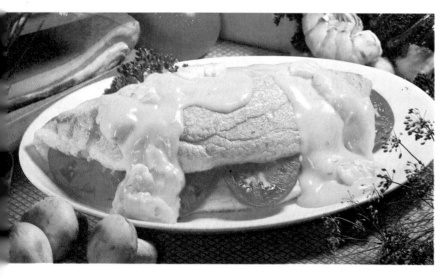

ways, such as *sole Mornay, sole meunière, sole Marguerite,* and *sole Normandie.* Fish is used in custard in France, as it is in the Scandinavian countries. Frogs' legs, snails, eels, and mussels are prepared in homes throughout France. Oysters on the half shell are served as a first course or as hors d'oeuvres.

Bread. The bread most generally eaten in France is a long, slender, crusty loaf. Rolls and flaky croissants and brioches are served for breakfast. The French loaf is popular around the world. It is often sliced to the bottom crust, spread with garlic butter, and heated for serving at dinner or lunch.

Milk and cheese. Milk is not widely drunk in France. Only small children drink it regularly. Coffee is served at breakfast as *café au lait*—coffee with hot milk. Instead of milk, the French use a great deal of cheese, accompanied by fresh fruit, as dessert. Cheese is also used in soufflés and rabbits.

Eggs. The French omelet is a world-famous dish. So are eggs scrambled in meat drippings. Eating eggs for breakfast is unusual in France, but it is becoming more common as the French learn more about nutrition. Eggs are an important part of soufflés.

Desserts. For dessert, the French may serve something as sweet as petits fours, meringues, fruit tarts, puff pastry, mousses, ices, custards, *crêpes Suzette*, and soufflés. Or they may simply serve cheese and fresh fruit with or without bread.

DEVELOPING GOURMET STYLE

We have used our own country and France to illustrate how people develop a gourmet style. Such a style usually develops in a home in which an imaginative person cares a great deal about making a lot out of little.

Great cooks are not born but made. You can read all the books about the values in foods and cooking. You can own the latest cookbooks. But the learning comes when you get in the kitchen with the food and your pots and pans! You must try out your ideas until they are perfected.

One person may be more sensitive than another to the flavor of foods, but even a sensitive taste can be learned. Success in the kitchen does not happen immediately. Learning to cook is, in some ways, like learning to write. Expert writers must often write a page over and over again before they are finally satisfied with it. Cooks, too, will try out recipes again and again until they succeed in producing perfect results.

The first step is to master the basic principles of simple, nutritious cooking. You may then develop a few food specialties for which you become noted. Most cooks throughout the world begin with the same basic foods. Then they creatively transform basic foods into dishes with a special character of their own.

To learn about gourmet dishes, go to restaurants of different nationalities. Ask for the specialty of the house—or *plat maison,* as they say in French restaurants.

What makes a certain dish of gourmet quality? It does not matter how popular it is. What matters is that the food be distinctive.

True gourmets do not eat merely because they are hungry. They savor each bit of food to feel the pleasure of its taste in their mouths. Eating is mingled with

Good cooks are made, not born, through practice, patience, and perseverence.

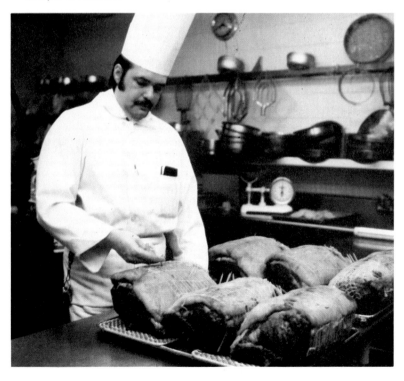

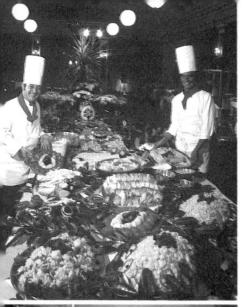

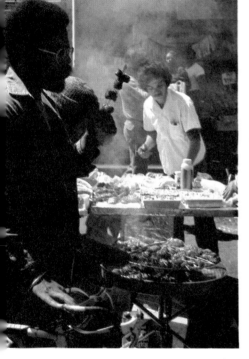

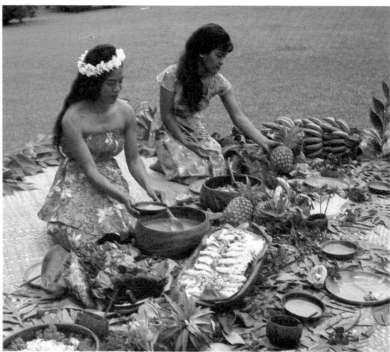

One of the best ways of learning about gourmet dishes is to sample them in restaurants and at food fairs.

good friendship and good conversation. It cannot be rushed. With good food that is well prepared, the most inexpensive meal tastes perfect.

The people of India have an admirable attitude about preparing food. Traditionally, they believe the cooking of food is "one of God's revelations to people" and a divine art. Thus, the Indian homemaker approaches cooking with pleasure and devotion.

By all means, seek to master the art of gourmet cooking. At the same time, use your knowledge of nutrition to keep yourself in good health.

THINKING AND EVALUATING

1. How have you interpreted the word "gourmet" in the past? Has your interpretation changed since reading this chapter? Explain.

2. What is the modern challenge to gourmet cooking?

3. What are the objectives of the modern gourmet?

4. As a nation, why is the United States so unique in its culinary offerings?

5. What have you learned in this chapter that can stimulate you to a wider exploration of the food of other nations?

6. How would you go about creating a gourmet dish?

APPLYING AND SHARING

1. In a bookstore, look over cookbooks that present foods of other nations. Make a list of those you might like as gifts.

2. Look up in your library the food customs and cultural origins of the foods of different nations in which you are interested. Try some of their recipes in your kitchen.

3. Select moderately priced restaurants that specialize in foreign foods and try them according to your financial ability to eat out. Study their menus and the flavor of each food you eat. Discuss in class.

4. Plan menus and prepare meals at your home typical of at least three other nations. Evaluate your results. Make a plan for improvement. Repeat the best one for guests. Discuss the results in class.

5. Organize a gourmet club that meets in the homes of members once a month for a gourmet meal. Help lead the group in preparing healthful, attractive, and delectable meals at a price you can afford.

CAREER CAPSULES

Chef Works in kitchen of restaurant, cafeteria, hospital, other institution; usually has responsibility for preparation and cooking of one kind of food—for example, the fried items or the pastries. Vocational education and on-the-job training required.

Cooking school teacher Works in own kitchen, other people's kitchens, or cooking school kitchen; teaches cooking, often ethnic (French, Chinese) or otherwise specialized (pastry, chocolate). Required education varies; cooking experience essential.

VOCABULARY

boeuf à la mode
bouillabaisse
bouquet garni
café au lait
gourmet
hors d'oeuvres
pot-au-feu

RELATED READING

Belinke, Helen. *The New Gourmet in the Low-Calorie Kitchen Cookbook.* New York: David McKay, 1971. Features low-calorie gourmet recipes; includes chapter on entertaining and popular dishes of other countries.

Better Homes and Gardens Holiday Cookbook. New York: Meredith Press, 1967. Contains recipes, menus, and table settings for holidays, birthdays, anniversaries, parties; includes some foreign fare.

Pellaprat, Henri-Paul. *Everyday French Cooking for the American Home,* adapted by Avanelle S. Day. Ampersand Press, 1965. A treasury of French recipes.

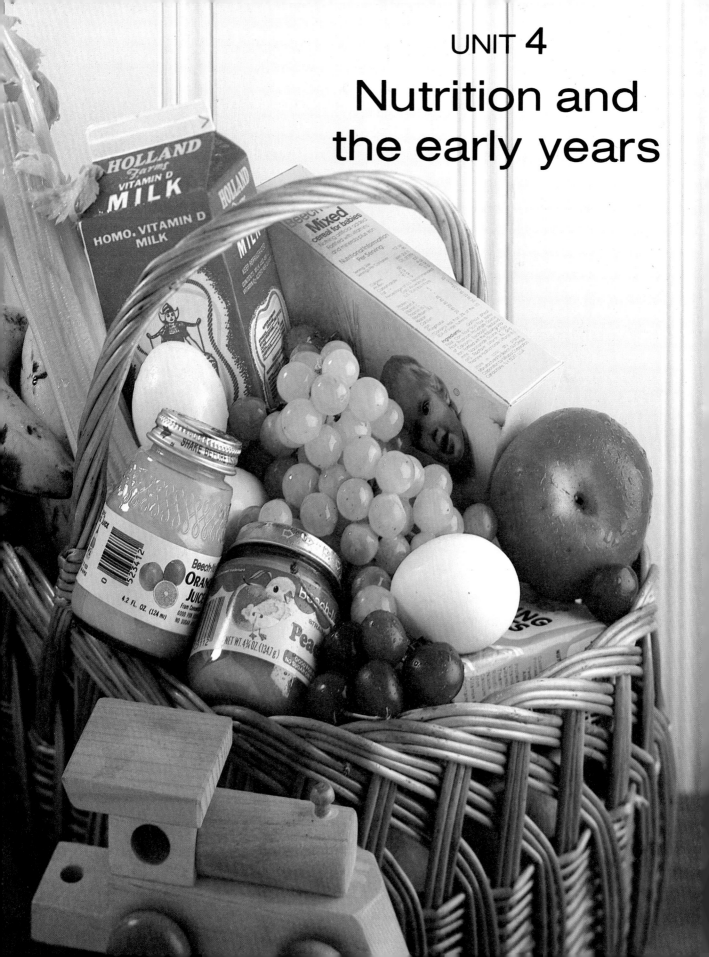

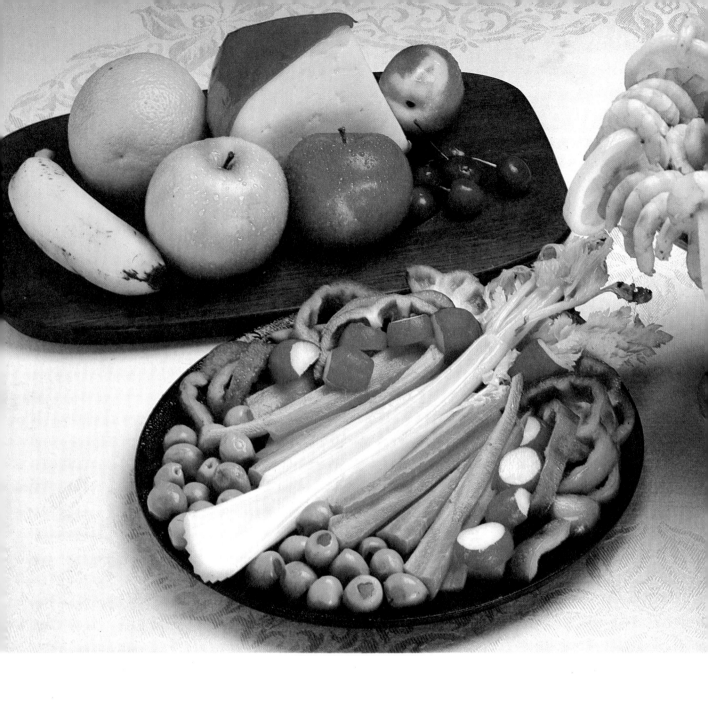

CHAPTER **20**

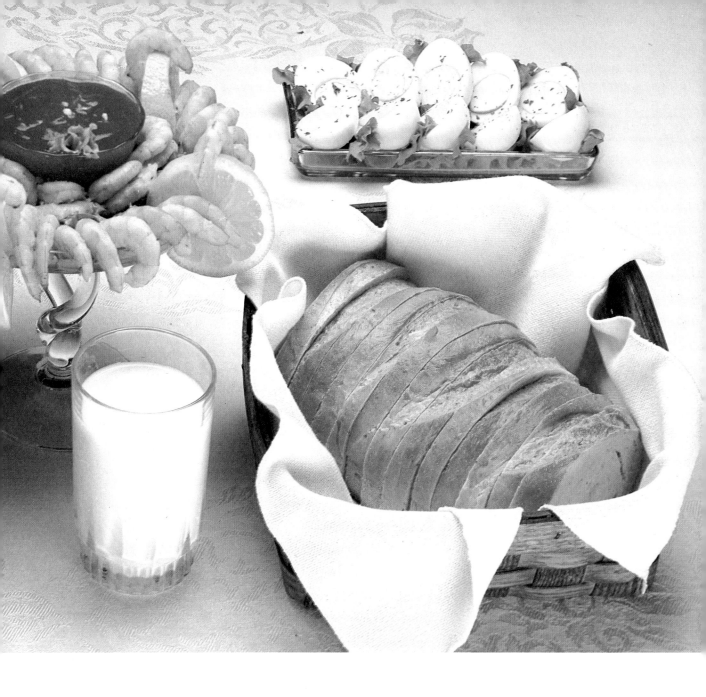

Food during pregnancy

After studying this chapter, you will be able to

- list examples showing how the mother's good diet aids in the development of a healthy baby.
- describe how the mother nourishes the embryo.
- list some nutrition-related complications that may arise during pregnancy.
- explain the importance of additional protein during pregnancy.

Information about the correct diet essential to the health of an expectant mother and her developing baby is available from many sources, including prenatal clinics and training courses, publications, and the attending physician.

Every person benefits from good eating habits. Perhaps a pregnant woman benefits most of all. If she is healthy and well-nourished she is less likely to have complications during her pregnancy. She is also more likely to give birth to a healthy infant that is carried a full term.

One young woman in ten is a mother before she is 18 years old. Unfortunately, adolescents are the least likely of any age group to have the good eating habits they need. Many young people are not prepared to care for the nutritional needs of a family. They may eat poorly for many reasons. They may deprive themselves of proper food just to keep slender. They may either lack information about nutrition or simply ignore it. Young people often have strong food prejudices that contribute to their poor eating habits.

Dr. Genevieve Stearns, former Research Professor of Pediatrics at the University of Iowa, studied

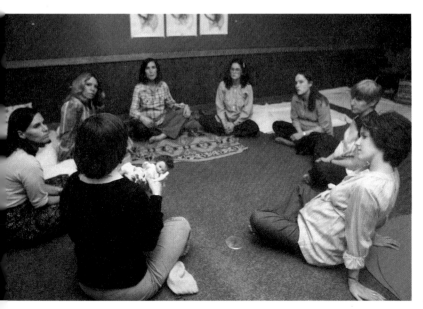

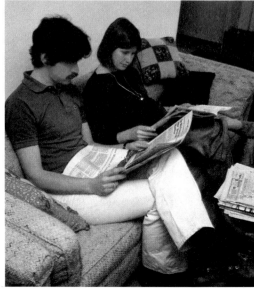

two groups of pregnant women. The first group had been eating an excellent diet for at least the previous four years. The second group had only a fair diet. Each group did have three glasses of milk daily. Both groups were then given a series of increasingly good diets. The women who had good eating habits were able to utilize the nutrients in the diet more rapidly than women with poor eating habits. The second group took five months to reach the nutritional level of the first.

Proper eating habits are essential for the development of a healthy infant. Following are just a few examples of the development processes dependent on proper nutrition.

1. The uterus must enlarge until it is big enough to hold a 2.7-kg to 4.1-kg (6-lb to 9-lb) baby 47.5 to 52.5 cm (19 to 21 in) long. A balanced diet aids this process. Dr. Ray Hepner states that the length of the baby is better measurement of true growth and good nutrition than weight. An "average" baby is 50 cm (20 in) long and weighs slightly over 3.2 kg (7 lb).

2. A balance of high-quality nutrients is needed to build and maintain the constantly changing placenta.

3. The mother must provide enough iron for several purposes. First, she must build a complete blood supply for her baby for life outside the womb. Second, because milk is low in iron, she must supply reserves of iron for the baby's body to last about four months after birth. Third, she must avoid becoming anemic herself either during pregnancy or afterwards. Fourth, she must build up a reserve to protect herself from any undue loss of blood at delivery.

4. The mother must provide the nutrients required to form and maintain the protective membrane that surrounds the growing baby. The umbilical cord that connects the baby to the mother by way of the placenta must be well formed and maintained.

5. An adequate diet is essential for the mother to nurse the baby.

6. From one cell at the beginning, the baby grows to 200 million cells. From a microscopic fertilized ovum the baby grows to weigh 6 billion times more. All this results from the nutrients that a mother supplies. If she doesn't eat what is needed, nutrients are taken from her body reserves. If they are not available in either her food or her own body tissues, the baby may be harmed before birth and afterwards.

NOURISHMENT OF THE BABY DURING GESTATION

Nourishment of the baby in the womb occurs through a remarkable filter–transfer system. Nutrients that enter into the mother's bloodstream are passed on to the baby an hour or two after she eats them. The mother also passes on immunity to certain diseases.

The transfer system unfortunately passes other substances besides nutrients from the mother's bloodstream. If the mother takes a drink of alcohol, the baby gets some. If she smokes a cigarette, the baby gets some nicotine. Large substances, such as protein and whole blood, as well as most bacteria, are filtered out by the walls of the umbilical blood vessels. But smaller substances, including the anesthesia used at childbirth, pass into the baby's bloodstream.

The mother's use of drugs may interfere with the normal formation of new life. This was illustrated dramatically during the early 1960s. At this time a tranquilizer called thalidomide was widely used. Many babies born to mothers who had used this drug in the early stages of pregnancy were found to have imperfectly developed arms and legs. The drug had interfered with the normal development of the fetus.

Function of the placenta

The placenta is vitally important to the life of a baby before it is born. It is a powerful organ made of spongy tissue and a network of large and small blood vessels. The placenta is attached to the mother at the wall of the uterus and to the baby by the umbilical cord.

The mother's blood never directly enters the baby's body. Nor does the baby's blood enter the mother's body. The placenta is the intermediary. It functions as adult lungs do. It supplies oxygen from the mother's blood and re-

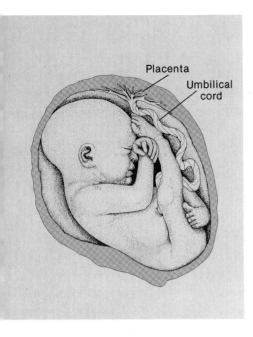

Figure 20-1　The fetus in the womb is nourished by the mother through the placenta and the umbilical cord.

moves carbon dioxide from the baby's blood.

The placenta has other important functions, as well. Through it the baby's waste is picked up and eliminated by the mother's blood. The placenta acts as an adult liver does. It makes iron from the mother's blood cells available to the baby. It also acts as adult intestines do. Nutrients from the mother's blood are absorbed through the placenta into the baby's blood. The placenta processes food molecules with the aid of digestive enzymes so that the baby's blood vessels can pick up the nutrients. It even produces hormones.

To summarize, the placenta serves as (1) a storehouse from the mother's diet to meet the nutrient needs of the baby, (2) a superb transport system between mother and baby, and (3) the medium for disposing of the baby's wastes.

Function of the umbilical cord

The umbilical cord is the baby's lifeline to the mother by way of the placenta. Its main task is to supply vitamins, minerals, fat, proteins, and carbohydrates from the mother's diet or from her body reserves. In the first stage of life, the umbilical cord is a short, stemlike connection. By birth it varies in length from 12.5 cm (5 in) to 3.6 m (4 ft).

All people closely associated with an expectant mother should try to make her pregnancy as free from stress and tension as possible.

The umbilical cord is a masterpiece of engineering. It has a closed blood system in which blood travels at the rate of 6.4 km (4 mi) an hour. The force of blood is so great that the cord rarely becomes knotted or tangled. It takes only 30 seconds for the blood to make a round trip through the baby and the cord. Inside the cord are two arteries. These arteries carry the used blood from the baby to the placenta. In the placenta wastes are traded for sustenance. Fresh nutrients and oxygen are then carried back to the baby. They travel through a large blood vessel that enters the baby's body at the navel, where the umbilical cord is connected. From this point, the baby's blood vessels take over. They supply each expanding tissue with fresh supplies of food and oxygen.

Function of hormones

Hormones are closely related to every stage of successful pregnancy. Hormones are made from food. They work as a team with enzymes, nutrients, and one another. Hormone secretions are stimulated by progesterone. Progesterone comes from the adrenal cortex and during pregnancy from the placenta. Progesterone signals other glands to get busy as a new life starts. For example, it signals the change that begins to take place in the breasts of the expectant mother. Two other hormones—gonadotropin and estrogen—are especially concerned with reproduction. Among other things, they regulate the nutrition of developing tissues.

The Nutrition and Pregnancy Symposium of the Council on Foods and Nutrition of the American Medical Association has stated that pregnancy complications are the third leading cause of death in the United States. The symposium has further suggested that birth defects can arise from nutritional deficiencies.

Pregnancy complications include sterility, spontaneous abortion, premature or immature birth, stillbirth, toxemia, labor problems, and anemia of the mother during pregnancy and of the baby during the first year. The defects in children that may be related to nutritional factors are convulsions, mental deficiency, and so-called cerebral palsy.

The lack of any particular nutrient in the mother's diet may produce different harmful effects at different stages of pregnancy. The time clock for the development of each of the baby's organs and parts of the body is set at the time of conception. Hence the expectant mother and her baby have an enormous advantage if she is well-nourished.

Anemia

Anemia is a common condition during pregnancy. It is often caused by iron deficiency. Expectant mothers should eat a well-balanced diet with a good supply of iron-rich foods. Babies born to anemic mothers may lack sufficient iron reserves, resulting in infant anemia.

Another form of anemia common to pregnant and lactating women and their infants is macrocytic anemia (also called megablastic anemia), caused by a deficiency in folacin (refer to Chapter 5). In this form of anemia, the red blood cells are too few in number and much too large. They also contain too little hemoglobin. Treatment with folic acid can cure this condition.

Toxemia

Toxemia—a combination of symptoms—sometimes develops in pregnancy. It results from malfunction of the kidneys, which are under a strain during pregnancy. Symptoms include high blood pressure and edema—the retention of fluid in tissues—which results in the weight gain associated with toxemia. Albumin, a protein in the urine that does not occur normally, is another sign of toxemia. Toxemia often occurs in excessively overweight women, especially those whose excess weight has been gained during pregnancy.

In studying pregnant women, B. S. Burke and his associates found that not one who ate a good diet had toxemia. On the other hand, 44 percent of those on poor diets and 8 percent on fair diets developed it. When a poor diet was supplemented by high-quality proteins and increased vitamins, less toxemia resulted.

Constipation

Constipation may occur during pregnancy, especially in the later

The expectant mother's diet should include high-quality protein foods.

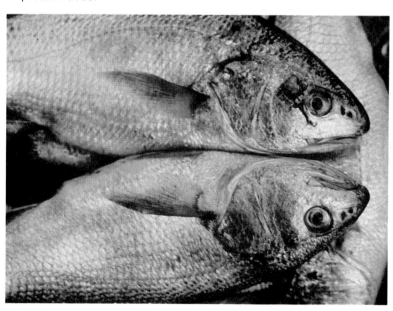

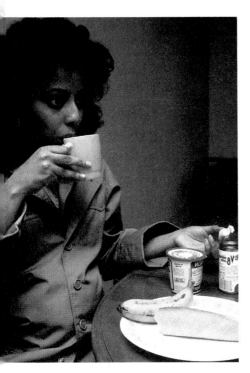

Morning sickness, which may be caused by a shortage of carbohydrates, can be prevented by a simple breakfast.

stages. In most cases, the mother can control constipation without the aid of laxatives by eating a well-balanced diet. She can eat vegetables, fruits, whole-grain breads, and cereals for their fiber. It also helps to drink fluids daily, exercise regularly, and get enough rest and sleep. Freedom from unusual stress or tension is also important in avoiding constipation.

Edema

Edema occurs when water is retained in the tissues. It can be partially or completely controlled by a low-sodium diet, if there is no toxemia. (Sometimes this diet is incorrectly referred to as "salt free.")

Morning sickness

Morning sickness is the name often given to nausea or vomiting that sometimes occurs in pregnant women. It usually occurs upon getting up in the morning.

Why does morning sickness occur? One theory is that during the night the embryo in the womb uses up the carbohydrate (glycogen) stored in the liver. This leaves the mother with a shortage of carbohydrate. If she then eats no breakfast for fear of nausea or vomiting, the shortage of carbohydrate is increased. The carbohydrate loss should, of course, be replaced in the morning. Moving quietly instead of vigorously and eating a simple breakfast of cereal, fruit or fruit juice, and skim milk will replace the carbohy-

Whole-grain cereals and fruits are natural laxatives.

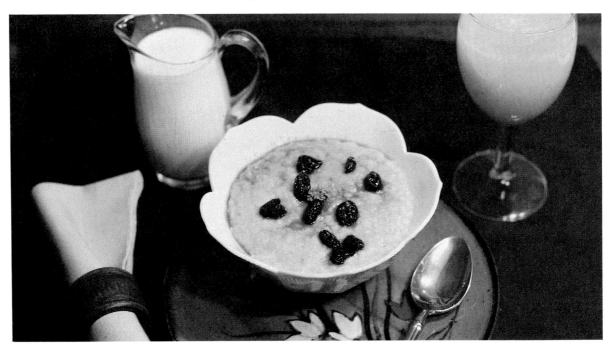

drates and prevent morning sickness. Tests show that even dry toast taken before arising helps prevent nausea.

Pernicious vomiting

When vomiting is severe and persistent, it is called pernicious vomiting. It can lead to serious nutritional disturbance if the woman does not seek medical attention. For some women, vitamin B_6 relieves the symptoms. Others need to be fed intravenously every two hours with a high-carbohydrate low-fat diet. Each feeding consists of glucose mixed with vitamins and other nutrients. Other foods are added gradually, until a balanced diet is resumed (Table 20-1). Small amounts of liquid are taken frequently to avoid dehydration.

Birth defects

Birth defects have been surrounded by mystery for centuries.

Table 20-1 Examples of meals for pernicious vomiting

CEREAL WITH MILK AND SUGAR	MEAT BROTH (ALL FAT REMOVED)
DRY TOAST WITH JELLY	BAKED POTATO (WITHOUT FAT)
CRACKERS WITH JELLY	PLAIN RICE WITH MILK AND SUGAR
TOMATO JUICE	PLAIN GELATIN (OR FRUIT AND VEGETABLE PURÉE)

In the Middle East, anthropologists have unearthed drawings on clay rocks, dating from four thousand or more years ago, showing dwarfism and other birth defects. Dr. Lucille S. Hurley of the University of California at Davis has compared birth defects of ancient times with those of today. She has found them to be identical. Here is what she says about the problem today.

Today, birth defects loom as one of the major health problems. For example, the percent of infant deaths due to congenital malformations has shown a steady increase since 1910. But not all congenital malformations are fatal. They often produce a living but handicapped child. In the infants' ward of a large children's hospital, it was found that over a period of five months, more than one-third of the children were in the ward because of structural congenital malformations. Today it is recognized that congenital malformations can be caused by genetic factors, by radiation, by viruses, by drugs and by other environmental factors such as nutrition.[1]

---

[1] Lucille S. Hurley, "Nutrition and Birth Defects," speech given at meeting of American Home Economics Association, San Francisco, 1966.

WEIGHT CONTROL DURING PREGNANCY AND LACTATION

Some women fear retaining fat after pregnancy. But women who understand the meaning of a balanced diet have no fears about controlling their weight.

Caloric intake

Women should increase their intake of calories only after the fourth month of pregnancy. Even then they should have only 300 calories more than the normal daily allowance (Table 20-2). The calorie intake is increased by 500 per day during lactation (nursing). The baby, in turn, uses up these calories in rapid growth before and after birth.

The normal weight gain during pregnancy is from 7.2 to 10.8 kg (16 to 24 lbs). The extra weight is only partly from the weight of the baby. The increased size of the uterus and the breasts adds weight. So do the placenta, the extra fluid in which the baby floats, and the extra blood for mother and baby.

Rate of weight gain

An expectant mother should gain weight gradually during the first six months. Research shows that this reduces the likelihood of premature birth or toxemia.

Table 20-2 Daily balanced diets for pregnant and lactating mothers

| FOOD | PREGNANCY DIET[1] | | LACTATION DIET[1] |
	NORMAL + 300 CALORIES Measure	LOW-CALORIE[2] Measure	NORMAL + 500 CALORIES Measure
MILK	1 L (1 qt) whole, vitamin D-fortified	1 L (1 qt) whole, vitamin D-fortified[3]	1½–2 L (1½–2 qts) whole, vitamin D-fortified
MEAT, FISH, POULTRY Liver and seafood at least once per week	112–168 g (4–6 oz), lean	112 g (4 oz), lean	168 g (6 oz), lean
EGG	1 whole	1 whole	1 whole
VEGETABLES Dark green leafy or deep yellow, potato, others— 1 raw	At least 4 servings	At least 4 servings, succulent	At least 4–5 servings
FRUIT 1 or more servings citrus, 1–2 other	3 servings	3 servings	3 servings
BREAD-CEREALS Whole-grain or enriched	4 servings	4 servings	4–6 servings
BUTTER OR MARGARINE	15 mL (3t)	15 mL (3t)	15–45 mL (1–3T)
OTHER FOODS Desserts, vegetable oil to season, fruit juices, other foods desired from recommended group. Lactating mothers should avoid fats, concentrated sweets, highly seasoned foods	To meet calorie need	To meet calorie need	To meet calorie need

[1]Depends on age.
[2]Low-calorie pregnancy and lactation diets should be supervised by a physician.
[3]Diet can be reduced by 300 calories by substituting 1 L (1 qt) skim milk for whole milk and taking vitamin A supplement under physician's directions.

Underweight during pregnancy hurts both the mother and the baby. Studies have revealed more premature births after severe loss of weight during the first three months. Underweight may be caused by disease. If so, a physician can treat it. But it can also be caused by a false concept of what is beautiful in a figure. It can be caused by psychological factors, such as depression and inability or unwillingness to eat. The cure for underweight is a balanced diet with a larger calorie intake. The foods eaten should be rich in protein of good quality and high in vitamins and minerals.

The concept to remember is simple. An expectant mother should gain weight gradually and not lose weight unless she is advised to do so by her physician. The mother returns to her normal weight after the baby's birth, provided she eats wisely during pregnancy and afterwards. The RDA for expectant and lactating mothers are given on pages 402-403.

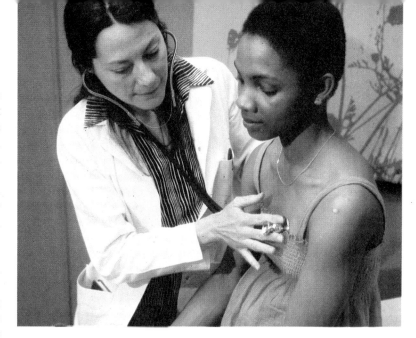

Weight gain—or loss—during pregnancy should be supervised by the physician.

NUTRIENTS REQUIRED DURING PREGNANCY AND LACTATION

A good diet for the whole family and a good diet for the expectant mother hardly differ. Good eating habits help us enjoy good health at any time during the life cycle.

Protein

Adequate protein in the diet improves the health of the expectant or lactating mother and her baby. It also helps prevent miscarriages. The recommended increase in protein is 30 grams daily during pregnancy and 20 grams during lactation.

Why does a mother need more protein? Protein is used to build every cell of her baby's body. A mother must also develop new tissues in her own body to take care of the baby. These tissues must serve her during pregnancy, delivery, and lactation. The baby's need for protein continues after birth. If the mother breast feeds, her milk must supply the needed protein.

The expectant mother should have a generous amount of animal protein divided about equally among her meals and snacks. Table 20-3 shows the protein content of the normal-plus-300-calorie diet.

Minerals

Calcium. During pregnancy and lactation, the need for calcium increases. (See the RDA table, page 403.) The extra calcium is needed for the developing fetus and later for breast milk. All kinds of milk except the condensed kind will supply generous amounts of calcium

Table 20-3 **Protein content of foods in Table 20-2 (grams)**

FOOD	PROTEIN
1 L (1 qt) of milk	36
1 egg at breakfast or lunch	6
42 g (1½ oz) tuna fish or 45 g (3 T) peanut butter at lunch	12
4 servings of bread-cereal	8
4 servings of vegetables	8
3 servings of fruit or juice	3
84 g (3 oz) lean cooked meat, fish, or poultry	16–20
Total daily protein	89–93

Table 20-4 **Meals providing increased daily intake of iron for pregnant women**

FOOD	IRON (MG)	CALORIES
BREAKFAST		
1 egg	1.1	80
1 slice whole-grain bread	0.8	65
½ grapefruit	0.5	45
5 mL (1 t) soft margarine	0.0	33
240 mL (3 oz) skim milk	0.1	90
Total	2.5	313
LUNCH		
56 g (2 oz) ham	1.6	135
120 mL (½ c) cooked spinach	2.0	20
1 raw tomato[1]	0.9	40
¼ head Boston lettuce[1]	1.1	8
1 slice enriched bread	0.6	65
5 mL (1 t) soft margarine	0.0	33
120 mL (½ c) dried cooked apricots	2.6	120
240 mL (8 oz) skim milk	0.1	90
Total	8.9	511
DINNER		
84 g (3 oz) pot roast (beef)	2.9	245
1 potato	0.7	90
120 mL (½ c) cooked peas	1.5	58
½ head Boston lettuce[1]		
1 slice enriched bread	0.6	65
5 mL (1 t) soft margarine	0.0	33
½ cantaloupe	0.8	60
240 mL (8 oz) skim milk	0.1	90
Total	8.8	656
SNACK		
60 mL (2 oz) prune juice	3.0	50
Day's total	23.2	1530[2]

[1]A total of 30 mL (2 T) of safflower oil or 45 mL (3 T) of corn, soybean, or cottonseed oil may be used as salad dressing or seasoning during the day to provide linoleic acid. Safflower oil will add 250 calories to the day's total. One of the other oils will add 375 calories.

[2]To meet the day's total calorie need, foods may be added to these menus as desired.

and phosphorus. To build the bony structure of the baby, calcium must be teamed with vitamins D, C, and A, amino acids, and other nutrients.

Iodine. If the mother's diet is deficient in iodine, simple goiter sometimes results because of the extra demand on the mother for iodine during pregnancy and lactation. Iodine is readily available in seafoods and iodized salt.

Iron. Anemia during pregnancy can be prevented by in-

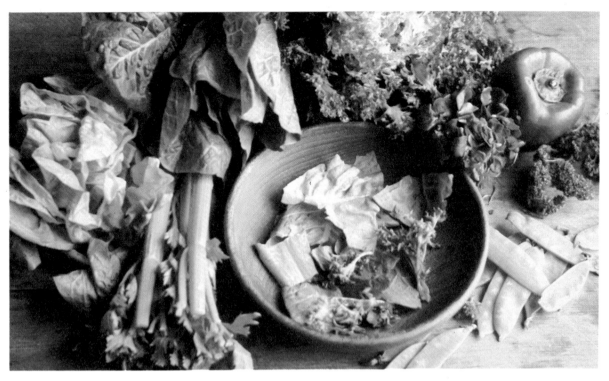

Green leafy vegetables are among the best sources of vitamins for the expectant mother.

creasing the amount of daily iron intake. The table opposite shows a day's menus rich in iron. But more iron is usually needed than even a carefully planned diet can supply. The woman's doctor decides how much iron she needs and prescribes a supplement.

Vitamins

Vitamin D. The vitamin-D requirement is 400 IU daily during pregnancy and lactation. Vitamin D is essential for absorbing calcium and phosphorus from the digestive tract. These minerals are needed to build the skeletal frame and the future teeth of the baby.

Vitamin A. An expectant mother should consume an extra 1000 to 2000 IU daily of vitamin A. This vitamin is essential for the formation of the epithelial cells that line every organ, gland, and membrane inside both the baby's body and the body of the mother.

Vitamin C. Vitamin C is involved in the life processes of every tissue. Fifteen mg more of it is needed daily during pregnancy and 35 mg more during lactation.

B vitamins. It is not difficult to provide the increase needed of the many B vitamins when the recommended variety of foods is eaten.

Vitamin K. Vitamin K has been called the coagulation vitamin. It is indispensable for the normal clotting of blood. It is therefore essential for a normal pregnancy and delivery, as well as for recovery afterwards.

Human babies are born with no vitamin K reserve. That is why many hospitals give vitamin K to the mother just before delivery or to the infant just after birth. Mothers who eat a balanced diet will have enough of this vitamin. It is widely distributed in foods, especially liver, leafy green vegetables, tomatoes, cauliflower, soybean oil, and egg yolk.

Young mothers who maintain good eating habits throughout the entire childbearing period of life have the best chance of producing healthy, strong, full-term babies. The mothers themselves are healthier. They suffer less loss of maternal tissues during and after birth. A well-nourished mother is less likely to suffer depression and fatigue after the birth of a child. Finally, the baby of a well-nourished mother will have a better chance to reach its full hereditary mental and physical potential.

Effect of diet on the expectant mother

Nourishment of the baby during gestation
Function of the placenta   Function of the umbilical cord   Function of hormones

Pregnancy complications related to diet
Anemia   Toxemia   Morning sickness   Pernicious vomiting   Constipation   Edema   Birth defects

Weight control during pregnancy and lactation
Caloric intake   Rate of weight gain

Nutrients required during pregnancy and lactation
Protein   **Minerals** *Calcium   Iodine   Iron*
Vitamins *Vitamin D   Vitamin A   Vitamin C   B vitamins Vitamin K*

1. Why is proper nutrition for the expectant mother important to the development of the baby?

2. Why is it important to avoid drugs and alcohol during pregnancy?

3. Describe how the placenta functions.

4. Name the hormones that are important during pregnancy, and briefly explain what they do.

5. Is it necessarily true that women must gain a great deal of weight during pregnancy? Explain.

6. Summarize the role of nutrition during pregnancy. Include the need for protein, and specific vitamins and minerals.

1. Invite a qualified nutritionist to address the class on the subject of the expectant mother and her baby.

2. Question your mother or another woman in your family who has children about the nutritional advice she received from her doctor during her pregnancy. Does it vary from the information given today? Discuss your findings in class.

3. As a class project, request from various agencies literature, pamphlets, charts, and other such material on nutrition and pregnancy. Exhibit them in your classroom, school library, or health classes.

VOCABULARY

anemia

edema

hormone

placenta

progesterone

toxemia

umbilical cord

Public health nutritionist Works in a clinic, often in a special area of nutrition: obstetrical, pediatric, geriatric; advises patients on sensible nutritional practices for specific health conditions. R.D. certification and advanced degree in nutrition required.

Field representative for farmers' organization Works for organization that represents farmers' views on relevant local and national events, prices, scientific developments; recruits members, arranges meetings, disseminates information on new developments. Four-year college education and on-the-job training required; knowledge of farming helpful.

RELATED READING

Flanagan, Geraldine Lux. *The First Nine Months*. New York: Simon & Schuster, 1962. Discusses the growth of life before birth.

Food and Nutrition Board, Committee on Maternal Nutrition. *Maternal Nutrition and the Course of Pregnancy*. Washington, D.C.: National Research Council—National Academy of Sciences, 1970. Discusses basic nutritional needs of mother and fetus.

Williams, P. S. *Nourishing Your Unborn Child*. Los Angeles: Nash Publishing, 1974. Presents the basic facts of food, nutrition, and health during pregnancy; contains practical suggestions, menus, and recipes.

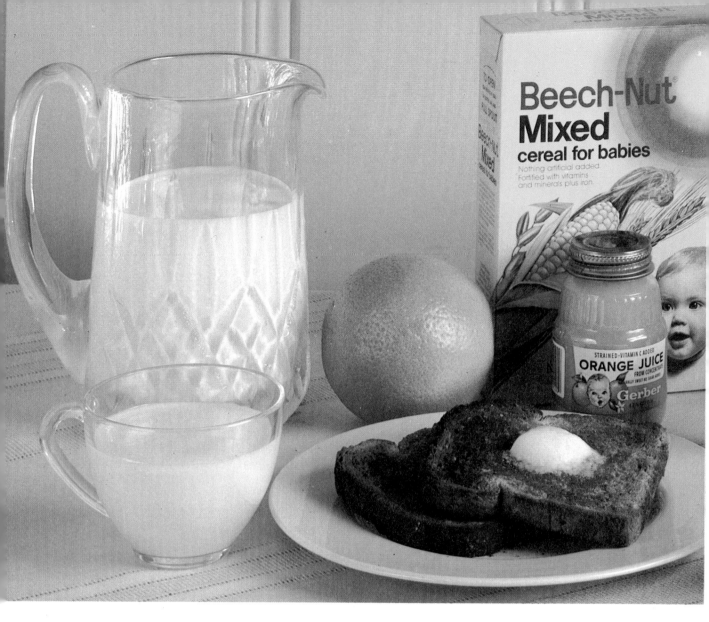

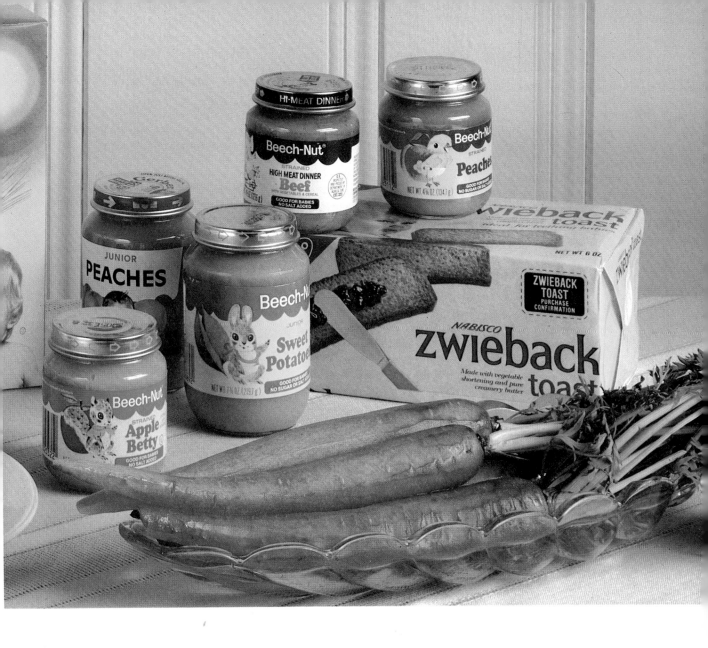

Feeding the young child

FEEDING INFANTS FROM BIRTH TO ONE YEAR OLD

Why do you like some foods and not others? Taste is only part of the answer. Your food preferences are influenced by your emotions. Since infancy and childhood, your food habits have also been influenced by parents and family, and by the emotional climate of the home, especially at mealtime.

Childrens' eating habits are set long before they enter school. As babies, they learn to like new foods.

Some children develop dislikes for foods for psychological reasons. Our knowledge of how likes and dislikes of food develop is growing. Parents can draw upon this knowledge—and their knowledge of food and nutrition—to help their children develop good eating habits.

Characteristics of infants

Full-term babies. Full-term babies average 50 cm (20 in) in length and 3.2 kg (7 lbs) in weight. They are overweight if they are heavier than 4.5 kg

(10 lbs) and probably premature if under 2.5 kg (5½ lbs). The birth weight of a baby should double in five months and triple in about one year. Of course, weight increase depends on the type of feeding and the individual baby.

Newborn full-term healthy babies can cry vigorously, suckle, and digest and absorb food. They are lively, have a good color, respond to stimuli, and sleep well. They have a good reserve of iron. Up to 75 percent of their weight is water. The proportion of water decreases until about the age of 10, when the average amount of water levels off at 55 to 70 percent—the same as an average adult. The bony structure of babies, most of which is cartilage, is one-fifth their weight. Compared to older children, their heads are large, and their arms and legs are short.

Premature babies. Premature babies have many more problems to overcome than full-term babies. Besides being premature, they are also immature. Their skulls are softer than those of full-term babies, because of inadequate bone mineralization.

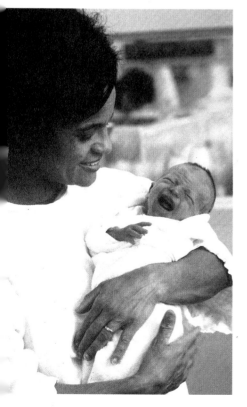

Newborn full-term healthy babies are physically active and cry lustily.

Premature babies are more likely to hemorrhage and be brain injured at birth because of pressure on the soft skull. They have a lower iron reserve and are more likely to be anemic, with weak muscles and little fat. Their digestion and absorption of food are poor because their enzymes do not function well and their stomachs are small. They may not be able to suckle well. While eating they may become fatigued quickly. Their underdeveloped respiratory system may present breathing problems. Since their sweat glands are immature, it is hard for them to regulate their body temperature.

Breast-feeding

Breast-feeding is a natural method of nourishing an infant. It has advantages for both the baby and the mother even if it is continued for only a few months. When breast-feeding is not possible, the alternative is properly managed formula-feeding.

Colostrum. Colostrum is the first thin, yellowish fluid that comes from the mother's breast after the child is born. It is not milk, but it is rich in protein, minerals, and vitamin A. It is well suited to the needs of a newborn. At first, colostrum is lower in sugar, fat, and other vitamins than milk, but these levels become comparable to mature milk by about the tenth day. By the end of two weeks the mother's milk no longer contains any colostrum.

Nutrients. According to H. H. Williams of Cornell University, mother's milk contains an ideal

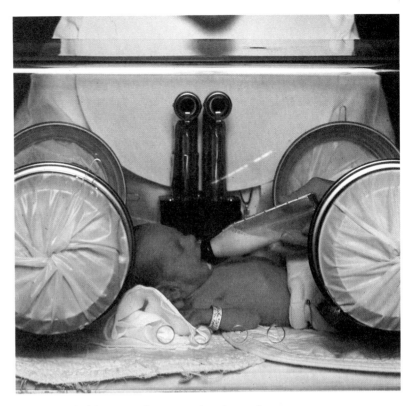

Premature babies sometimes need prolonged professional care and the controlled environment of an isolette in order to thrive.

balance of chemicals and nutrients. Human milk has twice as much iron as cow's milk. It has more vitamins A, C, and E, niacin, and linoleic acid. Human milk has more milk sugar.

Digestion. The baby easily digests and absorbs human milk, thus getting the digestive tract off to a good start. Mother's milk is clean, fresh, pure, and the correct temperature. The breast-fed baby has few or no constipation problems. Studies show less thumb-sucking, less illness, and a lower mortality rate among breast-fed babies than among others.

Psychological benefits. Several studies show that babies and mothers derive psychological benefits from breast-feeding. Babies receive emotional satisfaction

from breast-feeding that has long-range effects even into adolescence and adulthood. They experience feelings of security and comfort by being held safely in their mothers' arms. Baby and mother begin to communicate at this early stage. They develop a bond that is richly rewarding to both.

Other benefits. When a mother breast-feeds, the uterus walls contract and return to normal size and position earlier than when the mother does not breast-feed. Breast-feeding saves both the money needed to buy formula and time needed to prepare it. It also eliminates errors in calculating and making formulas, and no special feeding equipment is needed.

Formula-feeding

In some circumstances, breast-feeding is not advisable.

1. The mother should not nurse if she has a serious illness, such as severe anemia, tuberculosis, epilepsy, chronic fever, insanity, serious heart disease, or some types of kidney disease, such as nephritis.

2. A nursing mother who becomes pregnant should discontinue breast-feeding.

3. When the mother works outside the home, she may have to depend on others to feed her baby at home, or she may have to feed the baby at work.

Parents who choose to feed their baby by formula should be guided by the baby's physician as to the kind and amount of formula to use. The physician will know the baby's changing needs.

Ready-to-use formulas in disposable containers are available. Before buying them, parents should compare the cost with that of home-prepared formula. Parents should read the labels carefully on ready-to-use formulas and check with their physician if they have any doubts or questions.

Formula-feeding has a few nutritional problems that you should know about. When water is added to formula, the proportion of vitamins and other nutrients is decreased. Other foods that supplement nutrients must be provided at an early age. Vitamin C and vitamin D are particularly recommended to supplement formula. The recommended daily nutrients

Left: Whether babies are breast-fed or bottle-fed, they should be held in a parent's arms. *Right:* Babies should be "burped" around the middle of a feeding and again at the end.

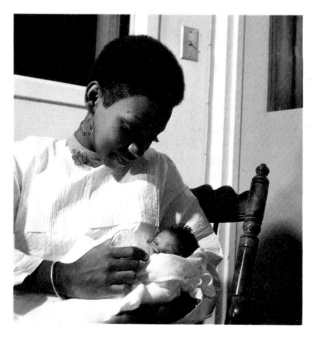
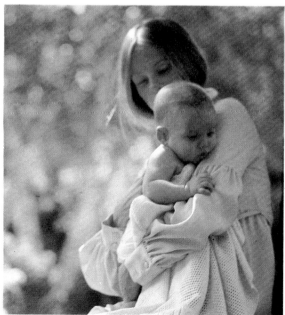

for a baby from birth to one year are given in the RDA table on pages 402–403.

Techniques of nursing

The same nursing techniques apply to both breast-feeding and formula-feeding.

1. Babies should be held in a parent's arms. The parent should select a comfortable chair and be prepared to sit for 15 to 20 minutes. Psychiatrists and psychologists have reported that the way a baby is fed affects the child's emotional development. When babies are fed with a propped-up bottle of formula, without closeness and human warmth, they may not develop well emotionally.

Holding babies while feeding helps them develop a normal capacity to give and receive love.

Infants can sense relaxation and love—or tension and anxiety. If parents cannot hold their babies at feeding time, they should select other regular periods in the day to hold and caress them.

2. Babies instinctively search for the nipple. Mothers can help by holding the nipple between two fingers and guiding it to the baby's mouth.

3. Some mothers become anxious and tense if the baby stops nursing. They worry that they perhaps have no milk. Usually there is no reason to be anxious. Each baby is different. Some stop nursing at intervals. Others nurse and swallow the milk very quickly. Premature infants often have difficulty nursing because of poor breathing and general underdevelopment.

4. As babies nurse, they swallow air along with the milk. To prevent discomfort and fussing, babies need to be "burped." Burping

should be done at the middle of the feeding and again at the end.

5. A 15- to 20-minute feeding period is recommended for both breast-fed and formula-fed babies. Hungry babies may drink quickly at the beginning of the feeding. They continue to drink even after satisfying their initial hunger. For successful breast-feeding, it is important to empty the breast completely. It often takes more than 20 minutes to breast-feed newborn full-term babies and still longer for those who are premature. If they fall asleep after the first hunger is satisfied, babies should be awakened with a gentle shake of their body and helped to start again.

Parents should not be discouraged if the formula-fed baby leaves milk in the bottle. Overfeeding during infancy or early childhood often leads to overeating and overweight as the child grows older.

INTRODUCING SOLID FOODS

Weaning

Some people wrongly believe that breast-fed babies are harder to wean than formula-fed babies. Weaning usually takes place easily as the mother's milk gradually diminishes. Breast-fed babies may go directly to drinking from a cup and eating solid food. But this depends on the age at weaning. The time for weaning a baby varies whether she or he is breast- or formula-fed. Weaning depends on the readiness of each baby.

While milk is the most important food in their diet, babies cannot live on milk alone. It is of

utmost importance that babies learn to like a variety of foods during the first year.

The manner in which new foods are introduced frequently determines the infant's acceptance or rejection of them. The first solid food should be in liquid form. Solid food can be liquified by adding formula or mother's milk. After the baby accepts the thin form, the mixture is gradually thickened to a semiliquid and finally to normal consistency. The first chopped food should be introduced when the baby has teeth and can chew (at about nine months of age).

A new food should be offered at the beginning of feeding, when the baby is hungry. The food should be held on the end of a baby spoon and placed in the center of the baby's mouth. The baby should be offered no more than 1.25 to 2.5 mL (¼ to ½ t) at a time. Parents should not be discouraged if the baby rejects the food at first. It is new in texture and flavor. The baby may spit it out. The parent should try again, showing no anxiety or tension, for three days. If the baby still rejects all the food after three days, the parent should wait for a few days, then try again.

Feeding the young child **337**

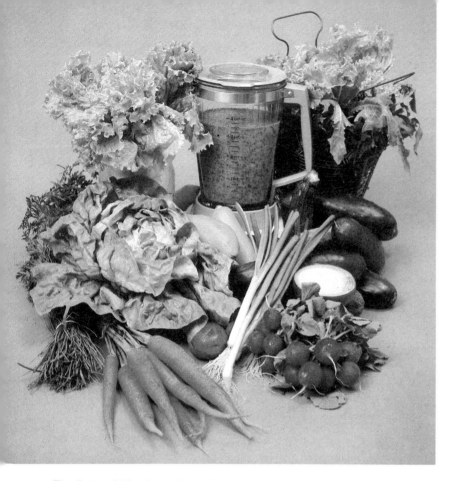

The first solid food to which babies are introduced should be in liquified form.

A new food should be offered to babies on the end of a spoon at the beginning of feeding, when they are hungry.

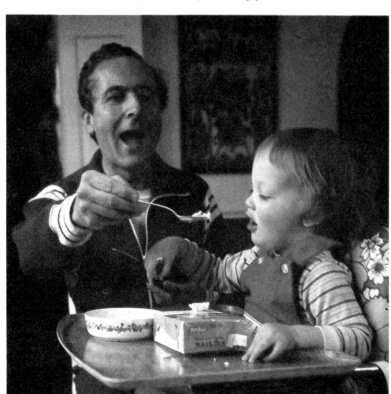

Only one food should be introduced at a time. The baby should learn to enjoy it thoroughly before the next one is introduced. Foods the baby already likes should accompany a new one.

Many babies reject food because it is too hot or too cold. A baby's food should be served at the same temperature as formula, about 38 °C (100 °F). Home-prepared baby food may be seasoned lightly.

Establishing good eating habits

The following guidelines—which all members of the family should observe—will help parents to establish good eating habits in babies. The guidelines assume an attitude in parents of confidence, relaxation, and cooperation.

1. Recognize that babies must get used to the different textures and flavors in foods and to eating from a spoon.
2. Praise babies immediately for success in doing what you want them to do. Praise encourages them to repeat desired behavior.
3. Make all remarks positive. Calling babies "bad" or scolding them with degrading names can do great emotional harm.
4. Avoid laughter or comments if babies do something that is "cute" but undesirable as permanent behavior.
5. Take quick and firm but relaxed action to stop unacceptable behavior. If babies refuse to eat or if they blow or throw food, they are either trying to get attention or they are not hungry. They

should be removed at once from the high chair or table and quietly told that they may return when they want to eat. They will understand that their behavior is not acceptable to those they love.

6. Don't feel you have to follow eating "rules" slavishly. Babies vary greatly in the times of development at which they will accept different foods and in the amount they eat.

FEEDING CHILDREN FROM ONE TO THREE YEARS OLD

Well-nourished one-year-olds are healthy, active, alert, happy children. They are firm but not fat. They have tripled their birth weight. They are also one and one-half times as tall as at birth. They have six or eight teeth, can stand well, and may walk or toddle. Some can say a few words, and most are making word sounds. They have been eating three meals a day for two to three months. Their hemoglobin and protein content is about the same as that of a well-nourished adult.

By the time children are one year old, psychological factors are already influencing what they eat. They are becoming more independent as they learn to walk and talk. They should be encouraged in this independence. Children at this age want to feed themselves and should be encouraged to do so. However, they may need some assistance, even if they themselves may not want any. Help can be given subtly by placing foods in bite sizes on a child's plate so that the pieces can be picked up with the fingers.

Children learn to become good eaters with good table manners through the example of sympathetic and mannerly parents who are relaxed and neither overly harsh nor overly protective. Children are great imitators. They also desire the love and approval of their parents.

Guidelines for parents

The following guidelines should help establish good eating habits in young children.

1. Provide well-balanced meals at regular times each day. Children who know when meals are to be served can plan for them. Hunger rhythms will develop a pattern. It is sometimes a good idea to let hungry young children eat before the rest of the family. When children are too tired or too hungry, they may eat poorly or throw temper tantrums.

2. Prepare food so that it looks and tastes good to the child.

3. Serve small portions according to childrens' individual needs. Being able to eat all of a small serving gives children a feeling of success. Don't force children to eat more than they want. Excuse children from the table as soon as they have stopped eating, and remove uneaten food from the table.

4. Avoid behavior at mealtime that may frustrate a child. Do not threaten or scold a child if he or she fails to eat. Threats and scolding set the stage for rebellion and revenge and may have harmful effects that go far beyond the eating of a particular food or meal.

5. Start meals early enough to allow time for even the slowest young eater. Rushing children through a meal causes them to feel frustrated.

6. Don't promise a child a present for good behavior. Bribing children for something they need to learn for their own sake does not help them develop emotionally. On the other hand, reward-

At about a year old, babies begin to want to feed themselves.

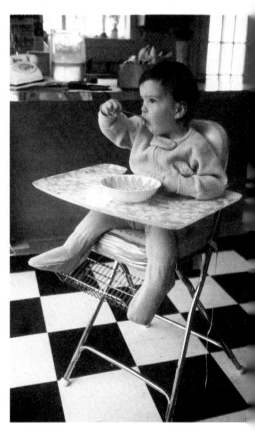

Showing children that shopping, gardening, cooking, and eating are enjoyable helps them to form good eating habits.

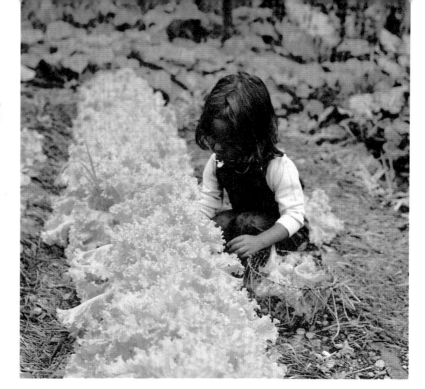

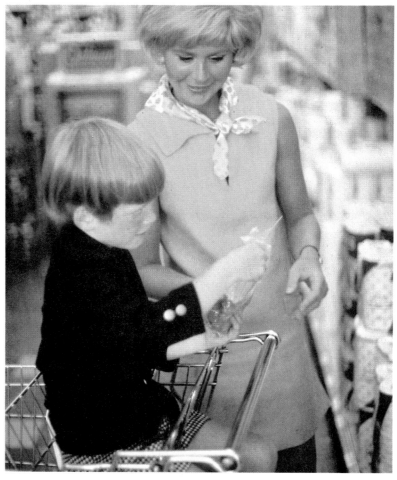

ing children afterward for something they have done well can reinforce desirable behavior. The reward does not have to be a concrete object. It may be a statement of praise.

7. Allow children between-meal snacks that fill genuine nutritional needs. The best snacks are fruit juice, fresh or dried fruit, milk or low-fat milk with a cracker or bread.

8. Teach table manners by setting a good example. Children who love their parents want to be like them.

Special food needs of children

The RDA table on pages 402–403 gives the daily amount of nutrients recommended for one-to three-year-olds. Parents should try to keep the diet balanced and the servings small.

Calories. Children do not grow evenly from month to month. They grow in spurts. Usually the appetite increases at the period of rapid growth, then levels off, as if the child wished to rest a bit from so much growth. Parents should realize that the child needs only a few more calories during growth-spurt periods. They should work on establishing good eating habits rather than forcing the child to eat large amounts.

Calcium. At one year or thereabouts, babies start to walk. Bones must be strong enough to support the weight of their muscles, which grow rapidly. When the bones are not properly mineralized, they bend, resulting in bowed legs and malformed joints.

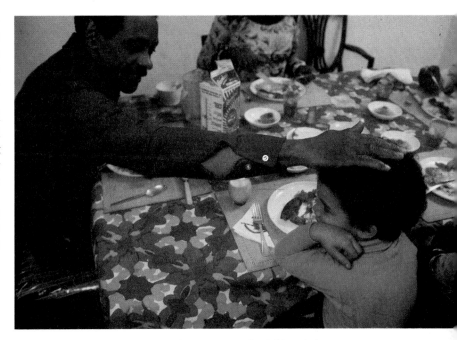

Praise from parents for good manners at the table reinforces desirable behavior in children.

Because their bones are growing, young children need as much calcium as adults need.

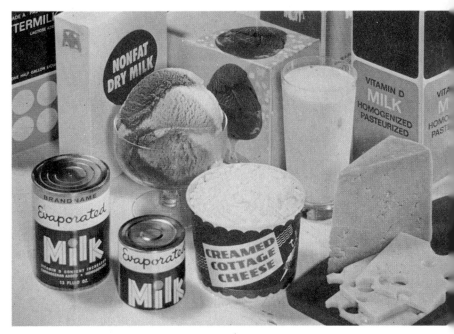

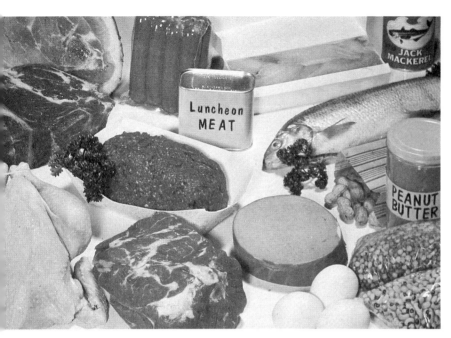

Children's muscles grow even faster than their bones and demand proportionate protein.

ding and from cheese cut into bite-size pieces. The milk intake may also be increased by adding nonfat dry milk to childrens' milk, cereal, and other foods.

Children from one to three years of age need as much calcium as adults. They need over half as much protein, vitamin C, riboflavin, thiamin, and niacin. They need more iron than an adult of 35 and over, and two-fifths the adult amount of vitamin A.

Protein. Children from one to three need about 1.5 g of protein per .45 kg (lb) of body weight. If they weigh 11.4 kg (25 lbs) they need about 38 g of protein. This is over half the protein need of a girl or woman from 15 years of age upward.

At about 18 months, the baby fat begins to disappear. Muscles grow rapidly in the next year and a half. Children's muscles grow faster than their bones and amount to one-half their weight. Muscle growth is particularly great in the thighs, hips, and back.

Calcium, other minerals, and vitamin D are laid down to harden the bones. Calcium comes mainly from milk, which should be part of every meal. The equivalent of 720 mL (1½ pints) of milk should be included in the child's diet at this age. Some milk can come from custard, rice or bread pud-

THINKING AND EVALUATING

1. Compare the characteristics of full-term and premature babies. Do you think most parents-to-be would try to eat good meals and snacks if they knew how much it would help their children and themselves? Explain.

2. What are the advantages of breast-feeding? List the reasons mother's milk is an excellent first food for the baby. Explain how a well-balanced diet on the part of the mother can help her breast-feed her baby well.

3. Why is breast-feeding psychologically beneficial to the baby?

4. Under what conditions should a mother not breast-feed?

5. Explain how to introduce new foods successfully into the diet of the baby.

6. List the guidelines for establishing good eating habits in babies and young children.

7. What are the physical and emotional characteristics of a well-nourished one-year-old?

8. Describe the food needs of the child from one to three years of age.

APPLYING AND SHARING

1. If you have a new baby in your family or can observe one, sit quietly and watch the way it nurses. If you can observe more than one infant, compare the way different babies take their milk. Discuss the differences in children in this respect with a mother who has more than one child. What did you learn? Share what you learn with the class.

2. Observe children from one to three years of age as they eat. Make notes on what they eat, the times of day they eat, and how they eat. How do the children compare?

3. Talk with the mother and the father of an infant and with the parents of a child one to three years old. Ask what feeding problems they have had and how they overcame them. Suggest ways to prevent feeding problems for toddlers. If possible, try out your plan when you baby sit.

4. Using the recommended diet for a lactating mother in Table 20-3, calculate the nutrients in each meal. Is each meal balanced? Do the nutrients for the whole day measure up? How would you adjust this menu to suit a low-cost diet for one day?

5. How would you plan to feed your baby so that the baby would be healthy and strong and like needed foods? How would you try to get your husband or wife to cooperate?

6. Visit the baby food section of your local supermarket and note the variety. Read the labels and compare the prices. Which do you think are "best buys" in each food category? Why?

VOCABULARY

cartilage
colostrum
full-term baby
premature baby
weaning

Feeding the young child **343**

7. Discuss with your teacher the possibility of having a pediatrician in your community talk to your class on feeding infants.

8. Plan, prepare, and feed a meal to a child one to three years old if you can. Evaluate your success.

Specialty shop worker Owns, manages, or clerks in a shop that specializes in one or a group of similar foods and/or equipment—for example, cheeses, candies and sweets, health foods, or pots and pans. Required education varies; some knowledge of food and business administration helpful.

Purchasing agent Works in food processing plant, food company, large supermarket, hospital, restaurant, school, other institution; responsible for budget control, ordering, bill paying. Four-year college education usually required; knowledge of mathematics and accounting essential.

Bogert, Jean, et al. *Nutrition and Physical Fitness*, 9th ed. Philadelphia, W. B. Saunders, 1973. The chapter "Nutrition in Infancy and the Preschool Years" focuses on general considerations for feeding infants, toddlers, and preschool children; considers the premature infant, food allergies, failure to thrive, overnutrition, lead poisoning, vegetarian diets, and child nutrition in developing countries.

McDonald, L. *Instant Baby Food,* 2d ed. Pasadena, Calif.: Oakland Press, ca. 1975. Focuses on developing good eating habits in children through variety of foods; includes practical information and recipes.

McWilliams, Margaret. *Nutrition for the Growing Years,* 2d ed. New York: John Wiley & Sons, 1975. Focuses on feeding children from infancy through adolescence.

UNIT 5

Research

Ruth Bennett White's

Low-calorie cookbook

RECIPES

ABOUT THIS COOKBOOK

This cookbook has been developed to enable you to put to use the principles of nutrition, food preparation, and meal management and economics. The recipes are arranged according to food groups. Each group contains a few selected basic recipes and suggested variations of the basic recipes. The recipes and their variations will help you to experience the culinary delights of different cultures, show you that gourmet cooking can be nutritious, and encourage you to create variations.

Most of the recipes have been adapted so that they are low in calories and fat content. Nonfat dry milk is used wherever possible as an economical and nutritious alternative to whole milk. When appropriate, polyunsaturated fats replace those high in saturated fatty acids.

Menu suggestions frequently accompany a recipe. In most menus, emphasis has been placed on the use of low-cost ingredients to produce economical, well-balanced meals.

Thirteen recipes are asterisked. This "baker's dozen" was specifically designed for preparation by one or more students within a classroom period of 30 to 45 minutes. As with all recipes in this book, you are encouraged to prepare these dishes at home.

Evaluating a recipe

Read the recipe through. Be sure you understand it before you use it. Refer to the Glossary on pages 431-440 for common cooking terms. Ask yourself the following questions.

1. Does it provide a fair share of the nutrients in the meal?

2. Is it consistent with our modern knowledge of nutrition? Can I change it, if necessary, to use the nutrients I need in place of those that are undesirable?

3. Does it fit within my food budget? If not, can I substitute less expensive ingredients for expensive ones?

4. Do I have on hand all the ingredients and utensils necessary? If not, can I make suitable substitutions?

5. Can I prepare this recipe in the time available?

6. Will my family and I enjoy eating it?

7. Am I making the best use of seasonal foods in using this recipe?

Using a recipe

Read the recipe critically all the way through before you begin.

Assemble in your mixing center all the ingredients and utensils required.

Do all preliminary preparation, such as chopping nuts or onions, peeling vegetables, oiling pans, or preheating the oven, before you start.

Measure accurately in standard cups or spoons.

Follow the recipe exactly, except in seasoning (which varies according to taste), until you are experienced in technique and understand the principles of food relationships in cooking.

Note any mistakes you may make. Review the recipe and your procedure. If necessary, make a plan to improve. Try the recipe again until you succeed, eliminating any previous mistakes, such as inaccurate measuring or failing to preheat the oven.

Experiment with herbs and spices to suit your taste. Note down what you do and the results.

Perfect each recipe to suit you, then broaden your experience by using others.

Useful food substitutes and equivalents[1]

1 T = 3 t or ½ fl oz
1 T all-purpose flour = 1½ t cornstarch, potato starch, rice starch, or arrowroot starch or 2 t quick-cooking tapioca
1 t baking powder = ¼ t baking soda + ½ c sour milk or buttermilk or ¼–½ c molasses
1 c = 16 T or 8 fl oz
1 c cake flour = 1 c less 2 T (⅞ c) all-purpose flour
⅓ c instant nonfat dry milk + ¾ c water = 1 c skim milk
1⅓ c instant nonfat dry milk + 3–3½ c water = 1 qt skim milk (see directions on package)
1 c whole milk = 1 c nonfat dry milk reconstituted + 2 t fat (this can be polyunsaturated, as in oil or soft margarine)
1 c buttermilk = 1 c milk + 1 T lemon juice or vinegar
1 14½-oz can evaporated milk (1⅔ c) + 1⅔ c water = 3⅓ c whole milk
1 6-oz can whole or skim evaporated milk = ⅔ c whole or skim milk
1 15-oz can sweetened condensed milk = 1⅓ c
1 lb grated cheddar cheese = 4 c
1 lb cottage cheese = 2 c
1 c butter, oleomargarine, or shortening = 1 c less 2 T vegetable oil or 1 c less 2 T lard + ½ t salt
1 c honey = 1½ c sugar + ¼ c liquid
1 c corn syrup = 1 c sugar + ¼ c liquid
1 c brown sugar, tightly packed = 1 c white granulated sugar
1 oz chocolate = 3 T cocoa + 1 T fat
8–10 graham crackers = 1 c crumbs
1 c whole large eggs (2 oz each) = 5 eggs
1 c egg whites = 8–9 eggs
1 c egg yolks = 12 eggs
2 c sifted egg powder + 2 c water = 12 large eggs

[1] Approximate customary measures. See table of metric conversion factors on page 400.

Sicilian Caponata
(Eggplant Antipasto)

(yield: 1.2 L [5 c] or about 20 servings)

Metric	Customary
80 mL	⅓ c vegetable oil
1	1 large eggplant, peeled and cubed
360 mL	1½ c diced celery
360 mL	1½ c diced onion
240 mL	1 c tomato paste
30 mL	2 T capers
60 mL	¼ c wine vinegar
120 mL	½ c diced black olives
30 mL	2 T sugar
5 mL	1 t salt
1.2 mL	¼ t coarse black pepper
60 mL	¼ c coarsely chopped walnut meats

Heat the oil in a large, thick-bottomed skillet and brown the peeled cubes of eggplant in it. Remove the cooked eggplant and drain on a paper towel.

Sauté the celery and onion in the skillet, stirring about 2 minutes.

Drain off the excess fat.

Add all the remaining ingredients and the cooked eggplant.

Cover and cook over low heat until mixture thickens (about 20 minutes), stirring occasionally to prevent sticking. Taste and adjust the seasoning according to your preference.

Store in a covered dish and refrigerate up to 10 days.

Serve at room temperature with warm French garlic bread as a first course.

Broiled Stuffed Mushrooms

Remove the stems from fresh or canned mushrooms and use them for a soup or a creamed dish.

Sauté the mushroom caps in a small amount of soft margarine, with salt and pepper to taste.

Stuff the inverted mushrooms with chicken or potted ham spread.

Broil and serve hot on circles of bread or crackers.

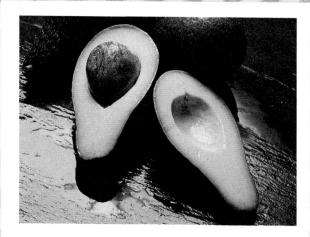

*Guacamole (Mexican)

(yield: 480 mL (2 c)

Metric	Customary
2	2 ripe avocados, mashed
1	1 clove garlic, crushed
30 mL	2 T lemon or lime juice
15 mL	1 T grated onion
2.5 mL	½ t chili pepper
1.2 mL	¼ t salt

Combine all the ingredients in a mixing bowl and blend thoroughly.

Serve in a bowl as a dip with raw vegetables or crackers, or as a salad dressing.

Top left: Mexican foods using tomatoes and other vegetables. *Top right:* Ingredients for tomato soup. *Bottom:* Vegetables.

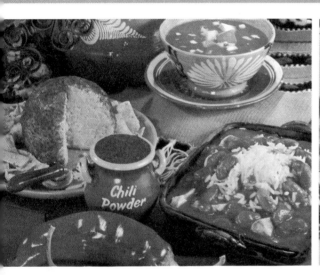

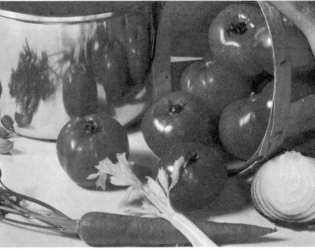

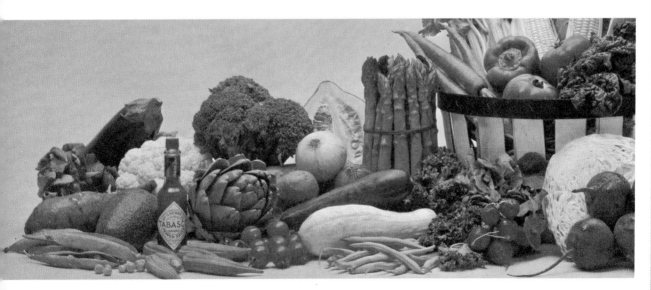

Left: Strawberries and whipped cream.
Top right: Finger vegetables and fruit.
Bottom right: Fruits.

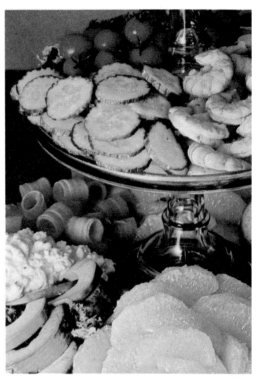

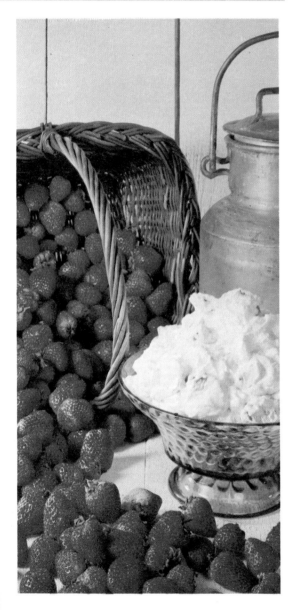

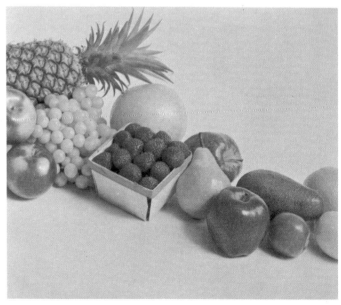

Winter Fruit Soup (Scandinavian)

(yield: 12 servings)

Metric	Customary
960 mL	**4 c water**
240 mL	**1 c seedless raisins**
240 mL	**1 c pitted prunes**
720 mL	**3 c sliced apples**
480 mL	**2 c sliced peaches**
1	**1 orange, sliced, with peel**
30 mL	**2 T lemon juice**
1.2 mL	**¼ t cloves**
1.2 mL	**¼ t nutmeg**
5 mL	**1 t cinnamon**
60 mL	**¼ c quick-cooking tapioca**
480 mL	**2 c pineapple juice**
	sugar to taste

Bring water to a boil.

Place uncooked fruits, lemon juice, spices, and 480 mL (2 c) of the boiling water in a 3.8-mL (4-qt) pressure saucepan; cook at 6.8 kg (15 lb) pressure 1 minute, allowing the pressure to return to normal. Or cook in a large covered saucepan until tender.

Mix the tapioca in the remaining hot water and add it to the hot fruit.

Cook over medium heat until slightly thickened.

Stir in pineapple juice and sugar to taste (not more than 60 mL [¼ c]).

Serve hot or cold as dessert, garnishing with a slice of lime or orange or a cherry.

Chef's Salad

(yield: 4 servings)

Metric	Customary
960 mL	**4 c bite-size torn green lettuce pieces (Bibb, Boston, bronze-tipped, Romaine)**
360 mL	**1½ c cubes or strips of any one or a combination of the following: chicken, turkey, ham, fish, or shellfish**
120 mL	**½ c sliced cucumber and/or green pepper strips**
120 mL	**½ c diced celery**
60 mL	**¼ c thinly sliced green onions**
360 mL	**1½ c thin strips of Swiss or sharp Cheddar cheese, or cottage cheese**
60 mL	**¼ c French dressing**
2	**2 tomatoes, sliced**

Combine all ingredients, except the cottage cheese (if used) and the tomatoes, in a large bowl, and toss lightly.

Arrange ingredients attractively in a salad bowl or individual bowls or plates. If cottage cheese is used, use a small mound for each serving and place the vegetables around it.

Garnish with the tomato slices.

Serve as the main dish for lunch, preceded by hot bouillon or lentil soup, and accompanied by popovers, hot muffins, hot rolls, or nut bread. For dessert, serve floating island or custard.

Variations on page 354.

VARIATIONS

1 / Tossed Salad

Omit the meat and cheese.

Use a combination of any fresh or cooked vegetables you like.

Garnish with watercress, radish roses, sliced hard-cooked eggs, avocado slices, or pepper strips, and any dressing you prefer.

2 / Citrus-Avocado Salad

Toss bite-size lettuce pieces with dressing and place on individual salad plates.

Arrange alternate sections of citrus fruit, apple slices, avocado slices, and/or pear slices over the lettuce.

Place 80–120 mL (⅓–½ c) cottage cheese in the center of each salad.

Top with a cherry tomato or a strawberry. When strawberries are in season, make a circle of fresh berries around the outside of the salad.

Serve, preceded by a French onion soup or split pea soup, and accompanied by hot bread and café au lait.

Cabbage-Carrot-Pineapple Mold

(yield: 8–10 servings)

Metric	Customary
23 mL	1½ T unflavored gelatin
240 mL	1 c water
240 mL	1 c pineapple juice, scalded (use amount drained from crushed pineapple)
2.5 mL	½ t salt
60 mL	¼ c sugar
60 mL	¼ c lemon juice
240 mL	1 c crushed pineapple, drained
480 mL	2 c grated cabbage
240 mL	1 c grated carrots
60 mL	¼ c mayonnaise
60 mL	¼ c sour cream
60 mL	¼ c chopped walnuts

Soften the unflavored gelatin in the water, then add it to the scalded pineapple juice, stirring until it is dissolved.

Add the salt and sugar, and stir until dissolved. Cool.

Add all but the last three ingredients, mixing thoroughly.

Rinse a 1.4-L (1½-qt) mold with cold water and pour the gelatin mixture into it.

Chill until firm.

Fresh Fruit Salad or Compote

Salad

Arrange a mixture of two or more fresh fruits in season on a bed of lettuce. The addition of cottage cheese or seafood in the center will provide protein and transform the salad into a main dish.

Compote

Arrange a mixture of fresh fruits in season in a tall sherbet dish and serve plain or top with sherbet for dessert. Use such fruits as melon balls, orange and grapefruit sections, avocado, pears, apples, strawberries, fresh pineapple, blueberries, peaches, grapes, and others.

Unmold by setting the mold into hot water for 10 seconds and turning it upside down on a flat plate.

Surround the mold with green lettuce.

Blend the mayonnaise, sour cream, and chopped walnuts. Place the mixture in the center hole of the mold.

Serve. If preferred, use individual small molds.

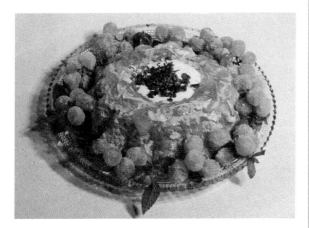

VARIATIONS

(yield: 4–6 servings)

1 / Cabbage-Fruit Salad

Toss lightly 480 mL (2 c) shredded cabbage, 240 mL (1 c) diced oranges, 240 mL (1 c) pineapple chunks with your favorite dressing. To make a molded salad, omit the dressing and add the ingredients to 1 package of orange-flavored gelatin prepared according to the package directions.

2 / Cabbage-Tomato-Onion Salad

Toss 960 mL (4 c) shredded cabbage, 2 tomatoes cut in wedges, 1 thinly sliced green onion, and oil-and-vinegar dressing.

3 / Cabbage-Apple-Peanut Salad

Mix 720 mL (3 c) shredded cabbage, 240 mL (1 c) diced apples, 120 mL (½ c) peanuts, 240 mL (1 c) diced celery, and just enough mayonnaise to moisten.

4 / Cabbage-Carrot-Orange Salad

Mix 480 mL (2 c) shredded cabbage, 240 mL (1 c) coarsely grated carrots, 240 mL (1 c) orange slices, 60 mL (¼ c) raisins, and mayonnaise.

VEGETABLE-FRUIT GROUP / COOKED VEGETABLES

Panned Vegetables (Oriental)

Shred finely any of the mixed greens mentioned on page 357 or slice thinly on the diagonal asparagus, cauliflower, any summer squash, green or snap beans, onions, Brussels sprouts, or broccoli.

Measure the vegetable after shredding and use 240 mL (1 c) of raw greens or 180 mL (¾ c) of the other vegetables per serving.

Heat 5 mL (1 t) of vegetable oil per serving in a heavy skillet with a tight cover.

Add the vegetable, stirring until all of it is coated with oil. Salt lightly and add other seasonings to taste. (See Table 10–7 for suggestions on herbs and seasonings to use.)

Stir thoroughly. Cover the pan.

Lower the heat and stir at intervals to prevent scorching.

Cook until just tender and serve at once as part of a balanced meal. Sauces may be added to panned vegetables as desired, but the vegetables are lower in calories when cooked and served simply.

VARIATION

Thinly sliced meat, poultry, or fish may be cooked first, then the vegetable if desired. Serve with hot rice. Serve cheese and fresh fruit for dessert.

Top: Molded gelatin and vegetable salad.
Bottom: Shrimp and rice salad.

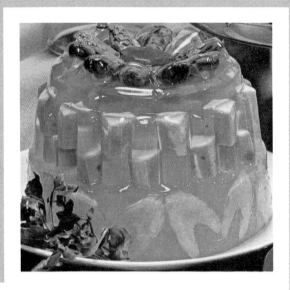

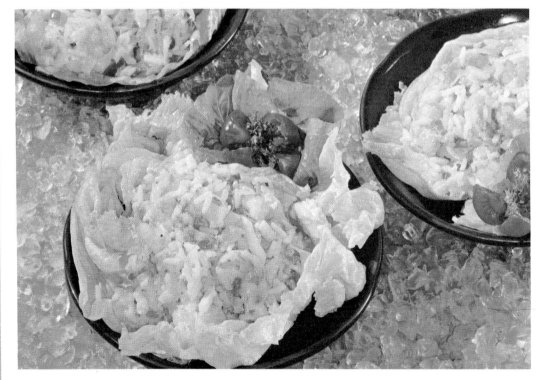

Sukiyaki (Japanese)

(yield: 6 servings)

Metric	Customary
.68 kg	1½ lb lean round steak
15 mL	1 T vegetable oil
45 mL	3 T soy sauce
120 ml	½ c water
2	2 chicken bouillon cubes
360 mL	1½ c celery, sliced diagonally (about 2.5 cm [1 in] thick)
	salt and pepper to taste
360 mL	1½ c sliced green onions
240 mL	1 c sliced mushrooms
140 g	5 oz canned bamboo shoots, drained and sliced
.45 kg or	1 lb chopped fresh spinach or
280 g	10 oz frozen chopped spinach, thawed
.96–1.44 mL	4–6 c cooked brown rice with ginger to taste

Trim all fat from the meat.

Cut meat into .63 x 5-cm (¼ x 2-in) diagonal strips, and brown in hot oil.

Push the meat to one side and add all the remaining ingredients except the spinach and rice.

Stir and simmer, uncovered, until the vegetables are tender, adding a small amount of liquid as needed. Add the spinach and cook until tender (about 1 minute).

Serve at once the hot meat-vegetable mixture over hot rice. Serve melon or citrus fruit as the first course and lemon cookies or meringues (recipe on page 381) as dessert, with tea.

*Southern Cooked Collard Greens

(yield: 4–6 servings)

Metric	Customary
.9 kg or	2 lb fresh collard greens or
560 g	20 oz frozen chopped collards, thawed
15 mL	1 T oil
4–6	4–6 bacon slices, uncooked and chopped
2.5 mL	½ t red dried pepper
1 medium	1 medium onion, chopped
5 mL	1 t salt
60–120 mL	¼–½ c boiling water

Remove all tough stems and damaged parts from fresh greens.

Wash thoroughly and chop.

Heat the oil.

Sauté the bacon with the red pepper and the onion in a 3.8-L (4-qt) saucepan or pressure cooker until it is soft, but not crisp; drain off fat.

Add the greens and the salt. If you are using a pressure saucepan, add 60 mL (¼ c) boiling water. Bring the pressure to 6.8 kg (15 lb) and cook 2–4 minutes. If you are using a regular saucepan, add 120 mL (½ c) of boiling water and boil until the greens are tender.

Garnish with sliced hard-cooked egg, if desired.

Serve with hot skillet corn bread (recipe on page 387), ham, black-eyed peas, sliced tomatoes, green onions, and cold milk or buttermilk, with nut pie or a pudding for dessert.

VARIATION

Mixed Greens

Mix equal amounts of two or more of the following greens: collards, Savoy cabbage, outer leaves of green or red cabbage, broccoli, turnip greens, kale, mustard greens, dandelion greens, Swiss chard, beet tops, endive, or spinach. These greens may also be cooked separately. Spinach or Swiss chard should be cooked only about 1 minute at boiling temperature. When mixing greens, add the spinach last.

*Spinach and Cheese Casserole Italian Style

(yield: 6–8 servings)

Metric	Customary
240 mL	1 c thick white sauce
15 mL	1 T soft margarine
.9 kg	2 lb fresh spinach
or	or
560 g	20 oz frozen chopped spinach, thawed and drained
3	3 eggs
180 mL	¾ c low-fat cottage cheese
120 mL	½ c nonfat dry milk
2.5 mL	½ t salt
1.25 mL	¼ t coarsely ground pepper
.63 mL	⅛ t nutmeg
1.25 mL	¼ t marjoram
180 mL	¾ c grated Parmesan or sharp Cheddar cheese
60 mL	¼ c slivered almonds or walnuts

Prepare the white sauce (recipe on page 365), and set aside.

Remove all damaged parts from the fresh greens; wash and chop.

Melt the margarine in a frying pan and cook the spinach over low heat until dry and just tender, stirring frequently to prevent burning. Remove from heat.

Beat eggs slightly in a mixing bowl.

Add the cooked, cooled spinach and all remaining ingredients, except 120 mL (½ c) of the grated cheese and the slivered almonds.

Mix thoroughly.

Blend the white sauce into this mixture.

Pour mixture into a 1.4-L (1½-qt) casserole.

Sprinkle top with the reserved cheese and the slivered almonds.

Bake in a preheated oven at 178 °C (350 °F) until mixture is firm and bubbly and cheese is golden brown (about 10 minutes).

Serve hot at once.

Note: Other greens may be used as an alternate to the spinach.

Succotash Mexican Style

(yield: 4–6 servings)

Metric	Customary
240 mL	1 c each corn, baby lima beans, and chopped tomatoes (fresh, frozen, or canned)
60 mL	¼ c diced onion
1	1 clove garlic, crushed
5 mL	1 t salt
5 mL	1 t chili powder
1.25 mL	¼ t black pepper
15 mL	1 T vegetable oil or margarine

Heat the corn, lima beans, and tomatoes in a thick-bottomed pan. Then add the onion, garlic, salt, chili powder, black pepper, and vegetable oil or margarine.

Bring to a boil and simmer until the vegetables are just tender.

Serve hot at once.

VARIATIONS

1 / Spinach and Cheese Soufflé

Separate the eggs. Use the yolks in the mixture and beat the whites to stiff, moist peaks. Before pouring the mixture into the casserole, fold in the egg whites.

Bake as above. Serve hot at once.

2 / Broccoli and Cheese Casserole or Soufflé

Use chopped broccoli instead of spinach for a casserole or a soufflé.

Cook the broccoli in 60 mL (¼ c) water and use the water as part of the liquid for the sauce. Proceed as above.

Creamed Peas, Carrots, and Onions

(yield: 4–6 servings)

Metric	*Customary*
240 mL	**1 c medium white sauce**
240 mL	**1 c sliced carrots**
60 mL	**¼ c water**
300 mL	**1¼ c fresh peas**
or	*or*
280 g	**10 oz frozen peas**
120 mL	**½ c diced onions**
5 mL	**1 t sugar**
	salt and white pepper to taste

Prepare a medium white sauce (recipe on page 365) and set aside.

Cook the carrots in the water for 2 minutes in the pressure saucepan at 6.8 kg (15 lb) pressure, or boil gently until tender in regular saucepan with water to cover. Drain.

Add the peas, onions, and white sauce and cook until vegetables are tender.

Blend in the sugar, salt, and white pepper.

Serve hot as part of a balanced meal.

VARIATIONS

1 / Other Creamed Vegetables

Cream any of the following vegetables (fresh, frozen, or canned): new potatoes, asparagus, cabbage, broccoli, spinach, cauliflower, lima beans, green or snap beans, turnips, rutabagas, or celery. Use 480 mL (2 c) of vegetables to 240 mL (1 c) of medium white sauce.

Add seasonings to taste (see Table 10–7 for herbs and spices appropriate for this purpose).

2 / Vegetable au Gratin (French)

Use any of the cooked vegetables suitable to creaming and place in a casserole.

Add 120 mL (½ c) grated cheese to the white sauce and top the casserole with strips of Cheddar, Swiss, or process cheese.

Sprinkle with paprika and bread crumbs, if desired, and bake at 178 °C (350 °F) until the cheese topping is melted and the mixture is hot and bubbly.

Serve hot at once as part of a balanced meal.

3 / Scalloped Potatoes

Alternate layers of thinly sliced potatoes with thin white sauce to within 2.5 cm (1 in) of the top of a casserole. Add sliced onion to middle layer, if desired.

Bake in a preheated oven at 178 °C (350 °F) until done.

Note: Any vegetable suitable for creaming may be scalloped.

4 / Potatoes and Ham

Add either slices of ham or pork strips to the top of the scalloped potato casserole and bake until done.

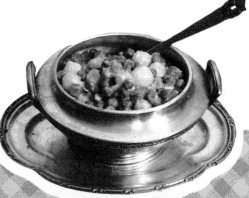

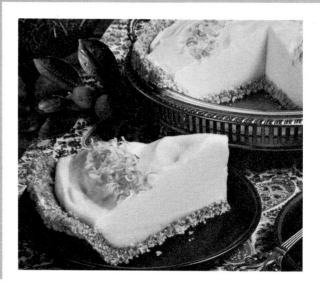

Top: Lemon cream pie with graham cracker crust. *Bottom:* Creamed seafood, saffron rice, mixed vegetables, herbed bread, warm fruit compote.

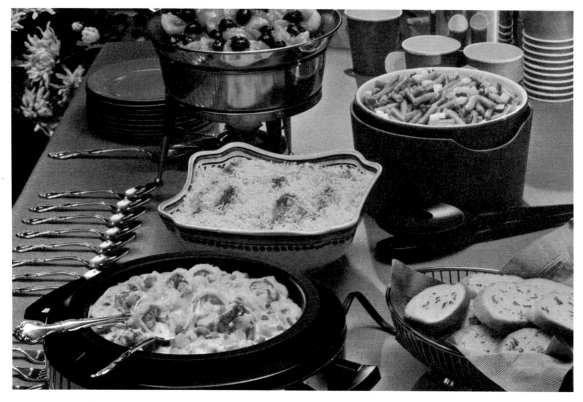

Yellow Winter Squash Casserole

(yield: 6–8 servings)

Metric	Customary
960 mL	**4 c cooked, mashed squash (butternut, Hubbard, acorn, banana)**
30 mL	**2 T soft margarine**
120 mL	**½ c nonfat dry milk**
120 mL	**½ c packed brown sugar**
5 mL	**1 t grated lemon peel**
5 mL	**1 t grated orange peel**
120 mL	**½ c orange juice**
1.25 mL	**¼ t nutmeg**
2.5 mL	**½ t mace**
2.5 mL	**½ t salt**

Combine all ingredients thoroughly and turn into a 1.4-L (1½-qt) casserole.

Bake in a preheated oven at 192 °C (375 °F) until bubbly and slightly brown.

Serve hot as a potato alternate. Squash blends well with any meat, vegetable, or salad as part of a balanced meal.

VARIATION

Pumpkin, Sweet Potato, or Yam Casserole

Use pumpkin, sweet potatoes, or yams and follow the squash recipe.

Top with marshmallows for the last few minutes of baking, if desired.

VEGETABLE-FRUIT GROUP/DESSERTS

Lime Pie

Metric	Customary
	graham cracker crust
295 mL	**14 oz sweetened, condensed milk**
120 mL	**½ c nonfat dry milk**
3	**3 egg yolks**
5 mL	**1 t grated lime or lemon rind**
120 mL	**½ c lime juice**
60 mL	**¼ c water**
3	**3 egg whites**
1.25 mL	**¼ t salt**
1.25 mL	**¼ t cream of tartar**
2.5 mL	**½ t vanilla**
2.5 mL	**½ t almond extract**
120 mL	**½ c sugar**

Prepare a graham cracker crust (recipe on page 395).

Mix the next six ingredients thoroughly, and set aside.

Place the egg whites into a mixing bowl.

Add the salt, cream of tartar, vanilla, and almond extract, and beat until foam begins to form.

Beat in the sugar, 15 mL (1 T) at a time, until thoroughly dissolved, and the whites are in moist shiny peaks.

Pour the pie filling into the crust, and top it with the meringue.

Bake in a preheated oven at 205 °C (400 °F) for 10 minutes. Turn off the heat and leave the pie in the oven for 20 minutes.

Remove from oven, and let cool.

Serve as part of a balanced meal.

Variations on page 362.

1 / Lime Fluff Pie

Beat the egg whites, omitting the sugar, and fold the custard into the stiffly beaten egg whites.

Pour into the crust and proceed as above. When ready to serve, cover each piece with a thin layer of sweetened and flavored yogurt or sour cream.

Top with fresh or thawed frozen berries or orange sections. If there is more filling than the crust will hold, cook it separately in a custard cup.

Note: This recipe has fewer calories than lime pie.

2 / Lemon Fluff Pie

Substitute 120 mL (½ c) lemon juice for the lime juice and proceed for either type of pie.

3 / Orange Fluff Pie

Substitute 180 mL (¾ c) orange juice for lime juice, add 5 mL (1 t) grated orange rind, and proceed as above.

MILK GROUP / HORS D'OEUVRES

Quick Cottage Cheese Pizza

Split English muffins. Oil them lightly. Brown in the broiler.

Spread each half with low-fat cottage cheese.

Spread about 15 mL (1 T) of canned pizza sauce over the cottage cheese.

Add chili pepper, if desired.

Top with finely diced chives or green onion tops and a generous sprinkling of grated Parmesan or sharp Cheddar cheese.

Garnish with 6 slices of stuffed olive and heat under the broiler until the cheese melts. (Omit olive for lower cost.)

Serve hot as the main dish for lunch or cut each muffin into six wedges and serve as an hors d'oeuvre at a party.

*Cottage Cheese Clam Dip

Metric	Customary
360 mL	1½ c low-fat cottage cheese
15 mL	1 T grated onion
15 mL	1 T minced parsley
15 mL	1 T lemon juice
15 mL	1 T horseradish
160 mL	⅔ c canned minced clams (drain, but save juice)
1.25 mL	¼ t salt
15 mL	1 T blue cheese
dash	dash hot sauce
	paprika

Blend all the ingredients except the paprika and clam juice until smooth.

Add enough clam juice to give the desired consistency.

Place in a covered container in the refrigerator overnight.

Bring to room temperature when ready to use.

Serve at once, garnished with paprika and accompanied by thin, crisp crackers.

Cheeses, solid and grated.

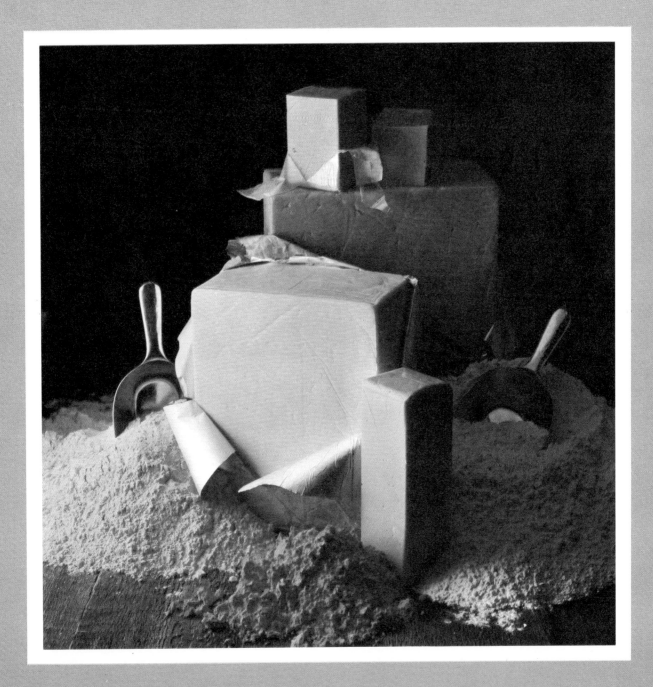

Cheese Soufflé (Swiss)

(yield: 4 servings)

Metric	Customary
120 mL	½ c flour
30 mL	2 T vegetable oil
480 mL	2 c skim milk
5	5 egg yolks, slightly beaten
240 mL	1 c grated Gruyère cheese
240 mL	1 c grated Swiss cheese
dash	dash nutmeg
.63 mL	⅛ t white pepper
5	5 egg whites
5 mL	1 t salt

Prepare a thick white sauce by placing the flour, vegetable oil, and skim milk in a heavy-bottomed 2.9-L (3-qt) saucepan.

Cook the sauce over low heat until it is thick and smooth, stirring to prevent lumps.

Add the slightly beaten egg yolks, grated cheeses, nutmeg, and white pepper; blend thoroughly. Let cool.

Beat the egg whites and salt in a large mixing bowl until moist, firm peaks are formed.

Fold the cheese mixture gradually into the egg whites until blended.

Pour into a buttered 1.4-L (1½-qt) casserole or small individual casseroles.

Bake in a preheated oven at 178 °C (350 °F) until golden brown (about 45–50 minutes).

Serve hot at once with cucumber, lettuce, and tomato salad, hot green beans, and warm French garlic bread, using fruit in season for dessert. This dish may be a main course for any meal.

VARIATIONS

1 / American Cheese Soufflé

Add a dash of cayenne pepper, 5 mL (1 t) dry mustard, and 15 mL (1 T) grated onion to the white sauce.

Use 224 g (½ lb) grated sharp Cheddar cheese instead of Swiss and Gruyère cheese.

Add 2.5 mL (½ t) cream of tartar to the egg whites before beating, to give a firmer texture.

2 / Scandinavian Cheese Soufflé

Poach .45 kg (1 lb) boneless fish with 1.25 mL (¼ t) each of fresh black pepper and thyme, a dash of cayenne pepper, 5 mL (1 t) grated lemon peel, 15 mL (1 T) lemon juice, and 60 mL (¼ c) boiling water. Cover and cook until tender (about 5 minutes).

Mash the fish and add it to the cheese, using the broth in which it is cooked as part of the liquid in making the sauce with nonfat dry milk.

Proceed as in the basic recipe. Serves 6–8.

3 / French Cheese Soufflé

Serve with a thin mushroom sauce, using 120 mL (½ c) sliced cooked mushrooms per cup of thin white sauce.

4 / Mexican Cheese Soufflé

Prepare the soufflé as the American version, but serve with a medium tomato sauce, using tomato juice instead of milk and adding 1 diced green pepper, 30 mL (2 T) diced onion, and 7.5 mL (1½ t) chili peppers. If desired, 120 mL (½ c) diced green chili peppers may be added for each 480 mL (2 c) sauce.

5 / Chicken or Turkey Soufflé

Add 480 mL (2 c) diced cooked chicken or turkey to the American variation.

Serve hot at once, with a mushroom sauce, as the main dish in a balanced meal.

*Cream of Vegetable Soup

(yield: 5–6 servings)

Metric	Customary
480 mL	2 c thin white sauce
240 mL	1 c vegetable purée
15 mL	1 T grated onion
5	5 chicken bouillon cubes
.63 mL	⅛ t celery salt
.63 mL	⅛ t garlic salt
	salt and pepper to taste

Prepare thin white sauce (recipe on this page) in a thick-bottomed 1.9-L (2-qt) saucepan.

Stir in remaining ingredients.

Heat until boiling; then simmer 1 minute.

Season to taste.

Serve hot in warm soup bowls or mugs, garnished with minced parsley, chopped chives, a slice of lemon or lime, or cheese croutons.

Note: Vegetables suited to cream soups include tomato, potato, spinach, watercress, kale, broccoli, lettuce, leek, onion, peas, beans, asparagus, celery, corn, carrot, squash, pumpkin, avocado, mushroom, cauliflower, beet, rutabaga, almond, or peanut. Other foods suited to cream soups are fish, ground poultry, ground meat, or a combination of some of these.

VARIATIONS

1 / Mexican Cream of Vegetable Soup.

Combine corn and beans and add 7.5 mL (1½ t) chili pepper.

2 / Italian Cream of Vegetable Soup

Add 1 clove of crushed garlic, 1.25 mL (¼ t) oregano, and 30 mL (2 T) minced parsley.

3 / Indian Cream of Vegetable Soup

Add 2.5 mL (½ t) curry powder.

*Basic Low-Fat, Low-Calorie White Sauce

THIN

Metric	Customary
15 mL	1 T flour
240 mL	1 c milk*
15 mL	1 T oil
1.25 mL	¼ t salt

MEDIUM

Metric	Customary
30 mL	2 T flour
240 mL	1 c milk*
15 mL	1 T oil
1.25 mL	¼ t salt

THICK

Metric	Customary
45 mL	3 T flour
240 mL	1 c milk*
15 mL	1 T oil
1.25 mL	¼ t salt

EXTRA THICK

Metric	Customary
60 mL	4 T flour
240 mL	1 c milk*
15 mL	1 T oil
1.25 mL	¼ t salt

Blend to a smooth paste equal amounts of flour and milk with the oil and salt.

Add seasonings and any additional ingredients called for by the specific recipe, such as herbs, spices, eggs, sugar.

Heat the remaining milk to scalding and add it gradually to the first mixture.

Cook in a 2.9-L (3-qt) pan at low heat until the desired smoothness and thickness are obtained, stirring constantly to prevent lumps. When extract is added for cream-type pies and the like, add it after the cooking is completed.

*For lower cost, substitute 120 mL (½ c) nonfat dry milk plus 240 mL (1 c) water per cup of liquid asked for in the sauce.

(yield: 10–12 servings)   (quick top-of-stove main dish)

Metric	Customary
30 mL	2 T oil
1 large	1 large green pepper, thinly sliced
1	1 clove garlic, crushed
30 mL	2 T grated onion
720 mL	3 c diced, cooked chicken or turkey
6	6 chicken boullion cubes
720 mL	3 c green celery, diagonally chopped
600 mL or 2 cans	2½ c medium white sauce or 2 cans cream of mushroom soup
	salt and pepper to taste
30 mL	2 T soy sauce
.45 kg can	1 lb can pineapple chunks (including juice)
960 mL	4 c hot cooked brown rice, noodles, macaroni or bulgur
60 mL	¼ c toasted almonds

Heat the oil in a 3.8-L (4-qt) saucepan.

Add the green pepper, garlic, and onion, and sauté for one minute.

Blend in all the remaining ingredients, except the almonds and rice, noodles, macaroni, or bulgur, stirring gently until well blended and bubbling hot.

Serve over rice, noodles, macaroni, or bulgur, and top with toasted almonds.

Note: This dish may be prepared the night before, poured into a casserole, covered tightly, and refrigerated. When it is to be used, heat in a preheated oven at 190 °C (375 °F) until it bubbles in the middle (about 25 minutes). Serve at once with a green vegetable, tossed salad, milk, and pumpkin nut bread (recipe on page 384) for dessert.

VARIATIONS

1 / Ham and Chicken Casserole

Use cooked leftover ham or fresh pork, or equal amounts of pork and chicken.

2 / Mexican Casserole

Add 120 mL (½ c) diced green chili peppers, removing the seeds, 240 mL (1 c) diced canned tomatoes, and 240 mL (1 c) grated sharp Cheddar cheese; blend in.

MILK GROUP/DESSERTS

Yogurt

(yield: 1.20–1.44 L [5–6 cups])

Metric	Customary
480 mL	2 c nonfat dry milk
240 mL	2 c water, warmed to 43 °C (110 °F)
60 mL	¼ c plain yogurt
720 mL	3 c water, boiled and cooled to 43 °C (110 °F)

Blend until smooth the nonfat dry milk, the warmed water, and the yogurt.

Add the boiled and cooled water, and mix thoroughly.

Pour mixture into a 1.4-L (1½-qt) bowl, or a casserole with a lid, and cover.

Set in a warm place out of drafts. Do not disturb until firm (about 5 to 7 hours). Then refrigerate.

Serve as an alternate for milk; or top with honey, sweetened strawberries, peaches, or other fruit; or sweeten, add 1.25 mL (¼ t) vanilla, and use as a dessert topping; or serve on any vegetable, meat, or salad.

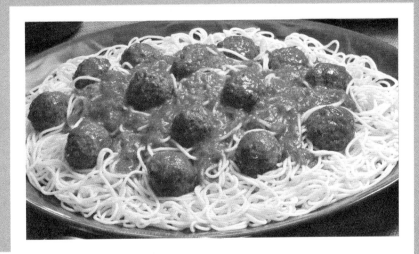

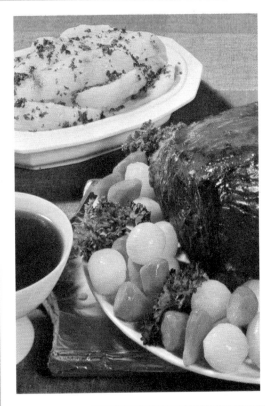

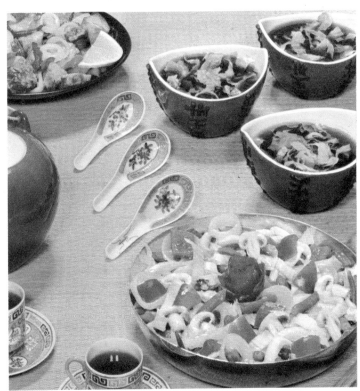

Top: Spaghetti and meatballs. *Bottom left:* Roast beef with gravy, baby carrots and pearl onions, parsley potatoes. *Bottom right:* Oriental vegetables, soup, and chicken.

(yield: 1 pie)

Metric	Customary
1 22.5-cm	1 9-in baked pie shell
120 mL	½ c packed brown sugar
60 mL	4 T flour
240 mL	1 c nonfat dry milk
15 mL	1 T soft margarine
540 mL	2¼ c water
3	3 egg yolks, slightly beaten
5 mL	1 t vanilla
3	3 egg whites
1.25 mL	½ t salt
1.25 mL	¼ t cream of tartar
120 mL	½ c granulated sugar

Prepare a baked pie shell (recipe on page 391) and set aside.

Mix in a thick-bottomed 1.9-L (2-qt) saucepan the brown sugar, flour, nonfat dry milk, margarine, and 120 mL (½ cup) of the water, to form a smooth paste.

Add the remaining water and the beaten egg yolks.

Cook over low heat, until mixture is smooth and thickened, stirring constantly to prevent lumps.

Remove from heat and blend in the vanilla. Set aside.

Prepare a meringue by beating the egg whites with the salt and cream of tartar until they start to foam, then beating in the granulated sugar, 30 mL (2 T) at a time, until all is dissolved and the meringue stands in firm, moist peaks.

Pour the hot filling into the baked crust.

Spread the meringue over the top of the pie to the edge of the outer crust (this helps the meringue hold to the crust), swirling for an attractive design.

Bake in a preheated oven at 234 °C (450 °F) until golden brown (7–10 minutes). Remove from oven.

Cool and serve as dessert in a balanced meal.

Note: Most cream pies may be made from this recipe. Fillings may be served as pudding without a crust, over cake, or topped with fruit, nuts, semisweet chocolate, sweetened yogurt, or whipped cream.

VARIATIONS

1 / Vanilla Pudding

Fold the beaten egg whites (without adding the white sugar) into the hot filling at once.

Cover and let stand until the egg whites have had time to cook. Do not place the pudding on the stove.

Pour into sherbet glasses or a large bowl.

Top with desired garnish and serve.

2 / Pineapple Cream Pie or Pudding

Add 240 mL (1 c) well-drained canned crushed pineapple just before the mixture is removed from the heat.

3 / Banana Cream Pie or Pudding

Add a thick layer of sliced ripe bananas over the pie crust before pouring in the cream filling.

4 / Coconut Cream Pie or Pudding

Add 60 mL (¼ c) shredded coconut to the cream filling.

Sprinkle 60 mL (¼ c) of shredded coconut over the meringue before browning.

5 / Chocolate Cream Pie or Pudding

Mix 75 mL (5 T) cocoa with 60 mL (¼ c) sugar and blend in at the first step.

Broiled Herbed Steak

(yield: 4–6 servings)

Metric	Customary
9–1.4 kg	**2–3 lb high-quality steak or tenderized round or rump**
1.25 mL	**¼ t crushed tarragon leaves**
1	**1 crushed clove garlic**
1 25 mL	**¼ t celery salt**
2.5 mL	**½ t coarsely ground black pepper**
60 mL	**¼ c soft margarine**

Trim the surplus fat from the outside of the steaks and wipe steaks with a clean damp cloth.

Place on a slightly oiled, preheated broiler rack and broil on each side 5–8 minutes, according to the thickness of the meat and the degree of rareness desired.

Mix the herbs with the margarine and spread lightly over each serving as it is served.

Broiled Chicken, Turkey, or Cornish Hen

Split broilers, chicken or turkey breasts or joints, or Cornish hens to make serving-size pieces. Wash and dry the meat.

Rub all sides with self-basting marinade (recipe on page 374) or herbed seasoning used for steak.

Place in a lightly oiled shallow oblong baking pan, skin side up, in broiler.

Broil on one side 20–30 minutes and turn, brushing the top with marinade. Broil until done (flesh is tender and no pink is showing).

Serve with a potato or alternate, a green or yellow vegetable, green salad, milk, and fruit cocktail cake (recipe on page 397).

*Broiled Fish Steaks With Almonds

(yield: 3 servings per .45 kg [1 lb])

Select fresh or thawed frozen salmon, filet of sole, halibut, haddock, red snapper, trout, shad, or other fish you prefer, boned.

Wash and dry the fish, if fresh.

Rub the fish on each side with self-basting marinade (recipe on page 374).

Sprinkle with slivered almonds.

Broil in a preheated broiler until the fish is lightly browned and flakes when tested with a fork (7–10 minutes, depending on thickness).

Serve hot at once, garnished with sliced lemon, lime, tomato, or greens. Complete the meal with brown rice, stewed tomatoes, okra and onion, cabbage salad, and café au lait, plus lime pie (recipe on page 361).

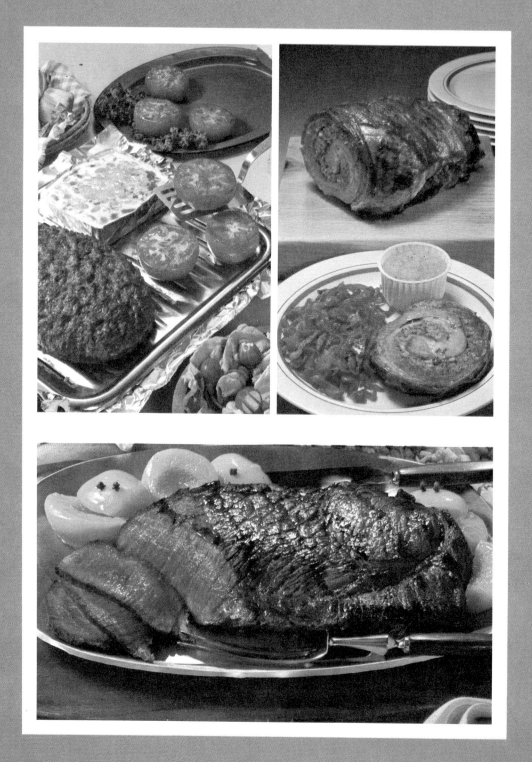

Top left: Broiled ground beef loaf, broiled tomatoes, scalloped potatoes *au gratin. Top right:* Roasted rolled stuffed veal with applesauce and red cabbage. *Bottom:* Grilled steak garnished with peaches and cloves.

Roast Lamb Turkish Style

(yield: 2–3 servings per .45 kg [1 lb])

Metric	Customary
1	1 boned leg of lamb
120 mL	½ c vegetable oil
68 mL	¼ c lemon juice
4	4 crushed garlic cloves
2	2 crushed bay leaves
10 mL	2 t fresh ground pepper
	salt to taste

Wipe the meat with a clean damp cloth and place it in a flat pan.

Mix the remaining ingredients and rub them well into the lamb on all sides.

Place meat in remaining marinade and allow to marinate in the refrigerator overnight, spooning the liquid over the meat at intervals. Three hours before roasting, remove the meat from the marinade and allow it to dry. Don't wipe.

Place meat on a rack in a shallow pan.

Insert a meat thermometer in the center of the thickest part.

Roast in a preheated oven at 94–150 °C (200–300 °F) to an internal temperature of 68–75 °C (150–165 °F). If preferred, reduce the oven heat to 94 °C (200 °F) after one-half hour and cook until the meat thermometer registers the desired degree of doneness. The lower cooking temperature takes about one and one-half times the cooking time, or more, but yields the best flavor, has the least loss of nutrients and juices, and has the least shrinkage.

Serve with pilaf, eggplant or squash, rye bread, lettuce and tomato salad, yogurt topped with strawberries or fresh fruit, and coffee.

VARIATIONS

1 / Shish Kabob (Turkish)

Cut the lamb into 2.5-cm (1-inch) cubes and marinate as roast (or use tender beef, if you prefer).

Place the meat on individual skewers, alternating with cubes of two or more of these vegetables: eggplant, summer squash, mushrooms, bell peppers, onions, cherry tomatoes.

Roast or broil until done.

Serve hot as part of a balanced meal.

2 / Ham Kabob With Pineapple (Turkish)

Cut precooked or canned ham in 2.5-cm (1-inch) cubes.

Place them on skewers, alternating with pineapple.

Roast or broil until done.

Serve hot with hot brown rice and scrambled eggs for breakfast or brunch, preceded by fresh fruit or juice, or for supper, accompanied by a salad and a baked caramel custard for dessert.

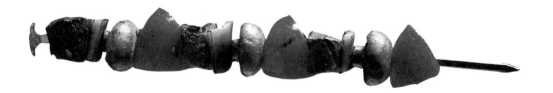

Standing rib, rolled sirloin, sirloin tip,
or crosscut
Salt and pepper to taste
Herbs and spices to taste

Wipe the meat carefully with a clean damp cloth or a paper towel.

Season it with salt, pepper, and other seasonings before, during, or after cooking. Seasoning penetrates only .63 cm (¼ in).

Place the meat on a rack in a shallow pan with the fat side up. Add no liquid.

Insert a meat thermometer in the center of the meat, not touching the fat or bone.

Roast in a preheated oven at 94–150 °C (200–300 °F) until the desired internal temperature is reached: 60 °C (140 °F) for rare, 70 °C (160 °F) for medium, 77 °C (170 °F) for well done.

Remove the meat from the oven 15–20 minutes before serving, for better cutting. Meat continues cooking for a few minutes out of the oven.

Serve hot with brown juice drippings (but not fat) on a hot platter, surrounded with vegetables, as part of a balanced meal.

VARIATIONS

1 / Lamb or Veal Roast

Use the leg, loin, or shoulder and follow above directions, roasting to an internal temperature of 68–75 °C (150–165 °F).

2 / Fresh Pork Roast

Use the loin, shoulder, ham, or picnic shoulder, and roast to an internal temperature of 84 °C (185 °F).

3 / Cured Pork Roast

Use cured ham or picnic shoulder, and roast to an internal temperature of 72–75 °C (160–165 °F).

Baked Stuffed Fish

Metric	Customary
1.4–1.8 kg	**3–4 lb whole fresh fish,** **drawn and scaled**
or	*or*
2	**2 large fish fillets**
1.25 mL	**¼ t salt**
1.25 mL	**¼ t pepper**
60–120 mL	**¼–½ c seasoned bread** **crumbs**
15 mL	**1 T vegetable oil**
	self-basting marinade

Wipe fish inside and out (both sides of fillet) with damp paper towels.

Combine salt and pepper, and sprinkle it inside whole fish. (If fillets are used, sprinkle one side of each fillet.)

Place stuffing inside the cavity of whole fish (in center length of the seasoned side of one fillet).

Drizzle vegetable oil over stuffing.

Close fish cavity (place seasoned side of second fillet over the first and secure with string around each end and in the center).

Cover fish with self-basting marinade (recipe on page 374).

Bake in a preheated oven at 150 °C (300 °F) until tender and fish flakes when touched with fork.

Serve hot as part of a balanced meal.

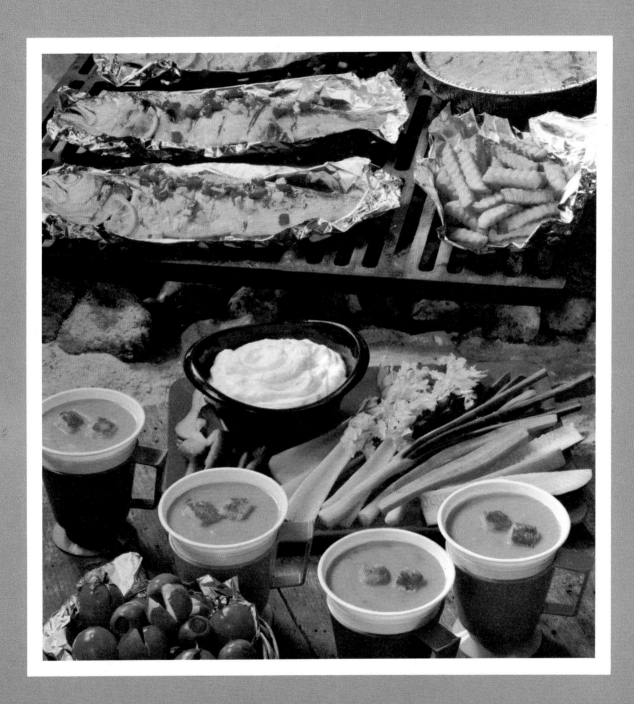

Baked stuffed fish, French fries, pea soup garnished with croutons and sour cream, finger vegetables.

Metric	Customary
120 mL	½ c flour
60 mL	¼ c lemon juice
60 mL	¼ c vegetable oil
30 mL	2 T grated onion
2	2 cloves garlic, crushed
2	2 thyme leaves, crushed
15 mL	1 T salt
2.5 mL	½ t black pepper
15 mL	1 T paprika

Blend all ingredients and rub the mixture on all sides of the poultry or fish (either whole or in pieces), spreading the mixture more thickly over the breast of poultry. The food needs no basting while cooking.

Baste with the juices that run off, just before serving.

Note: This marinade may also be used on a roast cooked at low temperture. For a thicker sauce, use more flour; less flour will make a thinner sauce.

MEAT GROUP / BRAISED MEAT

Pot Roast with Vegetables

(yield: 6 servings)

Metric	Customary
1.4–1.8 kg	3–4 lb lean meat
80 mL	⅓ c flour
30 mL	2 T vegetable oil
240 mL	1 c water
2.5 mL	½ t black pepper
1.25 mL	¼ t celery seed
10 mL	2 t salt
2	2 bay leaves
1	1 clove garlic, crushed
240 mL	1 c diced celery
120 mL	½ c diced onion
4	4 large white potatoes, quartered
6	6 small onions
8	8 carrots, quartered

Wipe the meat with a clean damp cloth.

Dredge meat in flour.

Heat the oil in a thick-bottomed pan, such as a Dutch oven or chicken fryer, and brown the meat on all sides.

Add the liquid, herbs, and spices. Cover tightly and allow to simmer until the meat is tender, or cook in a pressure saucepan at 6.8 kg (15 pounds) pressure for 12–15 minutes.

Remove the meat and skim off the excess fat from the liquid.

Add the vegetables, cover the pan, and cook the vegetables over low heat until just tender. If the pan is large enough, cook the vegetables with the meat the last 20 minutes (or in the pressure cooker about 3–5 minutes).

Serve the meat hot, surrounded by vegetables and covered with the nonfat drippings. Garnish with parsley or chopped green onions.

Accompany with bread, milk, green cabbage salad, and molasses cake or gingerbread.

VARIATIONS

1 / Boeuf à la Mode (French)

Add *bouquet garni* (bay leaf, thyme, rosemary, and parsley) to the liquid, following basic directions for pot roast. Omit the carrots.

Add 240 mL (1 c) sliced mushrooms with other vegetables.

Serve with warm French bread, green salad, small pastry, fresh fruit, and cheese.

*Nigerian Groundnut (Peanut) Stew

(yield: 8 servings)

Metric	Customary
1.44 L	6 c hot cooked white rice*
30 mL	2 T vegetable oil
240 mL	1 c finely diced onion
2	2 garlic cloves, crushed
1–3	1–3 dry red chili peppers, crushed
or	*or*
5–15 mL	1–3 t chili powder
2.5 mL	½ t nutmeg
480 mL	2 c cubed eggplant
960 mL	4 c cubed, cooked chicken
720 mL	3 c chicken broth
45 mL	3 T flour
336 g	12 oz canned tomato paste
180 mL	¾ c peanuts, crushed
10 mL	2 t salt

Prepare rice according to package directions.

Heat the oil in a 3.8-L (4-qt) saucepan.

Add the next five ingredients and cook over medium heat until eggplant is browned, stirring frequently to prevent sticking.

*Brown rice may be used, but it requires longer cooking time.

Add the remaining ingredients and stir to blend thoroughly.

Bring to a boil, cover, and let simmer 3–5 minutes.

Serve hot over hot rice, with any of the following toppings (in separate dishes): chopped peanuts; diced orange, pineapple, papaya; thin slices or small wedges of tomato; finely sliced green onions; diced green pepper; grated coconut; chutney or watermelon pickle.

Accompany with milk or café au lait and white coconut cake.

Note: Stew made the day before and stored in the refrigerator overnight has a better flavor. Heat only until bubbling hot and serve.

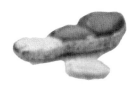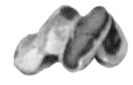

2 / Irish Stew

Use lean meat in 2.5-cm (1-in) cubes and omit the celery. Follow directions as in the basic recipe.

Serve with milk, bread, spread, green onions, and deep-dish apple pie.

3 / Mexican Stew

Use 2 cloves garlic, 2 crushed dried chili peppers, 240 mL (1 c) tomato paste; omit carrots.

Follow the basic method for braising.

Serve with tortillas, milk, and a whole orange.

Roast turkey garnished with spiced crabapples and celery frills, stuffing, glazed yams and apples.

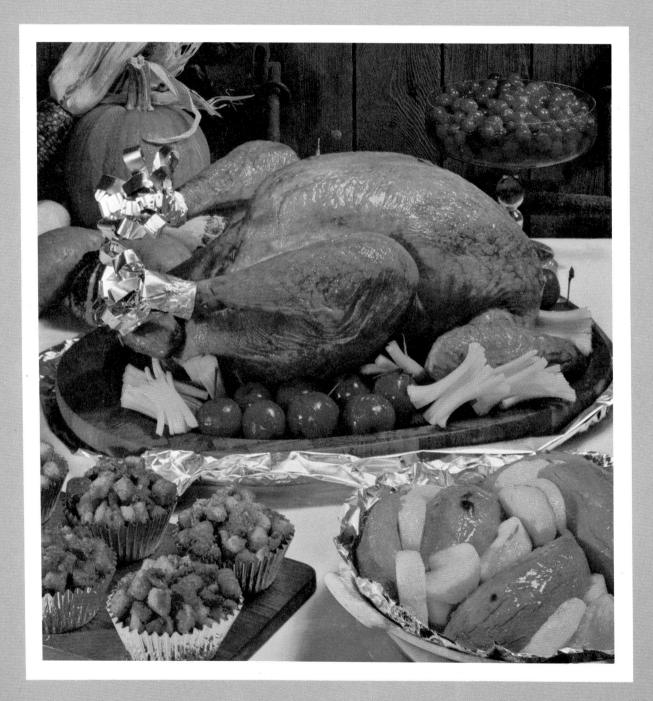

Baked Beans (American)

(yield: 8–9 servings)   (shortcut top-of-stove method)

Metric	Customary
.45 kg	1 lb dried pea beans
480 mL	2 c water
360 mL	1½ c tomato juice
15 mL	1 T vegetable oil
240 mL	1 c chopped onion
2	2 bacon strips, diced
.63–1.25 mL	⅛–¼ t crumbled red pepper
or	or
1–2	1–2 dried chili peppers
160 mL	⅔ c dark molasses
30 mL	2 T lemon juice or vinegar
5 mL	1 t dry mustard
15 mL	1 T salt

Precook the beans with the water, tomato juice, and vegetable oil for 2 minutes at 6.8 kg (15 lb) pressure, or boil them in a covered pot for at least 2 minutes. Then let the beans stand, covered, to soak for at least 2 hours.

Add all the remaining ingredients and cook in a pressure saucepan at 6.8 kg (15 lb) pressure for 5 minutes, letting the pressure return to normal gradually. Boiling in a regular pan requires 2½–3 hours. If desired, pour the beans into a casserole and brown under the broiler before serving.

Serve as a meat alternate with corn sticks, spinach-cheese casserole (recipe on page 358), sliced onion and orange salad, apple pie, and milk.

VARIATION

Boiled Beans

Omit the molasses and proceed as above.

MEAT GROUP/PAN-FRIED OR SAUTÉED MEATS

*Southern Fried Pork Chops and Yams

(yield: 4 servings)

Metric	Customary
4	4 thick pork chops
60 mL	¼ c flour
15 mL	1 T vegetable oil
30 mL	2 T flour
240 mL	1 c skim milk
	salt and pepper to taste
2	2 large yams, peeled and halved, fresh or canned

Parboil raw yams about 15 minutes; remove from heat and drain.

Trim the excess fat from the pork chops.

Dredge pork chops in flour. Reserve excess flour.

Heat the vegetable oil in a large ovenproof skillet.

Brown the chops quickly on both sides.

Remove chops from the pan.

Drain any excess fat from the pan and add the remaining flour, stirring over low heat until it is brown.

Stir in the skim milk, and continue stirring until smooth.

Add salt and pepper to taste.

Return the chops to the gravy.

Place one yam section on each chop.

Cover tightly and simmer, or bake in moderate oven until the chops and yams are tender (10–15 minutes).

Serve hot with collards, turnip greens, or another green leafy vegetable, corn bread, margarine, milk, fresh green onions, and applesauce.

*Liver and Onions Italian Style

(yield: 6 servings)

Metric	Customary
.45 kg	1 lb liver
60 mL	¼ c flour
2.5 mL	½ t salt
2.5 mL	½ t thyme
.63 mL	⅛ t pepper
30 mL	2 T vegetable oil
2	2 medium onions, thinly sliced
80 mL	⅓ c water
80 mL	⅓ c white wine
30 mL	2 T minced parsley
2	2 beef bouillon cubes

Slice the liver into thin strips.

Combine the next four ingredients in a brown paper bag or a clear plastic bag.

Add liver strips and shake vigorously until all the strips are coated with the seasoned flour.

Heat the oil in a large skillet.

Add the onions and sauté until soft (about 3 minutes).

Add the liver to the onions and cook, stirring frequently, over medium heat until just done.

Remove mixture from pan, and hold in an 80-°C (175-°F) oven until needed.

Combine the remaining ingredients in the skillet and bring to a boil.

Stir to blend thoroughly.

Reduce heat to a simmer; cook for 1 minute.

Place liver in a warm serving dish; pour hot sauce over liver and onions.

Serve with panned green beans, baked potatoes, green lettuce salad, fruit cocktail, and skim milk.

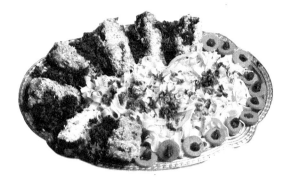

Veal Cordon Bleu

(yield: 4 servings)

Metric	Customary
.45 kg	1 lb veal slice
1.25 mL	¼ t salt
1.25 mL	¼ t pepper
10 mL	2 t lemon juice
4	4 thin slices cooked ham
4	4 slices Emmenthaler (Swiss) or sharp Cheddar cheese
	flour
1	1 egg, beaten
	bread crumbs
45 mL	3 T oil

Flatten the veal, pounding it with a heavy knife or a meat hammer, or ask your butcher to do this.

Cut the veal into four equal pieces.

Combine salt, pepper, and lemon juice, and rub over veal slices.

Place a slice of ham and a slice of cheese in the center of each piece of veal.

Roll the veal and fasten it with a toothpick.

Dredge the veal rolls in flour.

Dip the meat into the egg and then roll it in the bread crumbs.

Heat oil in large skillet.

Add the veal rolls and cook over medium heat until evenly browned and tender (about 10–15 minutes).

Drain on doubled paper towels and serve immediately, or keep warm in a flat pan in an 80-°C (175-°F) oven.

Serve hot with brown rice or noodles, broccoli, tomato and cucumber salad, whole-wheat French bread, café au lait, and vanilla cream pie or pudding (recipe on page 368).

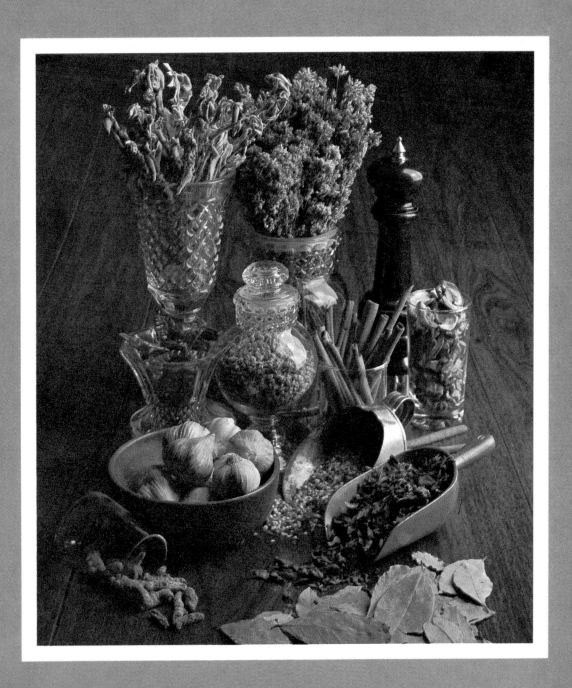

Seasonings: dried whole sage, dried whole marjoram, pepper mill, dried chili peppers, dried camomile flowers, cinnamon sticks, dried mushroom slices, garlic, crushed dried chili peppers, dried basil leaves, dried ginger root, dried bay leaves.

Basic Beef Vegetable Soup

(yield: 8–10 servings)

Metric	Customary
1	**1 marrow bone (split)**
.9 kg	**2 lb lean meat, cubed**
720 mL	**3 c water**
15 mL	**1 T salt**
1.25 mL	**¼ t black pepper**
1	**1 dried chili pepper, crushed (optional)**
1	**1 onion**
240 mL	**1 c diced potatoes**
240 mL	**1 c sliced carrots**
240 mL	**1 c sliced celery**
120 mL	**½ c diced turnips**
240 mL	**1 c diced onion**
240 mL	**1 c minced parsley**
240 mL	**1 c thinly sliced okra (optional)**
600 mL	**3½ c canned tomatoes**
1	**1 clove garlic, crushed**

Combine the first six ingredients in a 3.8-L (4-qt) saucepan.

Bring to a boil; reduce heat and simmer 2 hours, or until meat is tender.

Remove and discard marrow bone.

Remove meat from pan and set aside; skim off fat from liquid.

Add remaining ingredients to the liquid, and cook over moderate heat until vegetables are just tender.

Stir in additional boiling water to desired thinness, if needed.

Return meat to pot, and bring just to boiling point.

Serve hot with crackers or corn sticks, a tossed salad, milk, and lemon fluff pie (recipe on page 362).

Store one meal of leftover soup in the refrigerator.

Freeze the remainder.

VARIATIONS

1/Mexican Vegetable Soup

Omit the potatoes and turnips.

Add 240 mL (1 c) each of fresh or canned kernel corn and red beans, 2 cloves garlic, and 15 mL (1 T) chili pepper.

2/Fish Chowder

Skin and bone .9 kg (2 lb) fresh or frozen fish.

Wash and cut it into 2.5-cm (1-in) cubes.

Add 45 mL (3 T) of lemon juice and proceed as in the basic recipe, simmering the fish until tender (about 5 minutes). If a thickened soup is desired, blend 120 mL (½ c) flour with 240 mL (1 c) water until smooth. Add the mixture to the soup, stirring until it is slightly thickened.

Return the fish to the chowder. Add .96 L (4 c) skim milk, heating until hot, but do not boil.

Serve as the main dish in a balanced meal, garnished with a slice of lemon or lime.

3/Ham and Bean Soup

Use a ham bone or hock with about 480 mL (2 c) of cubed lean ham, instead of the beef.

Add 30 mL (2 T) vegetable oil, 2 whole cloves, and 2 whole allspice.

Wash 240 mL (1 c) dried beans (any type), split peas, black-eyed peas, or lentils. Add to the meat with 1.7 L (7 c) water (1.2 L [5 c] for pressure cooking), 10 mL (2 t) dry mustard, and seasonings to taste.

Boil for 2 minutes. Turn off the heat and let the mixture soak for at least 2 hours. This tenderizes the beans, cuts down the cooking time, and makes the beans hold their shape better.

Cook about 2½ hours, or until tender. If using a pressure saucepan, remove the bone and bring the pressure to 6.8 kg (15 lb). With the exception of navy and pinto beans (which require only 10 minutes' cooking time), all beans, peas, and lentils should be cooked for 5 minutes at 6.8 kg (15 lb) pressure. Let the pressure return to normal, then add boiling water until the soup is the desired thickness.

Serve as the main dish in a balanced meal, garnished with diced fresh green pepper or onions, or both.

Quiche Lorraine (French)

(yield: 6 servings)

Metric	Customary
1 22.5-cm	1 9-inch unbaked pie shell
4	4 large eggs
360 mL	1½ c grated Swiss or sharp Cheddar cheese
120 mL	½ c milk
30 mL	2 T flour
2.5 mL	½ t dry mustard
.63 mL	⅛ t nutmeg
120 mL	½ c sautéed mushrooms, fresh or canned
	salt and pepper to taste
6	6 strips bacon, fried crisp and crumbled (optional)

Prepare an unbaked pie shell (recipe on page 391) and set aside.

Beat the eggs until foamy and blend in all remaining ingredients, except the bacon.

Sprinkle half the bacon over the shell and pour the egg mixture into the shell.

Bake in a preheated oven at 190 °C (375 °F) until the custard is firm (about 30 minutes).

Garnish the top with the remaining bacon crumbs.

Serve hot as the main dish for lunch, supper, breakfast, or brunch, preceded by French onion soup and accompanied by fresh spinach and tomato salad, plain white cake (recipe on page 396) topped with fresh or thawed frozen strawberries, and café au lait.

Basic Meringues

Metric	Customary
2	2 egg whites (large eggs)
1.25 mL	¼ t salt
2.5 mL	½ t cream of tartar
2.5 mL	½ t almond extract
2.5 mL	½ t vanilla
160 mL	⅔ c fine granulated sugar

Place the egg whites in a mixing bowl.

Add the salt, cream of tartar, and flavorings and beat until foam begins to form.

Beat in the sugar, 15 mL (1 T) at a time, until thoroughly dissolved and the whites are in moist, shiny peaks.

Drop the meringue by teaspoonfuls onto a lightly oiled or nonstick cookie sheet, about 5 cm (2 in) apart.

Bake at 122 °C (250 °F) for about 50 minutes. While warm, remove the meringues with a pancake turner or spatula, being careful not to break them.

VARIATIONS

1 / Meringue Shells

Drop the meringue by teaspoonfuls onto cookie sheet, depressing the center of each meringue mound with the bowl of the spoon in order to form a shell.

Bake and allow to cool.

Fill the meringue shells with fresh or frozen fruits, such as peaches or strawberries; a chocolate, vanilla, or lemon sauce; or with fruited ice cream.

2 / Nut Chocolate Chip Meringues

Add 240 mL (1 c) each of semisweet chocolate chips and broken walnut meats, and gently fold into the meringue.

Drop by teaspoonfuls onto a lightly oiled cookie sheet and bake at 176 °C (350 °F) for 20 minutes. Yields 40–50 meringues.

Iç Pilav (Turkish)

(yield: 8–10 servings)

Metric	Customary
45 mL	**3 T vegetable oil**
112 g	**¼ lb liver (calf or lamb)**
240 mL	**1 c finely chopped onion**
120 mL	**½ c slivered almonds**
480 mL	**2 c uncooked white or brown rice**
960 mL *or*	**4 c meat or chicken stock *or***
6 *plus*	**6 bouillon cubes *plus***
960 mL	**4 c water**
1	**1 large tomato, chopped**
30 mL	**2 T sugar**
5 mL	**1 t salt**
2.5 mL	**½ t coarsely ground pepper**
2.5 mL	**½ t allspice**
1.25 mL	**¼ t thyme leaves**
60 mL	**¼ c currants**

Heat the oil in a 1.9-L (2-qt) saucepan. Cut the liver into cubes, and fry it with the onion in the hot oil over moderate heat.

Remove the liver and onion to drain on a paper towel. Reserve it.

Add the almonds and rice to the saucepan, and fry for 5 minutes, stirring constantly to prevent sticking.

Drain off the excess fat. Add the stock or the bouillon cubes and water and all the remaining ingredients except the liver.

Stir to blend thoroughly.

Bring to a boil, then lower heat to simmer.

Cover and cook until all the liquid is absorbed and the rice is tender (about 45 minutes). Do not stir. Turn off the heat and allow the mixture to stand in a warm place 20 minutes.

Add the liver and onions; gently toss to mix all ingredients.

Garnish with chopped parsley, and serve with roast lamb or chicken, an eggplant casserole, and a cucumber salad. Add yogurt and fresh fruit for dessert, followed by café au lait, demitasse, or Turkish coffee.

Chicken Tetrazzini (Italian)

(yield: 4–6 servings)

Metric	Customary
480 mL	**2 c cooked noodles or spaghetti**
480 mL	**2 c diced cooked chicken**
240 mL	**1 c broken walnut meats or slivered almonds**
240 mL	**1 c sautéed sliced mushrooms**
480 mL	**2 c medium white sauce**
4	**4 chicken bouillon cubes**
	salt and pepper to taste
15 mL	**1 T grated onion**
dash	**dash nutmeg**
15 mL	**1 T sherry**
80 mL	**⅓ c grated Parmesan cheese**

Mix all ingredients except the cheese gently in a mixing bowl and spoon into a buttered 1.9-L (2-qt) casserole.

Top with cheese and bake in a preheated oven at 190 °C (375 °F) until golden brown and bubbly.

Serve hot with green peas, tossed salad, milk, and pumpkin chiffon cake.

Note: May be made ahead and refrigerated or frozen before adding cheese and baking.

VARIATIONS

1 / Shellfish Tetrazzini

Substitute lobster, shrimp, crab, or tuna for the chicken.

2 / Mexican Chicken Tetrazzini

Add 1–2 chili peppers and 1.25 mL (¼ t) oregano, if desired.

Tamale Pie (Mexican)

(yield: 6 servings)

Crust

Metric	Customary
300 mL	1¼ c yellow cornmeal
240 mL	1 c nonfat dry milk
5 mL	1 t baking powder
5 mL	1 t salt
5 mL	1 t chili pepper
15 mL	1 T vegetable oil
600 mL	2½ c water

Mix all the ingredients in a 1.4-L (1½-qt) saucepan.

Bring to a boil, stirring to prevent lumping or sticking.

Simmer until very thick (about 3 minutes).

Line the bottom and sides of an oiled pan 25 x 15 x 5 cm (10 x 6 x 2 in) with two-thirds of the dough, pressing to make it firm.

Bake in a preheated oven at 204 °C (400 °F) for 20 minutes, or until done.

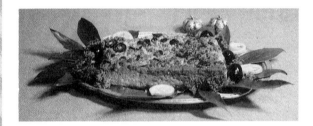

Filling

Metric	Customary
.45 kg	1 lb lean ground beef
120 mL	½ c diced onion
120 mL	½ c diced black olives (optional)
480 mL	2 c canned tomatoes
240 mL	1 c whole kernel corn
1	1 crushed clove garlic
2.5 mL	½ t salt
5–15 mL	1–3 t chili pepper
240 mL	1 c Cheddar cheese
30 mL	2 T diced red bell pepper, pimento, or mild chilis

Brown the beef and onion in a lightly oiled skillet.

Drain off all the fat and add the remaining ingredients, except the cheese and the bell pepper.

Pour the hot mixture into the cornmeal crust.

Spoon the remaining cornmeal dough around the outer edge of the tamale filling.

Sprinkle the top with grated cheese, then with the diced red pepper or pimento.

Bake in a preheated oven at 176 °C (350 °F) until the crust is brown and the tamale bubbles.

Serve hot with coleslaw or sauerkraut salad, milk, and sliced peaches.

GRAIN GROUP / BREAD

*Homemade Quick Bread Mix

Metric	Customary
2.4 L	10 c all-purpose flour
420 mL	1¾ c powdered sugar
60 mL	¼ c double-acting baking powder
22.5 mL	1½ T salt
480 mL	2 c nonfat dry milk
240 mL	1 c soft margarine

Measure and sift all dry ingredients into a 5.7-L (6-qt) pan or bowl, blending thoroughly.

Cut in the margarine with a pastry blender until the mixture is the consistency of coarse meal.

Store in a cool, dry place or in refrigerator in jars or cans with airtight lids.

"Using the mix" on page 384.

1 / Pancakes

Beat 1 egg in mixing bowl.

Add 240 mL (1 c) milk.

Add 240 mL (1 c) mix and blend until smooth. Makes 8–10 thin pancakes. Serve hot.

2 / Muffins

Beat 1 egg in a mixing bowl.

Stir in 180 mL (¾ c) milk.

Add 480 mL (2 c) dry mix and blend only until wet—about 15 strokes.

Fill oiled and floured muffin pans two-thirds full.

Bake at 218 °C (425 °F) about 20–25 minutes. Makes 12 muffins 5 cm (2 in) diameter.

3 / Waffles

Separate 3 eggs and beat the whites until they stand in stiff but moist peaks. In another mixing bowl, beat together the egg yolks and 240 mL (1 c) water.

Add about 300 mL (1¼ c) mix, according to the thickness desired, and stir until smooth.

Fold the mixture into the beaten whites. Do not beat.

Bake at once on a moderately hot waffle iron until golden brown. Serve hot.

4 / Biscuits

Measure 480 mL (2 c) of the mix into a bowl.

Add 160–180 mL (⅔–¾ c) milk, stirring to make a soft dough that will just cling together.

Sprinkle the board with flour and fold the dough over lightly into a ball until smooth.

Pat or roll the dough gently until it is about 1.25 cm (½ in) thick, and cut in the desired size.

Bake on a lightly oiled cookie sheet in a preheated oven at 232–260 °C (450–500 °F) 10–12 minutes, or until the biscuits are golden brown.

Serve at once.

Pumpkin Nut Bread

(yield: 1 large or 2 small loaves)

Metric	Customary	
80 mL	⅓ c nonfat dry milk	
400 mL	1⅔ c sifted all-purpose flour	
10 mL	2 t baking powder	
2.5 mL	½ t salt	
2.5 mL	½ t cinnamon	
2.5 mL	½ t nutmeg	
2.5 mL	½ t ginger	
2.5 mL	½ t vanilla	
15 mL	1 T grated orange rind	
80 mL	⅓ c vegetable oil	
320 mL	1⅓ c packed brown sugar	
3	3 eggs	
240 mL	1 c fresh or canned mashed pumpkin	
80 mL	⅓ c milk	
120 mL	½ c broken walnut meats	

Sift together the first seven ingredients.

Combine the remaining ingredients in another mixing bowl, and blend thoroughly.

Add these ingredients to the first mixture and blend until smooth.

Spoon into a greased and floured or non-stick loaf pan 22.5 x 12.5 x 7.5 cm (9 x 5 x 3 in).

Bake in a preheated oven at 176 °C (350 °F) until the loaf springs back when gently touched in the center (about 1 hour).

Slice and serve warm for breakfast or for dessert at other meals. (May be frozen and reheated, if desired.)

"Sticky buns," poppyseed rolls, Vienna bread, white bread, pumpernickel bread, raisin bread, croissants, French rolls, rye bread.

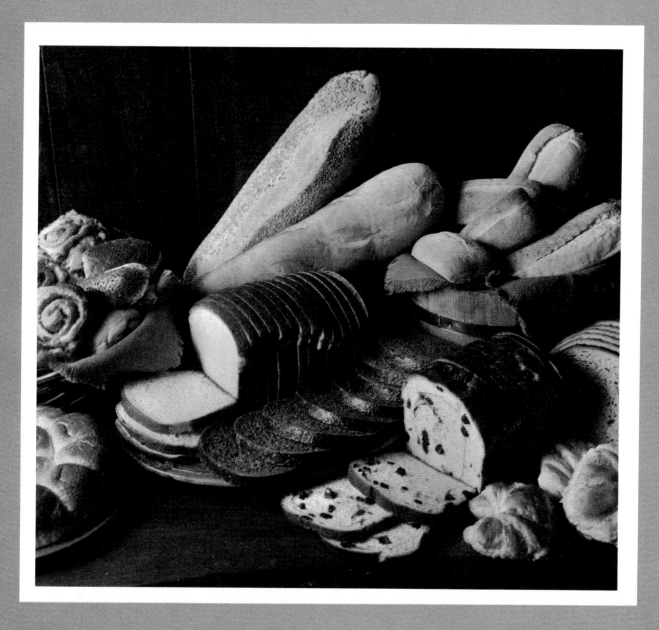

Top: Muffins and coffee cakes. *Bottom:* Macaroni chili.

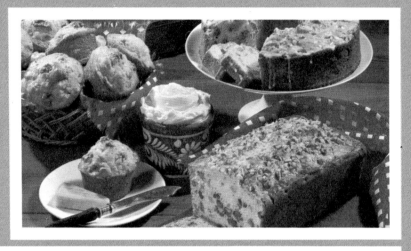

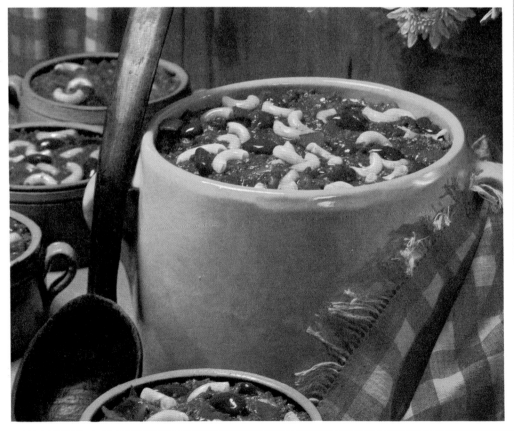

Skillet Corn Bread

(yield: 1 skillet of bread, 12 corn sticks, or 12 muffins)

Metric	Customary
1	**1 egg**
240 mL	**1 c buttermilk***
15 mL	**1 T sugar**
30 mL	**2 T vegetable oil**
360 mL	**1½ c yellow cornmeal**
120 mL	**½ c sifted all-purpose flour**
15 mL	**1 T baking powder**
2.5 mL	**½ t baking soda**
5 mL	**1 t salt**

Beat the egg in a large mixing bowl with the milk, sugar, and oil.

Sift the remaining ingredients together, blending thoroughly, and add to egg mixture. Mix gently. Do not beat.

*For lower cost, substitute 120 mL (½ c) nonfat dry milk plus 240 mL (1 c) water for the buttermilk.

Pour into a hot, lightly oiled and floured skillet and bake in a preheated oven at 218 °C (425 °F) until done (about 25 minutes), or pour into hot, oiled corn stick or muffin pans and bake.

Serve hot as part of a balanced meal.

VARIATIONS

Add any one of the following: 60 mL (¼ c) crisp cracklings, bacon crumbles, or diced ham; 120 mL (½ c) chopped green chili peppers; 60 mL (¼ c) grated onion; 60 mL (¼ c) chopped red or green sweet pepper; 5 mL (1 t) poultry seasoning, chili pepper, or thyme.

Sourdough Bread Starter

Metric	Customary
480 mL	**2 c flour**
360 mL	**1½ c warm milk**
15 mL	**1 T salt**
15 mL	**1 T vinegar**

Combine all ingredients in a nonmetal bowl and beat vigorously until smooth.

Cover tightly and let stand in a warm place 12 hours, leaving room enough for bubbles to rise.

Place 240 mL (1 c) of this starter in a mixing bowl and follow instructions for basic bread recipe on page 388. Add just enough extra flour to make a soft dough.

Note: Each time you remove a cup of sourdough starter, add 240 mL (1 c) of flour, 240 mL (1 c) of milk, 7.5 mL (½ T) salt, and 15 mL (1 T) sugar. Mix; let rise until bubbles form; cover, and store in refrigerator.

Sourdough Bran-Wheat Germ Bread

Metric	Customary
1	**1 pkg yeast**
240 mL	**1 c starter**
600 mL	**2½ c warm water**
240 mL	**1 c nonfat dry milk**
10 mL	**2 t salt**
80 mL	**⅓ c oil**
80 mL	**⅓ c dark molasses**
240 mL	**1 c 100% bran**
120 mL	**½ c wheat germ**
1.08–1.32 L	**4½–5½ c flour**
2	**2 eggs**

Proceed as for basic bread recipe on page 388.

Whole-Wheat Yeast Bread

(yield: 2 .45-kg [1-lb] loaves)

Metric	Customary
2	2 eggs
2	2 pkgs dry or compressed yeast
80 mL	⅓ c dark molasses
240 mL	1 c nonfat dry milk
480 mL	2 c water warmed to 43–46 °C (110–115 °F)
12.5 mL	2½ t salt
15 mL	1 T vegetable oil
480 mL	2 c sifted enriched white all-purpose flour
840 L	3½ c sifted whole-wheat flour

Beat the eggs slightly in a large bowl.

Add the next six ingredients, mixing until well blended and smooth.

Add the white flour and beat by hand, or in an electric mixer at medium speed, until mixture is elastic.

Beat in the whole-wheat flour, 240 mL (1 c) at a time, until 720 mL (3 c) have been added. The dough should now pull away from the sides of the bowl.

Cover and let rest about 10 minutes.

Sprinkle the remaining flour onto a bread-board.

Turn the dough out onto the board and shape into a ball.

Knead the dough gently on the board for 5 minutes or until small gas bubbles appear beneath the surface.

Return dough to a lightly oiled mixing bowl, and oil the exposed surface of the dough.

Cover with a towel, and set in a warm place away from drafts, allowing dough to rise to double its size (about 1 hour).

Punch dough down, turn out onto lightly floured board, shape into ball, and cut in half.

Shape each half into a loaf, place in greased loaf pans 22.5 x 12.5 x 7.5 cm (9 x 5 x 3 in).

Cover with a towel, set in warm place, and allow loaves to rise to double their bulk.

Bake at 190 °C (375 °F) for about one hour or until done (bread will spring back when pressed in center with finger).

Remove bread from oven; let stand for 2 minutes to "loosen."

Run a spatula around the edges to remove bread from pan; place on cake rack.

Rub crust with soft margarine.

Serve hot for best flavor.

VARIATIONS

1 / Bran-Wheat Germ Bread

Substitute 240 mL (1 c) 100 percent bran cereal and 120 mL (½ c) wheat germ for 360 mL (1½ c) of the whole-wheat flour, and use enriched white flour for the remaining flour in the recipe.

2 / Batter Bread

Proceed as for basic bread but use only .96–1.08 L (4–4½ c) flour and add it after the yeast has set with the liquid ingredients about 2 minutes. Mix until smooth. Then beat until the dough pulls from the side of the bowl (about 2 minutes). Cover. Let rise until the bulk doubles.

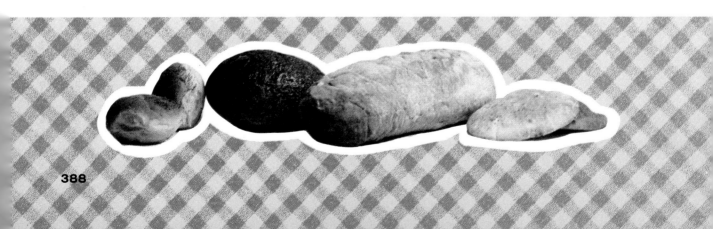

Stir and beat ½ minute, then turn into 2 greased casseroles or loaf pans. Let rise until bulk doubles, then bake at 190 °C (375 °F) for about 50 minutes.

3 / French-Style Bread

Divide the dough (whole-wheat or white) after the first rising to form two loaves 35 cm (14 in) long and 5 cm (2 in) wide, tapering at the ends.

Oil the loaves all over the outside and place them on a cookie sheet.

Cut seven diagonal slashes 31 mm (⅛ in) deep across the tops of the loaves.

Sprinkle the tops with cornmeal or sesame seed and let the loaves rise in a warm place until they are double in bulk.

Bake at 218 °C (425 °F) for 20 minutes. Then, reduce the heat to 176 °C (350 °F) and bake until done (5–10 minutes). Serve warm. Cut through the gashes for thick slices. If desired, spread the gashes with soft margarine blended with a crushed clove of garlic and warm the bread in the oven.

4 / Raisin Bread

Add 360 mL (1½ c) seedless raisins with the warm milk and proceed according to the basic recipe.

5 / Rolls

Shape the basic dough when it is ready to bake into rolls of any desired shape. Cloverleaf rolls are made by putting three small balls of dough into half the depth of a muffin tin. For Parker House rolls, the dough is rolled 63 mm (¼ in) thick and cut in circles with a biscuit or cookie cutter; the circles are folded in two and the edges pressed together. For crescent rolls, the dough is rolled 63 mm (¼ in) thick and cut in pie-shaped triangles, which are then rolled, beginning at the wide end and rolling toward the point; the ends are then curved in slightly.

Place the rolls on an oiled pan.

Brush the tops with melted soft margarine. Proceed as with the basic recipe, but bake at 218 °C (425 °F) for about 12–15 minutes or until golden brown.

6 / Low-Cholesterol Bread

Substitute for the 2 whole eggs 4 egg whites, beaten until they begin to foam.

Proceed with the basic recipe or its variations.

7 / Pizza Crust

Divide the basic dough into four equal parts. Set three aside for other uses. Divide the remaining part in two.

Roll each part to fit a 30-cm (12-in) pizza pan with a rim to stand above the pan.

Place the dough in the pan and fill it with your favorite pizza filling. Let stand 15 minutes.

Bake at 176 °C (350 °F) 30 to 35 minutes, or until done.

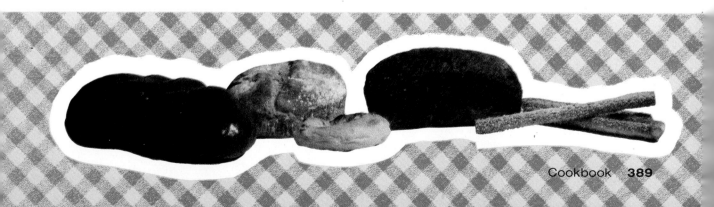

Mushroom-Onion-Cheese Pizza

(yield: 1 30-cm [12-in] pizza)

Metric	Customary
1 30-cm	**1 12-in unbaked pizza crust**
30 mL	**2 T vegetable oil**
240 mL	**1 c finely chopped onions**
5 mL	**1 t salt**
5 mL	**1 t crushed oregano leaves**
5 mL	**paprika**
84 g	**3 oz sautéed sliced mushrooms, fresh or canned**
240 mL	**1 c grated sharp Cheddar or other cheese**
120–180 mL	**½–¾ c tomato sauce**
	sliced ripe olives (optional)

Prepare an unbaked pizza crust (recipe on page 389).

Sauté onions with vegetable oil, salt, oregano leaves, and paprika, cooking until onions are tender.

Add mushrooms and sauté 1 minute more.

Spread the mixture over the pizza dough, and sprinkle the top with cheese.

Drizzle the tomato sauce over the topping.

Garnish with sliced ripe olives, if desired.

Bake at 176 °C (350 °F) 15–20 minutes or until crust is brown.

Cut into pie-shaped slices and serve warm with a glass of milk and fresh fruit.

High-Nutrient Crêpes (French pancakes)

(yield: 2–3 servings)

Metric	Customary
3	**3 egg yolks**
180 mL	**¾ c cottage cheese**
80 mL	**⅓ c nonfat dry milk**
80 mL	**⅓ c lime or lemon juice**
5 mL	**1 t grated orange rind or extract**
15 mL	**1 T vegetable oil**
15 mL	**1 T sugar**
3	**3 egg whites**
1.25 mL	**¼ t salt**
1.25 mL	**¼ t cream of tartar**
60 mL	**¼ c buckwheat pancake mix**

Blend the first seven ingredients in a blender. The mixture may be covered and refrigerated overnight.

Combine the next three ingredients, and beat until the egg whites stand in moist, firm peaks.

Blend the pancake mix into the egg yolk mixture.

Fold this mixture into the egg whites in three stages.

Cook on a lightly oiled, nonstick griddle at moderate heat in small-sized cakes.

Turn gently when bubbly (they are tender and break easily) and brown on the other side.

Serve hot for breakfast or dessert with orange marmalade or heated syrup to which some marmalade has been added.

Hawaiian Quick Fruit Bread

(yield: 1 loaf)

Metric	Customary
3	3 large eggs
105 mL	½ c less 1 T vegetable oil
240 mL	1 c packed brown sugar
240 mL	1 c diced bananas
240 mL	1 c crushed pineapple with juice
80 mL	⅓ c orange juice
5 mL	1 t vanilla
15 mL	1 T grated orange rind
480 mL	2 c sifted all-purpose flour
80 mL	⅓ c nonfat dry milk
15 mL	1 T baking powder
2.5 mL	½ t salt
120 mL	½ c broken nut meats

Beat the eggs in a large mixing bowl until they are foamy.

Add the oil, brown sugar, bananas, pineapple, orange juice and rind, and vanilla.

Sift together all remaining ingredients except the nuts, and gradually stir into the liquid mixture.

Blend in the nuts.

Pour into an oiled and floured or nonstick loaf pan 22.5 x 12.5 x 7.5 cm (9 x 5 x 3 in) and bake in a preheated oven at 176° C (350 °F) for about 1–1¼ hours, or until center springs back when pressed with finger. Or bake in an oblong pan 32.5 x 22.5 x 5 cm (13 x 9 x 2 in) until done (about 35–40 minutes).

Let the loaf stand in the pan 15 minutes to "loosen," then remove to a cake rack to cool. If an oblong pan was used, leave the cake in the pan and cut in squares to serve.

Serve as dessert at lunch or dinner, as a breakfast bread, or for teas and parties.

GRAIN GROUP/PIES

Health Watchers' Oil Pastry

(yield: 2 22.5-cm [9-in] pie crusts)

Metric	Customary
480 mL	2 c sifted all-purpose flour
5 mL	1 t salt
120 mL	½ c vegetable oil
60 mL	4 T cold milk

Measure the sifted flour and sift it together with the salt into a mixing bowl.

Combine the oil and milk, and add to the flour.

Stir with a fork to mix quickly and form into a moist ball (more moist than the standard pastry).

Divide the dough equally to form two balls.

Roll one ball at a time between two 30-cm (12-in) squares of wax paper, to form a circle.

Remove the top wax paper and invert the crust over a 22.5-cm (9-in) pie pan, removing the other piece of paper and shaping the crust to fit snugly.

Flute the edges and prick the bottom and sides with the tines of a fork (unless a fruit filling is to be used).

Bake at 246 °C (475 °F) for 8–10 minutes.

Remove from oven and allow to cool.

Add any filling you prefer.

Note: For a two-crust pie with fruit, do not prick the bottom crust, but fill it with fruit (piling high in the center) and cover it with the top crust, pricking it or cutting a design on it to let steam escape. Then flute the two edges together. Bake at 232 °C (450 °F) until the top crust is golden brown and the fruit is cooked.

VARIATION

Standard Pastry

Use 160 mL (⅔ c) soft margarine instead of oil and work it with a pastry blender into the dry ingredients until it forms a coarse meal.

Proceed as for oil pastry.

Top left: Enriched white rice. *Top center:* Desserts made with dried pineapple, apricots, and raisins. *Top right:* Waffles and bacon, biscuits, French toast, pancakes and sausages. *Bottom left:* Macaroni casserole served with baked ham. *Bottom right:* Sandwich of cold cuts, Swiss cheese, lettuce, and tomato on sesame seed roll.

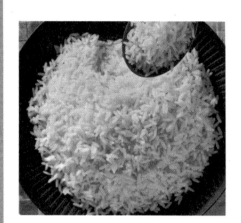

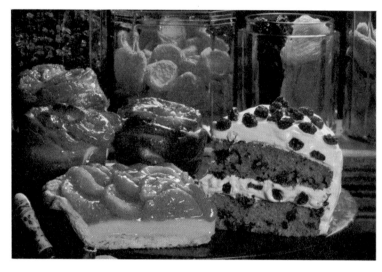

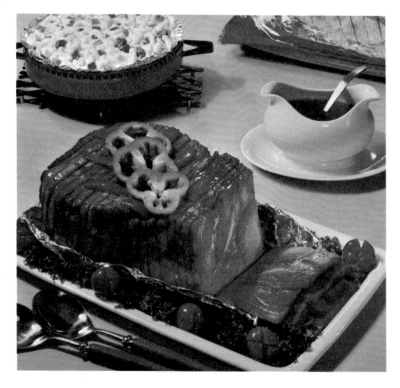

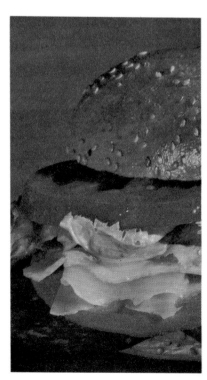

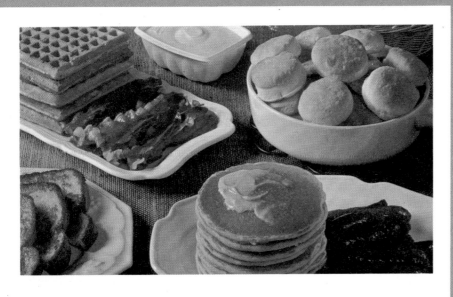

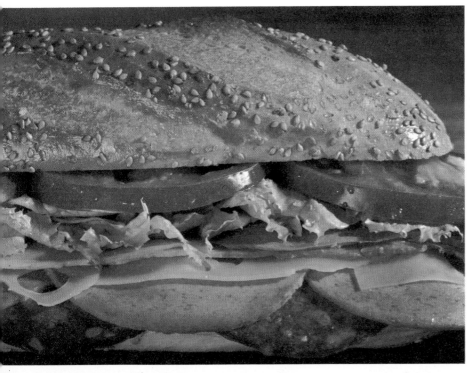

Apple Pie

(yield: 1 pie)

Metric	Customary
2 22.5-cm	**2 9-in unbaked pie crusts**
5–6	**5–6 tart apples, pared and sliced thin**
180 mL	**¾ c brown sugar**
15 mL	**1 T tapioca**
1.25 mL	**¼ t nutmeg**
1.25 mL	**¼ t allspice**
5 mL	**1 t cinnamon**
15 mL	**1 T lemon juice**

Prepare 2 unbaked pie crusts following one of the preceding recipes.

Chill standard crust (but not oil pastry) in the refrigerator until you are ready to use it.

Place the sliced apples on the unbaked bottom crust, piling them high in the center.

Mix the remaining ingredients and sprinkle over the apples.

Cover with the top crust.

Bake at 232 °C (450 °F) for 15 minutes, then reduce the heat to 190 °C (375 °F), and bake until the top crust is golden brown and the apples are tender (about 20–30 minutes).

Cherry Pie

(yield: 1 pie)

Metric	Customary
2 22.5-cm	**2 9-in unbaked pie crusts**
.45 kg	**1 lb canned sour cherries**
30 mL	**2 T quick-cooking tapioca**
160 mL	**⅔ c sugar**
15 mL	**1 T soft margarine**
5 mL	**1 t cinnamon**
15 mL	**1 T lemon juice**
2.5 mL	**½ t almond extract**

Prebake the bottom crust for 5 minutes at 232 °C (450 °F) with an inverted pie pan inside it.

Mix all the remaining ingredients except the almond extract in a saucepan, and bring the mixture to a boil.

Mix in the almond extract.

Pour the filling into the partially baked crust.

Place the top crust over the filling and flute the edges.

Bake in a preheated oven at 232 °C (450 °F) until the top crust is golden brown.

VARIATIONS

1 / Fresh Peach Pie

Pile about 750–840 mL (3–3½ c) thinly sliced peaches high and proceed as for cherry pie.

2 / Blueberry Pie

Use 720–840 mL (3–3⅓ c) of fresh blueberries and proceed as for cherry pie.

Low-Fat Graham Cracker Crust

(yield: 1 22.5-cm [9-in] crust)

Metric	Customary
240 mL	**1 c graham cracker crumbs**
45 mL	**3 T soft margarine**

Roll six graham crackers at a time between two squares of wax paper until the desired amount of crumbs is obtained.

Mix the crumbs with the fat in a 22.5-cm (9-in) pie pan until the mixture is like coarse meal.

Press it into place on the bottom and sides of the pan.

Chill for one hour before baking.

Bake in a preheated oven at 163 °C (325 °F) for 5 minutes.

VARIATIONS

1 / Spicy Graham Cracker Crust

Add 15 mL (1 T) of grated lemon or orange rind, 1.25 mL (¼ t) nutmeg, and 2.5 mL (½ t) cinnamon. Bake as usual.

2 / Vanilla Wafer Crust

Substitute vanilla wafers for graham crackers.

3 / Ginger Wafer Crust

Substitute ginger wafers for graham crackers. This is a good base for pumpkin or squash pie.

4 / Chocolate Wafer Crust

Substitute chocolate wafers for graham crackers, especially for lemon or lime chiffon pie.

Oklahoma Strawberry Pie

(yield: 1 pie)

Metric	Customary
1 22.5-cm	**1 9-in prebaked pie shell**
960 mL	**4 c fresh strawberries**
120–160 mL	**½–⅔ c granulated sugar**
30 mL	**2 T quick-cooking tapioca**

Prepare the pie shell.

Wash and hull the strawberries.

Mix together lightly in a saucepan the strawberries and the sugar. Let stand for 30 minutes.

Remove 240 mL (1 c) of berries and crush the remainder. Add the tapioca to the crushed berries and boil one minute, stirring slightly until thickened.

Add the reserved berries and mix lightly.

Pour into the pie shell.

Top with sweetened yogurt, whipped cream or ice cream, nonfat dry milk topping, if desired.

Cut in wedges and serve at once.

Note: Fresh uncooked berries may be piled into a freshly baked pie shell for an easy dessert.

Strawberry-Rhubarb Pie

(yield: 1 pie)

Metric	Customary
1 22.5-cm	**1 9-in unbaked pie shell**
480 mL	**2 c tender diced rhubarb**
480 mL	**2 c fresh strawberries**
300–360 mL	**1¼–1½ c sugar**
22 mL	**1½ T quick-cooking tapioca**
5 mL	**1 t soft margarine (optional)**
	graham cracker crumbs

Prepare pie shell.

Wash and hull the strawberries.

Mix together the rhubarb, strawberries, sugar, and tapioca. Let stand 15–30 minutes.

Pour into pie shell. Dot with margarine, if desired, and sprinkle with graham cracker crumbs.

Bake at 232 °C (450 °F) for 10 minutes. Reduce the heat to 190 °C (375 °F) and bake until the rhubarb is tender and the crust is golden brown.

GRAIN GROUP/CAKES AND COOKIES

Basic "Butter" Cake

(yield: 2 22.5-cm [9-inch] layers; 24 cupcakes)

Metric	Customary
480 mL	**2 c sifted all-purpose flour**
10 mL	**2 t double-acting baking powder**
360 mL	**1½ c sugar**
240 mL	**1 c skim milk**
80 mL	**⅓ c vegetable oil**
7.5 mL	**1½ t vanilla**
4	**4 egg yolks**
4	**4 egg whites**
2.5 mL	**½ t salt**
2.5 mL	**½ t cream of tartar**

Sift the flour, baking powder, and 240 ml (1 c) of the sugar three times into a large mixing bowl.

Make a hole in the center of the dry ingredients.

Mix in 120 mL (½ c) milk, the oil, and the vanilla. Beat for 1 minute at medium speed with an electric mixer or 150 strokes by hand, scraping the sides of the bowl constantly.

Add the egg yolks and the remaining milk and beat 1 minute more.

Beat the egg whites with the salt and cream of tartar until foamy.

Add the remaining 120 mL (½ c) of sugar, 30 mL (2 T) at a time, beating until glossy peaks form.

Fold the batter gradually into the meringue.

Pour the batter into two oiled and floured 22.5-cm (9-inch) cake pans and bake at 190 °C (375 °F) until done—about 30 minutes. If an oblong pan 7.5 x 22.5 x 6.3 cm (3 x 9 x 2½ in) is used, baking time is about 40–45 minutes. Cupcakes in muffin tins require about 20–25 minutes.

Remove from the oven when done and cool on a cake rack.

Top with your favorite frosting and serve.

VARIATIONS

1 / White Velvet Cake (no cholesterol)

Omit the egg yolks and proceed as for the basic recipe.

2 / Upside-Down Cake

Spread on the bottom of an oiled, oblong baking pan 37.5 x 27.5 x 6.3 cm (15 x 11 x 2½ in) 180 mL (¾ c) tightly packed brown sugar, 60 mL (¼ c) nut meats, and pineapple rings, peach slices, or other fruit. Arrange the fruit so that each serving will have some.

Fruit Cocktail Cake

(yield: 1 22.5-cm [9-in] square cake)

(low-calorie, low-fat, low-cholesterol)

Metric	Customary
1	1 large egg
240 mL	1 c tightly packed brown sugar
80 mL	⅓ c nonfat dry milk
320 mL	1⅓ c sifted all-purpose flour
5 mL	1 t baking powder
2.5 mL	½ t baking soda
2.5 mL	½ t salt
.45 kg	1 lb canned fruit cocktail, with syrup
180 mL	¾ c brown sugar
120 mL	½ c broken walnuts

Beat the egg in a mixing bowl.

Add the sugar and dry milk; mix until smooth.

Sift together the next four ingredients.

Stir dry ingredients into egg mixture.

Add the fruit cocktail with syrup, and blend. The batter will be thin.

Pour into a lightly oiled and floured 22.5-cm (9-in) square pan.

Combine the brown sugar and walnuts, and sprinkle evenly over top of batter.

Bake in a preheated oven at 176 °C (350 °F) until done (about 30–35 minutes).

Cut into squares and serve warm. Reheat leftover cake in a low oven and top with a scoop of ice cream, if desired.

Note: The only fat in this cake comes from the walnuts in the frosting, which are high in linoleic acid.

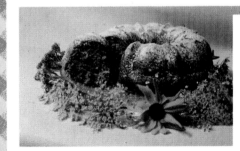

Pour either the basic or white cake batter evenly over the fruit and bake at 176 °C (350 °F) until done (about 40 minutes).

Cut into squares in the pan and serve with the fruit side up.

3/Chocolate Cake

Omit 120 mL (½ c) flour and add 120 mL (½ c) cocoa and 30 mL (2 T) oil at the first step.

Proceed as in basic recipe.

Poppy Seed Bundt Cake

(yield: 1 22.5-cm [9-in] cake)

Metric	Customary
1	1 pkg yellow cake mix
105 g	3¾ oz packaged butterscotch pudding mix
4	4 eggs
180 mL	¾ c vegetable oil
180 mL	¾ c orange juice
80 mL	⅓ c poppy seeds or chopped almonds

Combine all ingredients and beat 5 minutes with electric mixer. Pour into a lightly oiled and floured 22.5-cm (9-in) tube pan and bake in a 176 °C (350 °F) oven about 45 minutes, or until done. Let cool in pan about 5 minutes.

Remove to a cake rack.

Cool, and sift confectioner's sugar over top.

Note: Flavor is best when kept well covered in refrigerator 2–3 days.

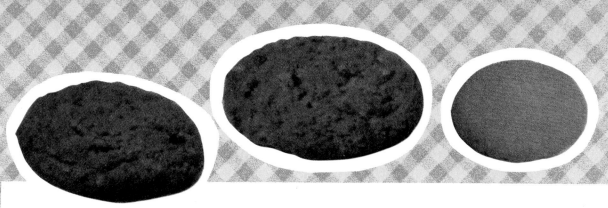

*Basic Drop Cookies

(yield: 7–8 dozen cookies)

Metric	Customary
80 mL	⅓ c orange juice
3	3 large eggs
90 mL	1 c less 2 T vegetable oil
15 mL	1 T grated orange rind
7.5 mL	1½ t vanilla
2.5 mL	½ t salt
480 mL	2 c packed brown sugar
960 mL	4 c sifted all-purpose flour
80 mL	⅓ c nonfat dry milk
20 mL	4 t baking powder
240 mL	1 c broken walnut meats

Mix the first seven ingredients thoroughly in a large bowl.

Add the next four ingredients and blend thoroughly.

Drop from the tip of a spoon onto a lightly oiled cookie sheet 5 cm (2 in) apart.

Bake in a preheated oven at 190 °C (375 °F) 10–12 minutes, or until done.

Remove with a spatula or pancake turner to cool on a rack.

Store cookies in a tightly covered jar or tin box. Reheating the cookies in a low-heat oven before serving improves the flavor.

VARIATIONS

1 / Raisin Cookies

Cook 240 mL (1 c) raisins in 120 mL (½ c) boiling water until plump. Drain.

Add the drained raisins last and use 80 mL (⅓ c) raisin water instead of the orange juice.

Proceed as for the basic recipe.

2 / Oatmeal Raisin Cookies

Substitute 480 mL (2 c) quick-cooking dry oats for 480 mL (2 c) of the flour and proceed as for raisin cookies.

3 / Chocolate Chip Cookies

Add 480 mL (2 c) semisweet chocolate chips to the basic recipe and proceed.

4 / Sesame Seed Cookies

Toast 240 mL (1 c) sesame seeds and 120 mL (½ c) shredded coconut by spreading thinly in a large shallow pan and heating at 149 °C (300 °F) until lightly browned (about 20 minutes).

Substitute the toasted seeds and coconut for the walnuts.

5 / Peanut Butter Cookies

Add 240 mL (1 c) chunk peanut butter at the first step in the basic recipe and omit the walnuts.

6 / Hermits

Add to the basic recipe 10 mL (2 t) cinnamon, 1.25 mL (¼ t) nutmeg, 1.25 mL (¼ t)

*Scones (Scottish Hot Biscuits)

(yield: 6–8 servings)

Metric	Customary
480 mL	2 c sifted all-purpose flour
45 mL	3 T double-acting baking powder
2.5 mL	½ t salt
2.5 mL	½ t cinnamon
60 mL	¼ c sugar
1	1 egg
120 mL	½ c dried raisins or currants
120 mL	½ c milk
60 mL	¼ c vegetable oil
30 mL	2 T sugar
2.5 mL	½ t cinnamon

Combine the first five ingredients and sift into a large mixing bowl.

Beat the egg slightly.

Make a hole in the middle of the dry ingredients and add the egg, raisins or currants, milk, and vegetable oil.

Mix gently until a soft dough is formed.

Turn dough out onto wax paper surface, and roll or pat out to a 1.9-cm (¾-in) thickness.

Cut scones with a cookie cutter.

Mix the remaining ingredients together, and sprinkle over the scones.

Place scones, well apart, on a lightly oiled cookie sheet.

Bake at 234 °C (450 °F) until golden brown (about 12 minutes).

Serve hot with margarine, butter, jam or honey.

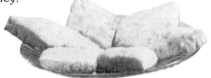

cloves, 1.25 mL (¼ t) mace, 240 mL (1 c) plumped raisins, 240 mL (1 c) diced dates, and 240 mL (1 c) glazed fruit, if desired.

7 / Refrigerator Cookies

Chill any of the above cookie doughs in the refrigerator for as long as two weeks. The flavors mellow as the dough stands. When ready to bake, drop from the tip of a spoon to an oiled cookie sheet.

8 / Rolled Cookies

Use a small amount of refrigerated dough at a time and roll it between two sheets of wax paper, sprinkling the paper with a little flour if necessary.

Cut in desired shapes and decorate, if you wish.

Lift carefully onto the cookie sheet with a spatula or pancake turner, as this dough is quite soft.

9 / Molasses Cookies

Omit the orange juice, orange rind, oil, vanilla, nuts, and 120 mL (½ c) of the brown sugar.

Add 160 mL (⅔ c) dark molasses, 5 mL (1 t) ginger, 5 mL (1 t) cinnamon, 2.5 mL (½ t) cloves, 2.5 mL (½ t) mace.

Proceed as for the basic recipe.

METRIC CONVERSION FACTORS (approximate)

SYMBOL	When you know number of	multiply by	to find number of	SYMBOL
	LENGTH			
in	inches	2.54	centimeters	cm
ft	feet	30.00	centimeters	cm
yd	yards	0.90	meters	m
mi	miles	1.60	kilometers	km
	AREA			
sq in	square inches	6.50	square centimeters	cm²
sq ft	square feet	0.09	square meters	m²
sq yd	square yards	0.80	square meters	m²
sq mi	square miles	2.60	square kilometers	km²
	acres	0.40	hectares	ha
	WEIGHT (mass)			
oz	ounces	28.00	grams	g
lb	pounds	0.45	kilograms	kg
	short tons (2000 pounds)	0.90	metric tons	t
	VOLUME			
t	teaspoons	5.00	milliliters	mL
T	tablespoons	15.00	milliliters	mL
cu in	cubic inches	16.00	milliliters	mL
fl oz	fluid ounces	30.00	milliliters	mL
c	cups	0.24	liters	L
pt	pints	0.47	liters	L
qt	quarts	0.95	liters	L
gal	gallons	3.80	liters	L
cu ft	cubic feet	0.03	cubic meters	m³
cu yd	cubic yards	0.76	cubic meters	m³
	TEMPERATURE (exact)			
°F	degrees Fahrenheit	5/9, after subtracting 32	degrees Celsius	°C

The metric system involves units of 10. Example: A kilogram is 1000 grams.

No periods are used after abbreviations. Example: mm, *not* mm.

No plurals are used with abbreviations. Example: 2 cm, *not* 2 cms

Spaces separate thousands, *not* commas. Example: 687 132, *not* 687,132

Decimals are used, *not* fractions. Example: 3.5, *not* 3½

WEIGHT-HEIGHT TABLE FOR AGES 7 TO 17

AGE years	Boys				Girls			
	AVERAGE WEIGHT pounds	RANGE IN WEIGHT pounds	AVERAGE HEIGHT inches	RANGE IN HEIGHT inches	AVERAGE WEIGHT pounds	RANGE IN WEIGHT pounds	AVERAGE HEIGHT inches	RANGE IN HEIGHT inches
7	52.5	45.4– 59.6	48.2	46.0–50.4	51.2	43.7– 58.7	47.9	45.7–50.1
8	58.2	49.5– 66.9	50.4	48.1–52.7	56.9	47.5– 66.3	50.0	47.7–52.3
9	64.4	54.6– 74.2	52.4	50.0–54.8	63.0	51.9– 74.1	52.0	49.6–54.4
10	70.7	59.2– 82.2	54.3	51.8–56.8	70.3	57.1– 83.5	54.2	51.6–56.8
11	77.6	64.5– 90.7	56.2	53.6–58.8	79.0	63.5– 94.5	56.5	53.7–59.3
12	85.6	69.8–101.4	58.2	55.3–61.1	89.7	71.9–107.5	59.0	56.1–61.9
13	95.6	77.4–113.8	60.5	57.3–63.7	100.3	82.3–118.3	60.6	58.0–63.2
14	107.9	87.8–128.0	63.0	59.6–66.4	108.5	91.3–125.7	62.3	59.9–64.7
15	121.7	101.1–142.3	65.6	62.5–68.7	115.0	98.8–131.2	63.2	60.9–65.5
16	131.9	113.0–150.8	67.3	64.5–70.1	117.6	101.7–133.5	63.5	61.3–65.7
17	138.3	119.5–157.1	68.2	65.6–70.8	119.0	103.5–134.5	63.6	61.4–65.8

From *Basic Body Measurements of School Age Children,* Office of Education, U.S. Department of Health, Education, and Welfare. The ranges given include the cases which fell within the middle two-thirds of those in the sample.

WEIGHT-HEIGHT TABLE FOR AGES 25 AND OVER

HEIGHT feet	inches	Men			HEIGHT feet	inches	Women		
		SMALL FRAME pounds	MEDIUM FRAME pounds	LARGE FRAME pounds			SMALL FRAME pounds	MEDIUM FRAME pounds	LARGE FRAME pounds
5	2	112–120	118–129	126–141	4	10	92– 98	96–107	104–119
5	3	115–123	121–133	129–144	4	11	94–101	98–110	106–122
5	4	118–126	124–136	132–148	5	0	96–104	101–113	109–125
5	5	121–129	127–139	135–152	5	1	99–107	104–116	112–128
5	6	124–133	130–143	138–156	5	2	102–110	107–119	115–131
5	7	128–137	134–147	142–161	5	3	105–113	110–122	118–134
5	8	132–141	138–152	147–166	5	4	108–116	113–126	121–138
5	9	136–145	142–156	151–170	5	5	111–119	116–130	125–142
5	10	140–150	146–160	155–174	5	6	114–123	120–135	129–146
5	11	144–154	150–165	159–179	5	7	118–127	124–139	133–150
6	0	148–158	154–170	164–184	5	8	122–131	128–143	137–154
6	1	152–162	158–175	168–189	5	9	126–135	132–147	141–158
6	2	156–167	162–180	173–194	5	10	130–140	136–151	145–163
6	3	160–171	167–185	178–199	5	11	134–144	140–155	149–168
6	4	164–175	172–190	182–204	6	0	138–148	144–159	153–173

Metropolitan Life Insurance Company. Weights include indoor clothing and shoes. Heights include 1-inch heels for men, 2-inch heels for women. For girls between 18 and 25, subtract 1 pound for each year under 25.

	AGE (years)	WEIGHT (kg)	(lb)	HEIGHT (cm)	(in)	Energy (kcal)[2]	Protein (gm)	Vitamin A Activity (RE)[3]	(IU)	Vitamin D (IU)	Vitamin E Activity[5] (IU)
INFANTS	0.0–0.5	6	14	60	24	kg × 117	kg × 2.2	420[4]	1400	400	4
	0.5–1.0	9	20	71	28	kg × 108	kg × 2.0	400	2000	400	5
CHILDREN	1–3	13	28	86	34	1300	23	400	2000	400	7
	4–6	20	44	110	44	1800	30	500	2500	400	9
	7–10	30	66	135	54	2400	36	700	3300	400	10
MALES	11–14	44	97	158	63	2800	44	1000	5000	400	12
	15–18	61	134	172	69	3000	54	1000	5000	400	15
	19–22	67	147	172	69	3000	54	1000	5000	400	15
	23–50	70	154	172	69	2700	56	1000	5000		15
	51+	70	154	172	69	2400	56	1000	5000		15
FEMALES	11–14	44	97	155	62	2400	44	800	4000	400	12
	15–18	54	119	162	65	2100	48	800	4000	400	12
	19–22	58	128	162	65	2100	46	800	4000	400	12
	23–50	58	128	162	65	2000	46	800	4000		12
	51+	58	128	162	65	1800	46	800	4000		12
PREGNANT						+300	+30	1000	5000	400	15
LACTATING						+500	+20	1200	6000	400	15

[1] The allowances are intended to provide for individual variations among most normal persons as they live in the United States under usual environmental stresses. Diets should be based on a variety of common foods in order to provide other nutrients for which human requirements have been less well defined.

[2] Kilojoules (KJ) = 4.2 × kcal. Abbreviation kcal = kilocalories.

[3] Retinol equivalents.

[4] Assumed to be all as retinol in milk during the first six months of life. All subsequent intakes are assumed to be one-half as retinol and one-half as β-carotene when calculated from international units. As retinol equivalents, three-fourths are as retinol and one-fourth as β-carotene.

Water-Soluble Vitamins | Minerals

Ascorbic Acid (mg)	Folacin[6] (µg)	Niacin[7] (mg)	Riboflavin (mg)	Thiamin (mg)	Vitamin B_6 (mg)	Vitamin B_{12} (µg)	Calcium (mg)	Phosphorus (mg)	Iodine (µg)	Iron (mg)	Magnesium (mg)	Zinc (mg)
35	50	5	0.4	0.3	0.3	0.3	360	240	35	10	60	3
35	50	8	0.6	0.5	0.4	0.3	540	400	45	15	70	5
40	100	9	0.8	0.7	0.6	1.0	800	800	60	15	150	10
40	200	12	1.1	0.9	0.9	1.5	800	800	80	10	200	10
40	300	16	1.2	1.2	1.2	2.0	800	800	110	10	250	10
45	400	18	1.5	1.4	1.6	3.0	1200	1200	130	18	350	15
45	400	20	1.8	1.5	2.0	3.0	1200	1200	150	18	400	15
45	400	20	1.8	1.5	2.0	3.0	800	800	140	10	350	15
45	400	18	1.6	1.4	2.0	3.0	800	800	130	10	350	15
45	400	16	1.5	1.2	2.0	3.0	800	800	110	10	350	15
45	400	16	1.3	1.2	1.6	3.0	1200	1200	115	18	300	15
45	400	14	1.4	1.1	2.0	3.0	1200	1200	115	18	300	15
45	400	14	1.4	1.1	2.0	3.0	800	800	100	18	300	15
45	400	13	1.2	1.0	2.0	3.0	800	800	100	18	300	15
45	400	12	1.1	1.0	2.0	3.0	800	800	80	10	300	15
60	800	+2	+0.3	+0.3	2.5	4.0	1200	1200	125	18+[8]	450	20
80	600	+4	+0.5	+0.3	2.5	4.0	1200	1200	150	18	450	25

Food and Nutrition Board, National Academy of Sciences—National Research Council, revised 1974.

[5] Total vitamin E activity, estimated to be 80 percent as α-tocopherol and 20 percent other tocopherols.

[6] The folacin allowances refer to dietary sources as determined by *Lactobacillus casei* assay. Pure forms of folacin may be effective in doses less than one-fourth of the RDA. Abbreviation µg = micrograms.

[7] Although allowances are expressed as niacin, it is recognized that on the average 1 mg of niacin is derived from each 60 mg of dietary tryptophan.

[8] This increased requirement cannot be met by ordinary diets, therefore, the use of supplemental iron is recommended.

NUTRITIVE VALUES OF FOODS

Adapted from *Nutritive Value of Foods*, USDA Home and Garden Bulletin 72 (revised 1977), and the more comprehensive tables in *Composition of Foods—Raw, Processed, Prepared*, USDA

Agriculture Handbook 8 (revised 1963). Both are for sale by the Superintendent of Documents, Washington, D.C. 20402.

ABBREVIATIONS   % = percent   cal = calories   g = gram   mg = milligram   IU = International Unit   tr = trace   — = lack of reliable data for a constituent believed to be present in measurable amount

NUTRIENTS IN INDICATED QUANTITY

NO.	FOOD AND APPROXIMATE MEASURE	Water %	Food energy cal	Protein g	Fat g	Fatty Acids Saturated g	Fatty Acids Unsaturated Oleic g	Fatty Acids Unsaturated Linoleic g	Carbohydrate g	Calcium mg	Phosphorus mg	Iron mg	Potassium mg	Vitamin A value IU	Thiamin mg	Riboflavin mg	Niacin mg	Ascorbic acid mg
	DAIRY PRODUCTS (CHEESE, CREAM, IMITATION CREAM, MILK; RELATED PRODUCTS)																	
	Butter. See items 103–108.																	
	Cheese, natural																	
1	Blue, 28 g (1 oz)	42	100	6	8	5.3	1.9	.2	1	150	110	.1	73	200	.01	.11	.3	0
2	Camembert, 38 g (1⅓ oz)	52	115	8	9	5.8	2.2	.2	tr	147	132	.1	71	350	.01	.19	.2	0
3	Cheddar, cut pieces, 28 g (1 oz)	37	115	7	9	6.1	2.1	.2	tr	204	145	.2	28	300	.01	.11	tr	0
4	cut pieces, 17.2 g (1 cu in)	37	70	4	6	3.7	1.3	.1	tr	124	88	.1	17	180	tr	.06	tr	0
5	shredded, 113 g (1 c)	37	455	28	37	24.2	8.5	.7	1	815	579	.8	111	1200	.03	.42	.1	0
	Cottage, curd not pressed down Creamed (4% fat)																	
6	large curd, 225 g (1 c)	79	235	28	10	6.4	2.4	.2	6	135	297	.3	190	370	.05	.37	.3	tr
7	small curd, 210 g (1 c)	79	220	26	9	6.0	2.2	.2	6	126	277	.3	177	340	.04	.34	.3	tr
8	Low fat (2%), 226 g (1 c)	79	205	31	4	2.8	1.0	.1	8	155	340	.4	217	160	.05	.42	.3	tr
9	Low fat (1%), 226 g (1 c)	82	165	28	2	1.5	.5	.1	6	138	302	.3	193	80	.05	.37	.3	tr
10	Uncreamed dry curd, less than ½% fat 145 g (1 c)	80	125	25	1	.4	.1	tr	3	46	151	.3	47	40	.04	.21	.2	0
11	Cream, 28 g (1 oz)	54	100	2	10	6.2	2.4	.2	1	23	30	.3	34	400	tr	.06	tr	0
12	Mozzarella, whole milk, 28 g (1 oz)	48	90	6	7	4.4	1.7	.2	1	163	117	.1	21	260	tr	.08	tr	0
13	part skim milk, 28 g (1 oz)	49	80	8	5	3.1	1.2	.1	1	207	149	.1	27	180	.01	.10	tr	0
14	Parmesan, grated, 100 g (1 c)	18	455	42	30	19.1	7.7	.3	4	1376	807	1.0	107	700	.05	.39	.3	0
15	5 g (1 T)	18	25	2	2	1.0	.4	tr	tr	69	40	tr	5	40	tr	.02	tr	0
16	28 g (1 oz)	18	130	12	9	5.4	2.2	.1	1	390	229	.3	30	200	.01	.11	tr	0
17	Provolone, 28 g (1 oz)	41	100	7	8	4.8	1.7	.1	1	214	141	.1	39	230	.01	.09	tr	0
18	Ricotta, whole milk, 246 g (1 c)	72	1790	28	32	20.4	7.1	.7	7	509	389	.9	257	1210	.03	.48	.3	0
19	part skim milk, 246 g (1 c)	74	340	28	19	12.1	4.7	.5	13	669	449	1.1	308	1060	.05	.46	.2	0
20	Romano, 28 g (1 oz)	31	110	9	8	—	—	—	1	302	215	—	—	160	—	.11	tr	0
21	Swiss, 28 g (1 oz)	37	105	8	8	5.0	1.7	.2	1	272	171	tr	31	240	.01	.10	tr	0
22	Cheese, pasteurized process American, 28 g (1 oz)	39	105	6	9	5.6	2.1	.2	tr	174	211	.1	46	340	.01	.10	tr	0

Table of nutritive values (milligrams, grams, and International Units per indicated portion):

Item No.	Food	Water (%)	Food energy (cal)	Protein (g)	Fat (g)	Saturated (g)	Oleic (g)	Linoleic (g)	Carbohydrate (g)	Calcium (mg)	Phosphorus (mg)	Iron (mg)	Potassium (mg)	Vitamin A (IU)	Thiamin (mg)	Riboflavin (mg)	Niacin (mg)	Ascorbic acid (mg)
23	Swiss, 28 g (1 oz)	42	95	7	7	4.5	1.7	.1	1	219	216	.2	61	230	tr	.08	tr	0
24	Cheese food, pasteurized process, American, 28 g (1 oz)	43	95	6	7	4.4	1.7	.1	2	163	130	.2	79	260	.01	.13	tr	0
25	Cheese spread, pasteurized process, American, 28 g (1 oz)	48	82	5	6	3.8	1.5	.1	2	159	202	.1	69	220	.01	.12	tr	0
	Cream, sweet																	
	Half-and-half (cream and milk)																	
26	242 g (1 c)	81	315	7	28	17.3	7.0	.6	10	254	230	.2	314	260	.08	.36	.2	2
27	15 g (1 T)	81	20	tr	2	1.1	.4	tr	1	16	14	tr	19	20	.01	.02	tr	tr
28	Light, coffee, or table, 240 g (1 c)	74	470	6	46	28.8	11.7	1.0	9	231	192	.1	292	1730	.08	.36	.1	2
29	15 g (1 T)	74	30	tr	3	1.8	.7	.1	1	14	12	tr	18	110	tr	.02	tr	tr
	Whipping, unwhipped (volume about double when whipped)																	
30	light, 239 g (1 c)	64	700	5	74	46.2	18.3	1.5	7	166	146	.1	231	2690	.06	.30	.1	1
31	15 g (1 T)	64	45	tr	5	2.9	1.1	.1	tr	10	9	tr	15	170	tr	.02	tr	tr
32	heavy, 238 g (1 c)	58	820	5	88	54.8	22.2	2.0	7	154	149	.1	179	3500	.05	.26	.1	1
33	15 g (1 T)	58	80	tr	6	3.5	1.4	.1	tr	10	9	tr	11	220	tr	.02	tr	tr
	Whipped topping, pressurized																	
34	60 g (1 c)	61	155	2	13	8.3	3.4	.3	7	61	54	tr	88	550	.02	.04	tr	0
35	3 g (1 T)	61	10	tr	1	.4	.2	tr	tr	3	3	tr	4	30	tr	tr	tr	0
36	Cream, sour, 230 g (1 c)	71	495	7	48	30.0	12.1	1.1	10	268	195	.1	331	1820	.08	.34	.2	2
37	12 g (1 T)	71	25	tr	3	1.6	.6	.1	1	14	10	tr	17	90	tr	.02	tr	tr
	Cream products, imitation (made with vegetable fat)																	
	Sweet																	
38	Creamers, liquid, frozen, 245 g (1 c)	77	335	2	24	22.8	.3	tr	28	23	157	.1	467	220¹	0	0	0	0
39	15 g (1 T)	77	20	tr	1	1.4	tr	0	2	1	10	tr	29	10¹	0	0	0	0
40	powdered, 94 g (1 c)	2	515	5	33	30.6	.9	tr	52	21	397	.1	763	190¹	0	.16¹	0	0
41	2 g (1 t)	2	10	tr	1	.7	tr¹	0	1	tr	8	tr	16	tr¹	0	tr¹	0	0
	Whipped topping																	
42	Frozen, 75 g (1 c)	50	240	1	19	16.3	1.0	.2	17	5	6	.1	14	650¹	0	0	0	0
43	4 g (1 T)	50	15	tr	1	.9	.1	tr	1	tr	tr	tr	1	30¹	0	0	0	0
44	powdered, made with whole milk 80 g (1 c)	67	150	3	10	8.5	.6	.1	13	72	69	tr	121	290¹	.02	.09	tr	1
45	4 g (1 T)	67	10	tr	tr	.4	tr	tr	1	4	3	tr	6	10¹	tr	tr	tr	tr
46	pressurized, 70 g (1 c)	60	185	1	16	13.2	1.4	.2	11	4	13	tr	13	330¹	0	0	0	0
47	4 g (1 T)	60	10	tr	1	.8	.1	tr	tr	tr	1	tr	1	20¹	0	0	0	0
48	Sour dressing (imitation sour cream), made with nonfat dry milk 235 g (1 c)	75	415	8	39	31.2	4.4	1.1	11	266	205	.1	380	20¹	.09	.38	.2	2
49	12 g (1 T)	75	20	tr	2	1.6	.2	.1	1	14	10	tr	19	tr¹	.01	.02	tr	tr
	Ice cream. See items 75–80.																	
	Ice milk. See items 81–83.																	
	Milk, fluid																	
50	Whole (3.3% fat), 244 g (1 c)	88	150	8	8	5.1	2.1	.2	11	291	228	.1	370	310²	.09	.40	.2	2
	Low-fat (2%)																	
51	no milk solids added, 244 g (1 c)	89	120	8	5	2.9	1.2	.1	12	297	232	.1	377	500	.10	.40	.2	2
52	milk solids added, label claim less than 10 g protein per c, 245 g (1 c)	89	125	9	5	2.9	1.2	.1	12	313	245	.1	397	500	.10	.42	.2	2
53	milk solids added, label claim 10 or more g protein per c (protein fortified), 246 g (1 c)	88	135	10	5	3.0	1.2	.1	14	352	276	.1	447	500	.11	.48	.2	3
	Low-fat (1%)																	
54	no milk solids added, 244 g (1 c)	90	100	8	3	1.6	.7	.1	12	300	235	.1	381	500	.10	.41	.2	2

¹Vitamin-A value is largely from beta-carotene used for coloring. Riboflavin value for items 40–41 apply to products with added riboflavin.

²Applies to product without added vitamin A. With added vitamin A, value is 500 IU.

NO.	FOOD AND APPROXIMATE MEASURE	Water %	Food energy cal	Protein g	Fat g	Fatty Acids Saturated g	Unsaturated Oleic g	Unsaturated Linoleic g	Carbohydrate g	Calcium mg	Phosphorus mg	Iron mg	Potassium mg	Vitamin A value IU	Thiamin mg	Riboflavin mg	Niacin mg	Ascorbic acid mg
	DAIRY PRODUCTS (CHEESE, CREAM, IMITATION CREAM, MILK; RELATED PRODUCTS)																	
55	milk solids added, label claim less than 10 g protein per c, 245 g (1 c)	90	105	9	2	1.5	.6	.1	12	313	245	.1	397	500	.10	.42	.2	2
56	milk solids added, label claim 10 or more g protein per c (protein fortified), 246 g (1 c)	89	120	10	3	1.8	.7	.1	14	349	273	.1	444	500	.11	.47	.2	3
	Nonfat (skim)																	
57	no milk solids added, 245 g (1 c)	91	85	8	tr	.3	.1	tr	12	302	247	.1	406	500	.09	.37	.2	2
58	milk solids added, label claim less than 10 g protein per c, 245 g (1 c)	90	90	9	1	.4	.1	tr	12	316	255	.1	418	500	.10	.43	.2	2
59	milk solids added, label claim 10 or more g protein per c (protein fortified), 246 g (1 c)	89	100	10	1	.4	.1	tr	14	352	275	.1	446	500	.11	.48	.2	3
60	Buttermilk, 245 g (1 c)	90	100	8	2	1.3	.5	tr	12	285	219	.1	371	80[3]	.08	.38	.1	2
	Milk, canned																	
61	Evaporated, unsweetened whole, 252 g (1 c)	74	340	17	19	11.6	5.3	.4	25	657	510	.5	764	610[3]	.12	.80	.5	5
62	skim, 255 g (1 c)	79	200	19	1	.3	.1	tr	29	738	497	.7	845	1000[4]	.11	.79	.4	3
63	Sweetened, condensed, 306 g (1 c)	27	980	24	27	16.8	6.7	.7	166	868	775	.6	1136	1000[3]	.28	1.27	.6	8
	Milk, dried																	
64	Buttermilk, 120 g (1 c)	3	465	41	7	4.3	1.7	.2	59	1421	1119	.4	1910	260[3]	.47	1.90	1.1	7
65	Nonfat instant, 91 g (3.2 oz)	4	325	32	1	.4	.4	tr	47	1120	896	.3	1552	2160[5]	.38	1.59	.8	5
66	68 g [7] (1 c)	4	245	24	tr	.3	.1	tr	35	837	670	.2	1160	1610[6]	.28	1.19	.6	4
	Milk beverages																	
	Chocolate milk (commercial)																	
67	regular, 250 g (1 c)	82	210	8	8	5.3	2.2	.2	26	280	251	.6	417	300[8]	.09	.41	.3	2
68	low-fat (2%), 250 g (1 c)	84	180	8	5	3.1	1.3	.1	26	284	254	.6	422	500	.10	.42	.3	2
69	low-fat (1%), 250 g (1 c)	85	160	8	3	1.5	.7	.1	26	287	257	.6	426	500	.10	.40	.2	2
70	Eggnog (commercial), 254 g (1 c)	74	340	10	19	11.3	5.0	.6	34	330	278	.5	420	890	.09	.48	.3	4
71	Malted milk, home-prepared chocolate, 265 g (1 c milk plus ¾ oz malted milk powder)	81	235	9	9	5.5	—	—	29	304	265	.5	500	330	.14	.43	.7	2
72	natural, 265 g (1 c milk plus ¾ oz powder)	81	235	11	10	6.0	—	—	27	347	307	.3	529	380	.20	.54	1.3	2
	Shakes, thick[9]																	
73	chocolate, 300 g (10.6 oz)	72	355	9	8	5.0	2.0	.2	63	396	378	.9	672	260	.14	.67	.4	0
74	vanilla, 313 g (11 oz)	74	350	12	9	5.9	2.4	.2	56	457	361	.3	572	360	.09	.61	.5	0
	Milk desserts, frozen																	
	Ice cream, regular (about 11% fat)																	
75	hardened, 1064 g (½ gal)	61	2155	38	115	71.3	28.8	2.6	254	1406	1075	1.0	2052	4340	.42	2.63	1.1	6
76	133 g (1 c)	61	270	5	14	8.9	3.6	.3	32	176	134	.1	257	540	.05	.33	.1	1
77	50 g (3 fl oz)	61	100	2	5	3.4	1.4	.1	12	66	51	tr	96	200	.02	.12	.1	tr

Item	Food, approximate measure, and weight (g)	Water (%)	Food energy (cal)	Protein (g)	Fat (g)	Saturated (g)	Oleic (g)	Linoleic (g)	Carbohydrate (g)	Calcium (mg)	Phosphorus (mg)	Iron (mg)	Potassium (mg)	Vitamin A (IU)	Thiamin (mg)	Riboflavin (mg)	Niacin (mg)	Ascorbic acid (mg)
78	soft serve (frozen custard), 173 g (1 c)	60	375	7	23	13.5	5.9	.6	38	236	199	.4	338	790	.08	.45	.2	1
79	Ice cream, rich (about 16% fat) hardened, 1188 g (½ gal)	59	2805	33	190	118.3	47.8	4.3	256	1213	927	.8	1771	7200	.36	2.27	.9	5
80	148 g (1 c)	59	350	4	24	14.7	6.0	.5	32	151	115	.1	221	900	.04	.28	.1	1
81	Ice milk, hardened (about 4.3% fat) 1048 g (½ gal)	69	1470	41	45	28.1	11.3	1.0	232	1409	1035	1.5	2117	1710	.61	2.78	.9	6
82	131 g (1 c)	69	185	5	6	3.5	1.4	.1	29	176	129	.1	265	210	.08	.35	.1	1
83	soft serve (about 2.6% fat) 175 g (1 c)	70	225	8	5	2.9	1.2	.1	38	274	202	.3	412	180	.12	.54	.2	1
84	Sherbet (about 2% fat), 1542 g (½ gal)	66	2160	17	31	19.0	7.7	.7	469	827	594	2.5	1585	1480	.26	.71	1.0	31
85	193 g (1 c)	66	270	2	4	2.4	1.0	.1	59	103	74	.3	198	190	.03	.09	.1	4
86	Milk desserts, other — Custard, baked, 265 g (1 c)	77	305	14	15	6.8	5.4	.7	29	297	310	1.1	387	930	.11	.50	.3	1
87	Puddings (home recipe) — Starch base — chocolate, 260 g (1 c)	66	385	8	12	7.6	3.3	.3	67	250	255	1.3	445	390	.05	.36	.3	1
88	vanilla (blancmange), 255 g (1 c)	76	285	9	10	6.2	2.5	.2	41	298	232	tr	352	410	.08	.41	.3	2
89	Tapioca cream, 165 g (1 c)	72	220	8	8	4.1	2.5	.5	28	173	180	.7	223	480	.07	.30	.2	2
90	Puddings (chocolate mix with milk) — Regular (cooked), 260 g (1 c)	70	320	9	8	4.3	2.6	.2	59	265	247	.8	354	340	.05	.39	.3	2
91	Instant, 260 g (1 c)	69	325	8	7	3.6	2.2	.3	63	374	237	1.3	335	340	.08	.39	.3	2
92	Yogurt — With added low-fat milk solids — Fruit-flavored,[9] 227 g (8 oz)	75	230	10	3	1.8	.6	.1	42	343	269	.2	439	120[10]	.08	.40	.2	1
93	Plain, 227 g (8 oz)	85	145	12	4	2.3	.8	.1	16	415	326	.2	531	150[10]	.10	.49	.3	2
94	With added nonfat milk solids, 227 g (8 oz)	85	125	13	tr	.3	.1	tr	17	452	355	.2	579	20[10]	.11	.53	.2	2
95	Whole milk, 227 g (8 oz)	88	140	8	7	4.8	1.7	.1	11	274	215	.1	351	280	.07	.32	.2	1

EGGS

Item	Food, approximate measure, and weight (g)	Water (%)	Food energy (cal)	Protein (g)	Fat (g)	Saturated (g)	Oleic (g)	Linoleic (g)	Carbohydrate (g)	Calcium (mg)	Phosphorus (mg)	Iron (mg)	Potassium (mg)	Vitamin A (IU)	Thiamin (mg)	Riboflavin (mg)	Niacin (mg)	Ascorbic acid (mg)
96	Raw, large (24 oz per doz) — Whole, without shell, 1, 50 g	75	80	6	6	1.7	2.0	.6	1	28	90	1.0	65	260	.04	.15	tr	0
97	White, 1, 33 g	88	15	3	tr	0	0	0	tr	4	4	tr	45	0	tr	.09	tr	0
98	Yolk, 1, 17 g	49	65	3	6	1.7	2.1	.6	tr	26	36	.9	15	310	.04	.07	tr	0
99	Cooked, large (24 oz per doz) — Fried in butter, 1, 46 g	72	85	5	6	2.4	2.2	.6	1	26	80	.9	58	290	.03	.13	tr	0
100	Hard-cooked, shell removed, 1, 50 g	75	80	6	6	1.7	2.0	.6	1	28	90	1.0	65	260	.04	.14	tr	0
101	Poached, 1, 50 g	74	80	6	6	1.7	2.0	.6	1	28	90	1.0	65	260	.04	.13	tr	0
102	Scrambled (milk added) in butter, or omelet, 1, 64 g	76	95	6	7	2.8	2.3	.6	1	47	97	.9	85	310	.04	.16	tr	0

FATS, OILS; RELATED PRODUCTS

Item	Food, approximate measure, and weight (g)	Water (%)	Food energy (cal)	Protein (g)	Fat (g)	Saturated (g)	Oleic (g)	Linoleic (g)	Carbohydrate (g)	Calcium (mg)	Phosphorus (mg)	Iron (mg)	Potassium (mg)	Vitamin A (IU)	Thiamin (mg)	Riboflavin (mg)	Niacin (mg)	Ascorbic acid (mg)
	Butter																	
103	Regular, stick, 113 g (½ c)	16	815	1	92	57.3	23.1	2.1	tr	27	26	.2	29	3470[11]	.01	.04	tr	0
104	⅛ stick, 14 g (1 T)	16	100	tr	12	7.2	2.9	.3	tr	3	3	tr	4	430[11]	tr	tr	tr	0
105	pat, 5 g (1 x 1 x ⅓ in)	16	35	tr	4	2.5	1.0	.1	tr	1	1	tr	1	150[11]	tr	tr	tr	0
106	Whipped, stick, 76 g (½ c)	16	540	1	61	38.2	15.4	1.4	tr	18	17	.1	20	2310[11]	tr	.03	tr	0

[3]Applies to product without vitamin A added.
[4]Applies to product with added vitamin A. Without added vitamin A, value is 20 IU.
[5]Yields 1 qt fluid milk when reconstituted according to package directions.
[6]Applies to product with added vitamin A.
[7]Weight applies to product with label claim of 1 1/3 cups = 3.2 oz.
[8]Applies to products made from thick shake mixes and that do not contain added ice cream. Products made from milk shake mixes are higher in fat and usually contain added ice cream.
[9]Content of fat, vitamin A, and carbohydrate varies. Consult the label when precise values are needed for special diets.
[10]Applies to product made with milk containing no added vitamin A.
[11]Based on year-round average.

NUTRIENTS IN INDICATED QUANTITY

NO.	FOOD AND APPROXIMATE MEASURE	Water %	Food energy cal	Protein g	Fat g	Fatty Acids Saturated g	Fatty Acids Unsaturated Oleic g	Fatty Acids Unsaturated Linoleic g	Carbohydrate g	Calcium mg	Phosphorus mg	Iron mg	Potassium mg	Vitamin A value IU	Thiamin mg	Riboflavin mg	Niacin mg	Ascorbic acid mg
	FATS, OILS; RELATED PRODUCTS																	
107	⅛ stick, 9 g (1 T)	16	65	tr	8	4.7	1.9	.2	tr	2	2	tr	2	290[1]	tr	tr	tr	0
108	pat, 4 g (1¼ x 1¼ x ⅓ in)	16	25	tr	3	1.9	.8	.1	tr	1	1	tr	1	120[1]	tr	tr	tr	0
	Fats, cooking (vegetable shortenings)																	
109	200 g (1 c)	0	1770	0	200	48.8	88.2	48.4	0	0	0	0	0	—	0	0	0	0
110	13 g (1 T)	0	110	0	13	3.2	5.7	3.1	0	0	0	0	0	—	0	0	0	0
111	Lard, 205 g (1 c)	0	1850	0	205	81.0	83.8	20.5	0	0	0	0	0	0	0	0	0	0
112	13 g (1 T)	0	115	0	13	5.1	5.3	1.3	0	0	0	0	0	0	0	0	0	0
	Margarine																	
113	Regular, stick, 113 g (½ c)	16	815	1	92	16.7	42.9	24.9	tr	27	26	.2	29	3750[2]	.01	.04	tr	0
114	⅛ stick, 14 g (1 T)	16	100	tr	12	2.1	5.3	3.1	tr	3	3	tr	4	470[2]	tr	tr	tr	0
115	pat, 5 g (1 x 1 x ⅓ in)	16	35	tr	4	.7	1.9	1.1	tr	1	1	tr	1	170[2]	tr	tr	tr	0
116	Soft, 227 g (½ lb)	16	1635	1	184	32.5	71.5	65.4	tr	53	52	.4	59	7500[2]	.01	.08	.1	0
117	14 g (1 T)	16	100	tr	12	2.0	4.5	4.1	tr	3	3	tr	4	470[2]	tr	tr	tr	0
118	Whipped, stick, 76 g (½ c)	16	545	tr	61	11.2	28.7	16.7	tr	18	17	.1	20	2500[2]	tr	.03	tr	0
119	⅛ stick, 9 g (1 T)	16	70	tr	8	1.4	3.6	2.1	tr	2	2	tr	2	310[2]	tr	tr	tr	0
	Oils, salad or cooking																	
120	Corn, 218 g (1 c)	0	1925	0	218	27.7	53.6	125.1	0	0	0	0	0	—	0	0	0	0
121	14 g (1 T)	0	120	0	14	1.7	3.3	7.8	0	0	0	0	0	—	0	0	0	0
122	Olive, 216 g (1 c)	0	1910	0	216	30.7	154.4	17.7	0	0	0	0	0	—	0	0	0	0
123	14 g (1 T)	0	120	0	14	1.9	9.7	1.1	0	0	0	0	0	—	0	0	0	0
124	Peanut, 216 g (1 c)	0	1910	0	216	37.4	98.5	67.0	0	0	0	0	0	—	0	0	0	0
125	14 g (1 T)	0	120	0	14	2.3	6.2	4.2	0	0	0	0	0	—	0	0	0	0
126	Safflower, 218 g (1 c)	0	1925	0	218	20.5	25.9	159.8	0	0	0	0	0	—	0	0	0	0
127	14 g (1 T)	0	120	0	14	1.3	1.6	10.0	0	0	0	0	0	—	0	0	0	0
128	Soybean oil, hydrogenated (partially hardened), 218 g (1 c)	0	1925	0	218	31.8	93.1	75.6	0	0	0	0	0	—	0	0	0	0
129	14 g (1 T)	0	120	0	14	2.0	5.8	4.7	0	0	0	0	0	—	0	0	0	0
130	Soybean-cottonseed oil blend, hydrogenated, 218 g (1 c)	0	1925	0	218	38.2	63.0	99.6	0	0	0	0	0	—	0	0	0	0
131	14 g (1 T)	0	120	0	14	2.4	3.9	6.2	0	0	0	0	0	—	0	0	0	0
	Salad dressings, commercial																	
132	Blue cheese, regular, 15 g (1 T)	32	75	1	8	1.6	1.7	3.8	1	12	11	tr	6	30	tr	.02	tr	tr
133	low calorie, 16 g (1 T)	84	10	tr	1	.5	.3	tr	1	10	8	tr	5	30	tr	.01	tr	tr
134	French, regular, 16 g (1 T)	39	65	tr	6	1.1	1.3	3.2	3	2	2	.1	13	—	—	—	—	—
135	low calorie, 16 g (1 T)	77	15	tr	1	.1	.1	.4	2	2	2	.1	13	—	—	—	—	—
136	Italian, regular, 15 g (1 T)	28	85	tr	9	1.6	1.9	4.7	1	2	1	tr	2	—	tr	tr	tr	—
137	low calorie, 15 g (1 T)	90	10	tr	1	.1	.1	.4	tr	tr	1	tr	2	tr	tr	tr	tr	—
138	Mayonnaise, 14 g (1 T)	15	100	tr	11	2.0	2.4	5.6	tr	3	4	.1	5	40	tr	.01	tr	—
	Mayonnaise type																	
139	regular, 15 g (1 T)	41	65	tr	6	1.1	1.4	3.2	2	2	4	tr	1	30	tr	tr	tr	—
140	low calorie, 16 g (1 T)	81	20	tr	2	.4	.4	1.0	2	3	4	tr	1	40	tr	tr	tr	—
141	Tartar sauce, regular, 14 g (1 T)	34	75	tr	8	1.5	1.8	4.1	1	3	4	.1	11	30	tr	.01	tr	tr
	Thousand Island																	

FISH, SHELLFISH, MEAT, POULTRY; RELATED PRODUCTS

No.	Food	Water (%)	Food energy (cal)	Protein (g)	Fat (g)	Saturated (g)	Oleic (g)	Linoleic (g)	Carbohydrate (g)	Calcium (mg)	Phosphorus (mg)	Iron (mg)	Potassium (mg)	Vitamin A (IU)	Thiamin (mg)	Riboflavin (mg)	Niacin (mg)	Ascorbic acid (mg)
142	regular, 16 g (1 T)	32	80	tr	8	1.4	1.7	4.0	2	2	3	.1	18	50	tr	tr	tr	tr
143	low calorie, 15 g (1 T)	68	25	tr	2	.4	.4	1.0	2	2	3	.1	17	50	tr	tr	tr	tr
144	Salad dressings, home recipe, cooked type,[13] 16 g (1 T)	68	25	1	2	.5	.6	.3	2	14	15	.1	19	80	.01	.03	tr	tr
	Fish and shellfish																	
145	Bluefish, baked with butter or margarine, 85 g (3 oz)	68	135	22	4	—	—	—	0	25	244	.6	—	40	.09	.08	1.6	—
146	Clams, raw, meat only, 85 g (3 oz)	82	65	11	1	—	—	—	2	59	138	5.2	154	90	.08	.15	1.1	8
147	canned, solids and liquid, 85 g (3 oz)	86	45	7	1	—	—	—	2	47	116	3.5	119	—	.01	.09	.9	—
148	Crabmeat (white or king), canned, not pressed down, 135 g (1 c)	77	135	24	3	—	—	—	1	61	246	1.1	149	—	.11	.11	2.6	—
149	Fish sticks, breaded, cooked, frozen, 1 stick, 28 g (4 x 1 x ½ in or 1 oz)	66	50	5	3	—	—	—	2	3	47	.1	—	0	.01	.02	.5	—
150	Haddock, breaded, fried,[14] 85 g (3 oz)	66	140	17	5	1.4	2.2	1.2	5	34	210	1.0	296	—	.03	.06	2.7	2
151	Ocean perch, breaded, fried,[14] 1 fillet, 85 g	59	195	16	11	2.7	4.4	2.3	6	28	192	1.1	242	—	.10	.10	1.6	—
152	Oysters, raw, meat only, 240 g (1 c)	85	160	20	4	1.3	.2	.1	8	226	343	13.2	290	740	.34	.43	6.0	—
153	Salmon, pink, canned, solids and liquid, 85 g (3 oz)	71	120	17	5	.9	.8	.1	0	167[15]	243	.7	307	60	.03	.16	6.8	—
154	Sardines, Atlantic, canned in oil, drained solids, 85 g (3 oz)	62	175	20	9	3.0	2.5	.5	0	372	424	2.5	502	190	.02	.17	4.6	—
155	Scallops, frozen, breaded, fried, reheated, 6 scallops, 90 g	60	175	16	8	—	—	—	9	—	—	—	—	—	—	—	—	—
156	Shad, baked with butter or margarine, bacon, 85 g (3 oz)	64	170	20	10	—	—	—	0	20	266	.5	320	30	.11	.22	7.3	—
157	Shrimp, canned, meat, 85 g (3 oz)	70	100	21	1	.1	.1	tr	1	98	224	2.6	104	50	.01	.03	1.5	—
158	French fried,[16] 85 g (3 oz)	57	190	17	9	2.3	3.7	2.0	9	61	162	1.7	195	—	.03	.07	2.3	—
159	Tuna, canned in oil, drained solids, 85 g (3 oz)	61	170	24	7	1.7	1.7	.7	0	7	199	1.6	—	70	.04	.10	10.1	—
160	Tuna salad,[17] 205 g (1 c)	70	350	30	22	4.3	6.3	6.7	7	41	291	2.7	—	590	.08	.23	10.3	2
	Meat and meat products																	
161	Bacon, broiled or fried, crisp, (2 slices) 15 g	8	85	4	8	2.5	3.7	.7	tr	2	34	.5	35	0	.08	.05	.8	—
162	Beef,[18] braised, simmered, or pot roasted (piece, 2½ x 2½ x ¾ in): Lean and fat, 85 g (3 oz)	53	245	23	16	6.8	6.5	.4	0	10	114	2.9	184	30	.04	.18	3.6	—
163	Lean only, 72 g (2.5 oz)	62	140	22	5	2.1	1.8	.2	0	10	108	2.7	176	10	.04	.17	3.3	—
164	Beef, ground, broiled (patty 3 x ⅝ in): Lean with 10% fat, 85 g (3 oz)	60	185	23	10	4.0	3.9	.3	0	10	196	3.0	261	20	.08	.20	5.1	—
165	Lean with 21% fat, 82 g (2.9 oz)	54	235	20	17	7.0	6.7	.4	0	9	159	2.6	221	30	.07	.17	4.4	—
166	Beef, oven cooked, no liquid added (2 pieces, 4⅛ x 2¼ x ¼ in): Relatively fat, such as rib: Lean and fat, 85 g (3 oz)	40	375	17	33	14.0	13.6	.8	0	8	158	2.2	189	70	.05	.13	3.1	—
167	Lean only, 51 g (1.8 oz)	57	125	14	7	3.0	2.5	.3	0	6	131	1.8	161	10	.04	.11	2.6	—
168	Relatively lean, such as heel of round: Lean and fat, 85 g (3 oz)	62	165	25	7	2.8	2.7	.2	0	11	208	3.2	279	10	.06	.19	4.5	—
169	Lean only, 78 g (2.8 oz)	65	125	24	3	1.2	1.0	.1	0	10	199	3.0	268	tr	.06	.18	4.3	—

[12] Based on average vitamin-A content of fortified margarine. Federal specifications for fortified margarine require a minimum of 15000 IU of vitamin A per pound.
[13] Fatty acid values apply to product made with regular-type margarine.
[14] Dipped in egg, milk or water, and breadcrumbs; fried in vegetable shortening.
[15] If bones are discarded, value for calcium will be greatly reduced.
[16] Dipped in egg, breadcrumbs, and flour or batter.
[17] Prepared with tuna, celery, salad dressing (mayonnaise type), pickle, onion, and egg.
[18] Out layer of fat on the cut removed to within approximately 1/2 in of the lean. Deposits of fat within the lean not removed.

FISH, SHELLFISH, MEAT, POULTRY; RELATED PRODUCTS

NO.	FOOD AND APPROXIMATE MEASURE	Water %	Food energy cal	Protein g	Fat g	Fatty Acids Saturated g	Fatty Acids Unsaturated Oleic g	Fatty Acids Unsaturated Linoleic g	Carbohydrate g	Calcium mg	Phosphorus mg	Iron mg	Potassium mg	Vitamin A value IU	Thiamin mg	Riboflavin mg	Niacin mg	Ascorbic acid mg
	Beef, steak Relatively fat sirloin, broiled (piece, 2½ x 2½ x ¾")																	
170	Lean and fat, 85 g (3 oz)	44	330	20	27	11.3	11.1	.6	0	9	162	2.5	220	50	.05	.15	4.0	—
171	Lean only, 56 g (2 oz)	59	115	18	4	1.8	1.6	.2	0	7	146	2.2	202	10	.05	.14	3.6	—
	Relatively lean round, braised (piece, 4⅛ x 2¼ x ½")																	
172	Lean and fat, 85 g (3 oz)	55	220	24	13	5.5	5.2	.4	0	10	213	3.0	272	20	.07	.19	4.8	—
173	Lean only, 68 g (2.4 oz)	61	130	21	4	1.7	1.5	.2	0	9	182	2.5	238	10	.05	.16	4.1	—
	Beef, canned																	
174	Corned beef, 85 g (3 oz)	59	185	22	10	4.9	4.5	.2	0	17	90	3.7	—	—	.01	.20	2.9	—
175	Corned beef hash, 220 g (1 c)	67	400	19	25	11.9	10.9	.5	24	29	147	4.4	440	—	.02	.20	4.6	—
176	Beef, dried, chipped, 71 g (2.5 oz)	48	145	24	4	2.1	2.0	.1	0	14	287	3.6	142	—	.05	.23	2.7	0
177	Beef and vegetable stew, 245 g (1 c)	82	220	16	11	4.9	4.5	.2	15	29	184	2.9	613	2400	.15	.17	4.7	17
178	Beef potpie (home recipe), baked[19] 210 g (⅓ of 9-in pie)	55	515	21	30	7.9	12.8	6.7	39	29	149	3.8	334	1720	.30	.30	5.5	6
179	Chili con carne with beans, canned 255 g (1 c)	72	340	19	16	7.5	6.8	.3	31	82	321	4.3	594	150	.08	.18	3.3	—
180	Chop suey with beef and pork (home recipe), 250 g (1 c)	75	300	26	17	8.5	6.2	.7	13	60	248	4.8	425	600	.28	.38	5.0	33
181	Heart, beef, lean, braised, 85 g (3 oz)	61	160	27	5	1.5	1.1	.6	1	5	154	5.0	197	20	.21	1.04	6.5	1
	Lamb chop, rib, broiled																	
182	Lean and fat, 89 g (3.1 oz)	43	360	18	32	14.8	12.1	1.2	0	8	139	1.0	200	—	.11	.19	4.1	—
183	Lean only, 57 g (2 oz)	60	120	16	6	2.5	2.1	.2	0	6	121	1.1	174	—	.09	.15	3.4	—
	Lamb leg, roasted (2 pieces 1⅛ x 2¼ x ¼ in)																	
184	Lean and fat, 85 g (3 oz)	54	235	22	16	7.3	6.0	.6	0	9	177	1.4	241	—	.13	.23	4.7	—
185	Lean only, 71 g (2.5 oz)	62	130	20	5	2.1	1.8	.2	0	9	169	1.4	227	—	.12	.21	4.4	—
	Lamb shoulder, roasted (3 pieces, 2½ x 2½ x ¼ in)																	
186	Lean and fat, 85 g (3 oz)	50	285	18	23	10.8	8.8	.9	0	9	146	1.0	206	—	.11	.20	4.0	—
187	Lean only, 64 g (2.3 oz)	61	130	17	6	3.6	2.3	.2	0	8	140	1.0	193	—	.10	.18	3.7	—
188	Liver, beef, fried[20] 85 g (3 oz)	56	195	22	9	2.5	3.5	.9	5	9	405	7.5	323	45390[21]	.22	3.56	14.0	23
	Pork, cured, cooked																	
189	Ham, light cure, lean and fat, roasted[22] 85 g (3 oz)	54	245	18	19	6.8	7.9	1.7	0	8	146	2.2	199	0	.40	.15	3.1	—
	Luncheon meat																	
190	Boiled ham, slice, 28 g (1 oz)	59	65	5	5	1.7	2.0	.4	0	3	47	.8	—	0	.12	.04	.7	—
191	Canned, spiced or unspiced, slice, 60 g (3 x 2 x ½ in)	55	175	9	15	5.4	6.7	1.0	1	5	65	1.3	133	0	.19	.13	1.8	—
	Pork, fresh,[18] cooked Chop, loin, broiled																	

No.	Food	Water (%)	Food energy (cal)	Protein (g)	Fat (g)	Saturated (g)	Oleic (g)	Linoleic (g)	Carbohydrate (g)	Calcium (mg)	Phosphorus (mg)	Iron (mg)	Potassium (mg)	Vitamin A (IU)	Thiamin (mg)	Riboflavin (mg)	Niacin (mg)	Ascorbic acid (mg)
192	Lean and fat, 78 g (2.7 oz).	42	305	19	25	8.9	10.4	2.2	0	9	209	2.7	216	0	.75	.22	4.5	—
193	Lean only, 56 g (2 oz)	53	150	17	9	3.1	3.6	.8	0	7	181	2.2	192	0	.63	.18	3.8	—
	Oven cooked, no liquid added (piece, 2½ x 2½ x ¾ in.)																	
194	Lean and fat, 85 g (3 oz)	46	310	21	24	8.7	10.2	2.2	0	9	218	2.7	233	0	.78	.22	4.8	—
195	Lean only, 68 g (2.4 oz)	55	175	20	10	3.5	4.1	.8	0	9	211	2.6	224	0	.73	.21	4.4	—
	Shoulder cut, simmered (3 pieces, 2½ x 2½ x ¼)																	
196	Lean and fat, 85 g (3 oz)	46	320	20	26	9.3	10.9	2.3	0	9	118	2.6	158	0	.46	.21	4.1	—
197	Lean only, 63 g (2.2 oz)	60	135	18	6	2.2	2.6	.6	0	8	111	2.3	146	0	.42	.19	3.7	—
	Sausages (see also items 190–191)																	
198	Bologna, slice, 28 g (1 oz)	56	85	3	8	3.0	3.4	.5	tr	2	36	.5	65	—	.05	.06	.7	—
199	Braunschweiger, slice, 28 g (1 oz)	53	90	4	8	2.6	3.4	.8	1	3	69	1.7	—	1850	.05	.41	2.3	—
200	Brown and serve, browned, link 17 g (.75 oz)	40	70	3	6	2.3	2.8	.7	tr	1	—	—	—	0	—	—	—	—
201	Deviled ham, canned, 13 g (1 T)	51	45	2	4	1.5	1.8	.4	0	1	12	.3	—	0	.02	.01	.2	—
202	Frankfurter, cooked, 56 g (2 oz)	57	170	7	15	5.6	6.5	1.2	1	3	57	.8	—	—	.08	.11	1.4	—
203	Potted beef, chicken, turkey, canned, 13 g (1 T)	61	30	2	2	—	—	—	0	—	—	—	—	0	tr	.03	.2	—
204	Pork link, cooked, 13 g (1 oz)	35	60	2	6	2.1	2.4	.5	tr	1	21	.3	35	0	.10	.04	.5	—
205	Salami, dry type, slice, 10 g (.33 oz)	30	45	2	4	1.6	1.6	.1	tr	1	28	.4	—	0	.04	.03	.5	—
206	cooked type, slice 28 g (1 oz)	51	90	5	7	3.1	3.0	.2	tr	3	57	.7	—	—	.07	.07	1.2	—
207	Vienna sausage, 16 g (.45 oz)	63	40	2	3	1.2	1.4	.2	tr	1	24	.3	—	—	.01	.02	.4	—
	Veal, medium fat, cooked, bone removed																	
208	Cutlet, braised or broiled, 85 g (3 oz)	60	185	23	9	4.0	3.4	.4	0	9	196	2.7	265	—	.06	.21	4.6	—
209	Rib, roasted, 85 g (3 oz)	55	230	23	14	6.1	5.1	.6	0	10	211	2.9	259	—	.11	.26	6.6	—
	Poultry and poultry products																	
	Chicken pieces																	
210	Half breast, fried,[23] bones removed 79 g (2.8 oz)	58	160	26	5	1.4	1.8	1.1	1	9	218	1.3	—	70	.04	.17	11.6	—
211	Drumstick, fried,[23] bones removed 38 g (1.3 oz)	55	90	12	4	1.1	1.3	.9	tr	6	89	.9	—	50	.03	.15	2.7	—
212	Half broiler, broiled, bones removed 176 g (6.2 oz)	71	240	42	7	2.2	2.5	1.3	0	16	355	3.0	483	160	.09	.34	15.5	—
213	Chicken, canned, boneless, 85 g (3 oz)	65	170	18	10	3.2	3.8	2.0	0	18	210	1.3	117	200	.03	.11	3.7	3
214	Chicken a la king, cooked (home recipe) 245 g (1 c)	68	470	27	34	12.7	14.3	3.3	12	127	358	2.5	404	1130	.10	.42	5.4	12
215	Chicken and noodles, cooked (home recipe) 240 g (1 c)	71	365	22	18	5.9	7.1	3.5	26	26	247	2.2	149	430	.05	.17	4.3	tr
	Chicken chow mein																	
216	canned, 250 g (1 c)	89	95	7	tr	—	—	—	18	45	85	1.3	418	150	.05	.10	1.0	13
217	home recipe, 250 g (1 c)	78	255	31	10	2.4	3.4	3.1	10	58	293	2.5	473	280	.08	.23	4.3	10
218	Chicken potpie (home recipe), baked[19] 232 g (⅓ 9-in pie)	57	545	23	31	11.3	10.9	5.6	42	70	232	3.0	343	3090	.34	.31	5.5	5
	Turkey, roasted, flesh without skin																	
219	Dark meat, 4 pieces, 2½ x 1⅝ x ¼ in 85 g	61	175	26	7	2.1	1.5	1.5	0	—	—	2.0	338	—	.03	.20	3.6	—
220	Light meat, 2 pieces, 4 x 2 x ¼ in, 85 g	62	150	28	3	.9	.6	.7	0	—	—	1.0	349	—	.04	.12	9.4	—
	Light and dark meat																	
221	Chopped or diced, 140 g (1 c)	61	265	44	9	2.5	1.7	1.8	0	11	351	2.5	514	—	.07	.25	10.8	—
222	1 slice white meat, 2 slices dark meat, 85 g	61	160	27	5	1.5	1.0	1.1	0	7	213	1.5	312	—	.04	.15	6.5	—

[19] Crust made with vegetable shortening and enriched flour.
[20] Regular-type margarine used.
[21] Value varies widely.
[22] About one-fourth of the outer layer of fat on the cut removed. Deposits of fat within the cut not removed.
[23] Vegetable shortening used.

NUTRIENTS IN INDICATED QUANTITY

NO.	FOOD AND APPROXIMATE MEASURE	Water %	Food energy cal	Protein g	Fat g	Fatty Acids Saturated g	Unsaturated Oleic g	Unsaturated Linoleic g	Carbohydrate g	Calcium mg	Phosphorus mg	Iron mg	Potassium mg	Vitamin A value IU	Thiamin mg	Riboflavin mg	Niacin mg	Ascorbic acid mg
	FRUITS AND FRUIT PRODUCTS																	
	Apples, raw, unpeeled, without cores																	
223	Small, 1, 138 g (2¾-in diameter)	84	80	tr	1	—	—	—	20	10	14	.4	152	120	.04	.03	.1	6
224	Medium, 1, 212 g (3¼-in diameter)	84	125	tr	1	—	—	—	31	15	21	.6	233	190	.06	.04	.2	8
225	Applejuice, bottled or canned[24] 248 g (1 c)	88	120	tr	tr	—	—	—	30	15	22	1.5	250	—	.02	.05	.2	2[25]
	Applesauce, canned																	
226	Sweetened, 255 g (1 c)	76	230	1	tr	—	—	—	61	10	13	1.3	166	100	.05	.03	.1	3[25]
227	Unsweetened, 244 g (1 c)	89	100	tr	tr	—	—	—	26	10	12	1.2	190	100	.05	.02	.1	2[25]
	Apricots																	
228	Raw, without pits, 3, 107 g	85	55	1	tr	—	—	—	14	18	25	.5	301	2890	.03	.04	.6	11
229	Canned in heavy sirup, 258 g (1 c)	77	220	2	tr	—	—	—	57	28	39	.8	604	4490	.05	.05	1.0	10
230	Dried, uncooked, 130 g (1 c)	25	340	7	1	—	—	—	86	87	140	7.2	1273	14170	.01	.21	4.3	16
231	Dried, cooked, unsweetened, and liquid 250 g (1 c)	76	215	4	1	—	—	—	54	55	88	4.5	795	7500	.01	.13	2.5	8
232	Apricot nectar, canned, 251 g (1 c)	85	145	1	tr	—	—	—	37	23	30	.5	379	2380	.03	.03	.5	36[26]
	Avocados, raw, whole, without skins and seeds																	
233	California, 1, 216 g (10 oz)	74	370	5	37	5.5	22.0	3.7	13	22	91	1.3	1303	630	.24	.43	3.5	30
234	Florida, 1, 304 g (1 lb)	78	390	4	33	6.7	15.7	5.3	27	30	128	1.8	1836	880	.33	.61	4.9	43
235	Banana without peel, 1, 119 g	76	100	1	tr	—	—	—	26	10	31	.8	440	230	.06	.07	.8	12
236	Banana flakes, 6 g (1 T)	3	20	tr	tr	—	—	—	5	2	6	.2	92	50	.01	.01	.2	tr
237	Blackberries, raw, 144 g (1 c)	85	85	2	1	—	—	—	19	46	27	1.3	245	290	.04	.06	.6	30
238	Blueberries, raw, 145 g (1 c)	83	90	1	1	—	—	—	22	22	19	1.5	117	150	.04	.09	.7	20
	Cantaloupe. See item 271.																	
	Cherries																	
239	Sour (tart), red, pitted, canned, water pack, 244 g (1 c)	88	105	2	tr	—	—	—	26	37	32	.7	317	1660	.07	.05	.5	12
240	Sweet, raw, without pits and stems, 10, 68 g	80	45	1	tr	—	—	—	12	15	13	.3	129	70	.03	.04	.3	7
241	Cranberry juice cocktail, bottled, sweetened, 253 g (1 c)	83	165	tr	tr	—	—	—	42	13	8	.8	25	tr	.03	.03	.1	81[27]
242	Cranberry sauce, sweetened, canned, strained, 277 g (1 c)	62	405	tr	1	—	—	—	104	17	11	.6	83	60	.03	.03	.1	6
243	Dates, whole, without pits, 10, 80 g	23	220	2	tr	—	—	—	58	47	50	2.4	518	40	.07	.08	1.8	0
244	chopped, 178 g (1 c)	23	490	4	1	—	—	—	130	105	112	5.3	1153	90	.16	.18	3.9	0
245	Fruit cocktail, canned, in heavy sirup 255 g (1 c)	80	195	1	tr	—	—	—	50	23	31	1.0	411	360	.05	.03	1.0	5
	Grapefruit																	
246	Raw, pink or red, ½ medium, with peel 241 g[28]	89	50	1	tr	—	—	—	13	20	20	.5	166	540	.05	.02	.2	44
247	Raw, white, ½ medium, with peel 241 g[28]	89	45	1	tr	—	—	—	12	19	19	.5	159	10	.05	.02	.2	44

No.	Food, approximate measure, and weight (g)	Water (%)	Food energy (cal)	Protein (g)	Fat (g)	Fatty acids Saturated (g)	Unsat. Oleic (g)	Linoleic (g)	Carbohydrate (g)	Calcium (mg)	Phosphorus (mg)	Iron (mg)	Potassium (mg)	Vitamin A (IU)	Thiamin (mg)	Riboflavin (mg)	Niacin (mg)	Ascorbic acid (mg)
248	Canned, sections with sirup, 254 g (1 c)	81	180	2	tr	—	—	—	45	33	36	.8	343	30	.08	.05	.5	76
	Grapefruit juice																	
249	Raw, pink, red, or white, 246 g (1 c)	90	95	1	tr	—	—	—	23	22	37	.5	399	(29)	.10	.05	.5	93
	Canned, white																	
250	unsweetened, 247 g (1 c)	89	100	1	tr	—	—	—	24	20	35	1.0	400	20	.07	.05	.5	84
251	sweetened, 250 g (1 c)	86	135	1	tr	—	—	—	32	20	35	1.0	405	30	.08	.05	.5	78
	Frozen concentrate, unsweetened																	
252	undiluted, 207 g (6 fl oz)	62	300	4	1	—	—	—	72	70	124	.8	1250	60	.29	.12	1.4	286
253	diluted with 3 parts water by volume 247 g (1 c)	89	100	1	tr	—	—	—	24	25	42	.2	420	20	.10	.04	.5	96
254	Dehydrated crystals, prepared with water, 247 g (1 c)	90	100	1	tr	—	—	—	24	22	40	.2	412	20	.10	.05	.5	91
	Grapes, European type (adherent skin), raw																	
255	Thompson seedless, 10, 50 g	81	35	tr	tr	—	—	—	9	6	10	.2	87	50	.03	.02	.2	2
256	Tokay and Emperor, seeded, 10, 60 g[30]	81	40	tr	tr	—	—	—	10	7	11	.2	99	60	.03	.02	.2	2
	Grapejuice																	
257	Canned or bottled, 253 g (1 c)	83	165	1	tr	—	—	—	42	28	30	.8	293	—	.10	.05	.5	tr[25]
	Frozen concentrate, sweetened																	
258	undiluted, 216 g (6 fl oz)	53	395	1	1	—	—	—	100	22	32	.9	255	40	.13	.22	1.5	32[31]
259	diluted with 3 parts water by volume 250 g (1 c)	86	135	1	tr	—	—	—	33	8	10	.3	85	10	.05	.08	.5	10[31]
260	Grape drink, canned, 250 g (1 c)	86	135	tr	tr	—	—	—	35	8	10	.3	88	—	.03[32]	.03[32]	.3	(32)
261	Lemon, raw, size 165, without peel and seeds, 74 g	90	20	1	tr	—	—	—	6	19	12	.4	102	10	.03	.01	.1	39
	Lemon juice																	
262	Raw, 244 g (1 c)	91	60	1	tr	—	—	—	20	17	24	.5	344	50	.07	.02	.2	112
263	Canned, or bottled, unsweetened 244 g (1 c)	92	55	1	tr	—	—	—	19	17	24	.5	344	50	.07	.02	.2	102
264	Frozen, single strength, unsweetened 183 g (6 fl oz)	92	40	1	tr	—	—	—	13	13	16	.5	258	40	.05	.02	.2	81
	Lemonade concentrate, frozen																	
265	Undiluted, 219 g (6 fl oz)	49	425	tr	tr	—	—	—	112	9	13	.4	153	40	.05	.06	.7	66
266	Diluted with 4⅓ parts water by volume 248 g (1 c)	89	105	tr	tr	—	—	—	28	2	3	.1	40	10	.01	.02	.2	17
	Limeade concentrate, frozen																	
267	Undiluted, 218 g (6 fl oz)	50	410	tr	tr	—	—	—	108	11	3	.2	129	tr	.02	.02	.2	26
268	Diluted with 4⅓ parts water by volume 247 g (1 c)	89	100	tr	tr	—	—	—	27	3	3	tr	32	tr	tr	tr	tr	6
	Lime juice																	
269	Raw, 246 g (1 c)	90	65	1	tr	—	—	—	22	22	27	.5	256	20	.05	.02	.2	79
270	Canned, unsweetened, 246 g (1 c)	90	65	1	tr	—	—	—	22	22	27	.5	256	20	.05	.02	.2	52
271	Muskmelons, raw Cantaloupe, orange-fleshed, ½ 477 g[33]	91	80	2	tr	—	—	—	20	38	44	1.1	682	9240	.11	.08	1.6	90
272	Honeydew, 1/10, 226 g[33]	91	50	1	tr	—	—	—	11	21	24	.6	374	60	.06	.04	.9	34

[24] Also applies to pasteurized apple cider.
[25] Applies to product without added ascorbic acid. For value of product with added ascorbic acid, refer to label.
[26] Based on product with label claim of 45% of U.S. RDA in 6 fl oz.
[27] Based on product with label claim of 100% of U.S. RDA in 6 fl oz.
[28] Weight includes peel and membranes between sections. Without these parts, the weight of the edible portion is 123 g for item 246 and 118 g for item 247.
[29] For white-fleshed varieties, value is about 20 IU per cup; for red-fleshed varieties, 1080 IU.
[30] Weight includes seeds. Without seeds, weight of the edible portion is 57 g.
[31] Applies to produce without added ascorbic acid. With added ascorbic acid, based on claim that 6 fl oz of reconstituted juice contain 45% or 50% of the U.S. RDA, value in milligrams is 108 or 120 for a 6-fl oz can (item 258), 36 or 40 for 1 cup of diluted juice (item 259).
[32] For products with added thiamin and riboflavin but without added ascorbic acid, values in milligrams would be 0.60 for thiamin, 0.80 for riboflavin, and trace for ascorbic acid. For products with only ascorbic acid added, value varies with the brand. Consult label.
[33] Weight includes rind. Without rind, weight of the edible portion is 272 g for item 271 and 149 g for item 272.

NO.	FOOD AND APPROXIMATE MEASURE	Water %	Food energy cal	Protein g	Fat g	Fatty Acids Saturated g	Unsaturated Oleic g	Unsaturated Linoleic g	Carbohydrate g	Calcium mg	Phosphorus mg	Iron mg	Potassium mg	Vitamin A value IU	Thiamin mg	Riboflavin mg	Niacin mg	Ascorbic acid mg
	FRUITS AND FRUIT PRODUCTS																	
	Oranges, raw																	
273	Whole, 1, 131 g (2⅝-in diameter)	86	65	1	tr	—	—	—	16	54	26	.5	263	260	.13	.05	.5	66
274	Sections without membranes 180 g (1 c)	86	90	2	tr	—	—	—	22	74	36	.7	360	360	.18	.07	.7	90
	Orange juice																	
275	Raw, 248 g (1 c)	88	110	2	tr	—	—	—	26	27	42	.5	496	500	.22	.07	1.0	124
276	Canned, unsweetened, 249 g (1 c)	87	120	2	tr	—	—	—	28	25	45	1.0	496	500	.17	.05	.7	100
	Frozen concentrate																	
277	undiluted, 213 g (6 fl oz)	55	360	5	tr	—	—	—	87	75	126	.9	1500	1620	.68	.11	2.8	360
278	diluted with 3 parts water by volume 249 g (1 c)	87	120	2	tr	—	—	—	29	25	42	.2	503	540	.23	.03	.9	120
279	Dehydrated crystals, prepared with water, 248 g (1 c)	88	115	1	tr	—	—	—	27	25	40	.5	518	500	.20	.07	1.0	109
	Orange and grapefruit juice, frozen concentrate																	
280	Undiluted, 210 g (6 fl oz)	59	330	4	1	—	—	—	78	61	99	.8	1308	800	.48	.06	2.3	302
281	Diluted with 3 parts water by volume 248 g (1 c)	88	110	1	tr	—	—	—	26	20	32	.2	439	270	.15	.02	.7	102
282	Papayas, raw, cubed, 140 g (1 c)	89	55	1	tr	—	—	—	14	28	22	.4	328	2450	.06	.06	.4	78
	Peaches																	
	Raw																	
283	Whole, peeled, pitted, 100 g (2½-in diameter)	89	40	1	tr	—	—	—	10	9	19	.5	202	1330[34]	.02	.05	1.0	7
284	Sliced, 170 g (1 c)	89	65	1	tr	—	—	—	16	15	32	.9	343	2260[34]	.03	.09	1.7	12
	Canned, yellow-fleshed, solids and liquid (halves or slices)																	
285	Sirup pack, 256 g (1 c)	79	200	1	tr	—	—	—	51	10	31	.8	333	1100	.03	.05	1.5	8
286	Water pack, 244 g (1 c)	91	75	1	tr	—	—	—	20	10	32	.7	334	1100	.02	.07	1.5	7
	Dried																	
287	Uncooked, 160 g (1 c)	25	420	5	1	—	—	—	109	77	187	9.6	1520	6240	.02	.30	8.5	29
288	Cooked, unsweetened, halves and juice, 250 g (1 c)	77	205	3	1	—	—	—	54	38	93	4.8	743	3050	.01	.15	3.8	5
	Frozen, sliced, sweetened																	
289	284 g (10 oz)	77	250	1	tr	—	—	—	64	11	37	1.4	352	1850	.03	.11	2.0	116[35]
290	250 g (1 c)	77	220	1	tr	—	—	—	57	10	33	1.3	310	1630	.03	.10	1.8	103[35]
	Pears																	
	Raw, with skin, cored,																	
291	Bartlett, 1, 164 g (2½-in diameter)	83	100	1	1	—	—	—	25	13	18	.5	213	30	.03	.07	.2	7
292	Bosc, 1, 141 g (2½-in diameter)	83	85	1	1	—	—	—	22	11	16	.4	83	30	.03	.06	.1	6
293	D'Anjou, 1, 200 g (3-in diameter)	83	120	1	1	—	—	—	31	16	22	.6	260	40	.04	.08	.2	8
294	Canned, solids and liquid, sirup pack, heavy (halves or slices), 255 g (1 c)	80	195	1	1	—	—	—	50	13	18	.5	214	10	.03	.05	.3	3

Item	Food, approximate measure, and weight (in grams)	Water (%)	Food energy (cal)	Protein (g)	Fat (g)	Saturated (total) (g)	Unsaturated Oleic (g)	Unsaturated Linoleic (g)	Carbohydrate (g)	Calcium (mg)	Phosphorus (mg)	Iron (mg)	Potassium (mg)	Vitamin A value (IU)	Thiamin (mg)	Riboflavin (mg)	Niacin (mg)	Ascorbic acid (mg)
	Pineapple																	
295	Raw, diced, 155 g (1 c)	85	80	1	tr	—	—	—	21	26	12	.8	226	110	.14	.05	.3	26
	Canned, heavy sirup pack, solids and liquid																	
296	Crushed, chunks, tidbits, 255 g (1 c)	80	190	1	tr	—	—	—	49	28	13	.8	245	130	.20	.05	.5	18
297	Slices and liquid, large, 1, 105 g	80	80	tr	tr	—	—	—	20	12	5	.3	101	50	.08	.02	.2	7
298	medium, 1, 58 g	80	45	tr	tr	—	—	—	11	6	3	.2	56	30	.05	.01	.1	4
299	Pineapple juice, unsweetened, canned 250 g (1 c)	86	140	1	tr	—	—	—	34	38	23	.8	373	130	.13	.05	.5	80[27]
	Plums																	
	Raw, without pits																	
300	Japanese and hybrid, 1, 66 g (2⅛-in diameter)	87	30	tr	tr	—	—	—	8	8	12	.3	112	160	.02	.02	.3	4
301	Prune-type, 1, 28 g (1½-in diameter)	79	20	tr	tr	—	—	—	6	3	3	.1	48	80	.01	.01	.1	1
302	Canned, heavy sirup pack, with pits and liquid, 272 g[36] (1 c)	77	215	1	tr	—	—	—	56	23	26	2.3	367	3130	.05	.05	1.0	5
303	140 g[36] (3 plums)	77	110	1	tr	—	—	—	29	12	13	1.2	189	1610	.03	.03	.5	3
	Prunes, dried, "softenized," with pits																	
304	Uncooked, 4 extra large or 5 large, 49 g[36]	28	110	1	tr	—	—	—	29	22	34	1.7	298	690	.04	.07	.7	1
305	Cooked, unsweetened, fruit and liquid 250 g[36] (1 c)	66	255	2	1	—	—	—	67	51	79	3.8	695	1590	.07	.15	1.5	2
306	Prune juice, canned or bottled, 256 g (1 c)	80	195	1	tr	—	—	—	49	36	51	1.8	602	—	.03	.03	1.0	5
	Raisins, seedless, not pressed down																	
307	145 g (1 c)	18	420	4	tr	—	—	—	112	90	146	5.1	1106	30	.16	.12	.7	1
308	14 g (.5 oz)	18	40	tr	tr	—	—	—	11	9	14	.5	107	tr	.02	.01	.1	tr
	Raspberries, red																	
309	Raw, capped, whole, 123 g (1 c)	84	70	1	1	—	—	—	17	27	27	1.1	207	160	.04	.11	1.1	31
310	Frozen, sweetened, 284 g (10 oz)	74	280	2	1	—	—	—	70	37	48	1.7	284	200	.06	.17	1.7	60
	Rhubarb																	
311	Raw, cooked, added sugar, 270 g (1 c)	63	380	1	tr	—	—	—	97	211	41	1.6	548	220	.05	.14	.8	16
312	Frozen, sweetened, cooked, 270 g (1 c)	63	385	1	1	—	—	—	98	211	32	1.9	475	190	.05	.11	.5	16
	Strawberries																	
313	Raw, whole, capped, 149 g (1 c)	90	55	1	1	—	—	—	13	31	31	1.5	244	90	.04	.10	.9	88
	Frozen, sweetened																	
314	sliced, 284 g (10 oz)	71	310	1	1	—	—	—	79	40	48	2.0	318	90	.06	.17	1.4	151
315	whole, 454 g (1 lb)	76	415	2	1	—	—	—	107	59	73	2.7	472	140	.09	.27	2.3	249
316	Tangerine, raw, size 176, without peel, 1, 86 g (2⅜-in diameter)	87	40	1	tr	—	—	—	10	34	15	.3	108	360	.05	.02	.1	27
317	Tangerine juice, canned, sweetened 249 g (1 c)	87	125	1	tr	—	—	—	30	44	35	.5	440	1040	.15	.05	.2	54
318	Watermelon, raw, 1 4 x 8-in wedge with rind and seeds, 926 g[37]	93	110	2	1	—	—	—	27	30	43	2.1	426	2510	.13	.13	.9	30
	GRAIN PRODUCTS																	
319	Bagel, egg, 1, 55 g (3-in diameter)	32	165	6	2	.5	.9	.8	28	9	43	1.2	41	30	.14	.10	1.2	0
320	water, 1, 55 g (3-in diameter)	29	165	6	1	.2	.4	.6	30	8	41	1.2	42	0	.15	.11	1.4	0
321	Barley, pearled, light, uncooked 200 g (1 c)	11	700	16	2	—	—	—	158	32	378	4.0	320	0	.24	.10	6.2	0

[34] Represents yellow-fleshed varieties. For white-fleshed varieties, value is 50 IU for 1 peach, 90 IU for 1 cup of slices.

[35] Value represents products with added ascorbic acid. For products without added ascorbic acid, value in milligrams is 116 for a 10-oz container, 103 for 1 cup.

[36] Weight includes pits. After removal of pits, weight of edible portion is 258 g for item 302, 133 g for item 303, 43 g for item 304, and 213 g for item 305.

[37] Weight includes rind and seeds. Without rind and seeds, weight of edible portion is 426 g.

NO.	FOOD AND APPROXIMATE MEASURE	Water %	Food energy cal	Protein g	Fat g	Fatty Acids Saturated g	Unsaturated Oleic g	Unsaturated Linoleic g	Carbohydrate g	Calcium mg	Phosphorus mg	Iron mg	Potassium mg	Vitamin A value IU	Thiamin mg	Riboflavin mg	Niacin mg	Ascorbic acid mg
	GRAIN PRODUCTS																	
	Biscuits, baking powder (enriched flour)[38]																	
322	Home recipe, 1, 28 g (2-in diameter)	27	105	2	5	1.2	2.0	1.2	13	34	49	.4	33	tr	.08	.08	.7	tr
323	Mix, 1, 28 g (2-in diameter)	29	90	2	3	.6	1.1	.7	15	19	65	.6	32	tr	.09	.08	.8	tr
	Breadcrumbs (enriched)[38]																	
324	Dry, grated, 100 g (1 c)	7	390	13	5	1.0	1.6	1.4	73	122	141	3.6	152	tr	.35	.35	4.8	tr
	Breads Soft. See items 349–350.																	
325	Boston brown bread, canned,[38] 1 slice 45 g (3¼ x ½ in)	45	95	2	1	.1	.2	.2	21	41	72	.9	131	0[39]	.06	.04	.7	0
	Cracked-wheat bread (¾ enriched wheat flour, ¼ cracked wheat)[38]																	
326	Loaf, 454 g (1 lb)	35	1195	39	10	2.2	3.0	3.9	236	399	581	9.5	608	tr	1.52	1.13	14.4	tr
327	Slice, 25 g (1 oz)	35	65	2	1	.1	.2	.2	13	22	32	.5	34	tr	.08	.06	.8	tr
	French or Vienna bread, enriched[38]																	
328	Loaf, 454 g (1 lb)	31	1315	41	14	3.2	4.7	4.6	251	195	386	10.0	408	tr	1.80	1.10	15.0	tr
329	Slice, French, 35 g (5 x 2½ x 1 in)	31	100	3	1	.2	.4	.4	19	15	30	.8	32	tr	.14	.08	1.2	tr
330	Vienna, 25 g (4¾ x 4 x ½ in)	31	75	2	1	.2	.3	.3	14	11	21	.6	23	tr	.10	.06	.8	tr
	Italian bread, enriched																	
331	Loaf, 454 g (1 lb)	32	1250	41	4	.6	.3	1.5	256	77	349	10.0	336	0	1.80	1.10	15.0	0
332	Slice, 30 g (4½ x 3¼ x ¾ in)	32	85	3	tr	tr	tr	.1	17	5	23	.7	22	0	.12	.07	1.0	0
	Raisin bread, enriched[38]																	
333	Loaf, 454 g (1 lb)	35	1190	30	13	3.0	4.7	3.9	243	322	395	10.0	1057	tr	1.70	1.07	10.7	tr
334	Slice, 25 g (1 oz)	35	65	2	1	.2	.3	.2	13	18	22	.6	58	tr	.09	.06	.6	tr
	Rye bread American, light (⅔ enriched wheat flour, ⅓ rye flour)																	
335	Loaf, 454 g (1 lb)	36	1100	41	5	.7	.5	2.2	236	340	667	9.1	658	0	1.35	.98	12.9	0
336	Slice, 25 g (4¾ x 3¾ x 7⁄16 in)	36	60	2	tr	tr	tr	.1	13	19	37	.5	36	0	.07	.05	.7	0
	Pumpernickel (⅔ rye flour, ⅓ enriched wheat flour)																	
337	Loaf, 454 g (1 lb)	34	1115	41	5	.7	.5	2.4	241	381	1039	11.8	2059	0	1.30	.93	8.5	0
338	Slice, 32 g (5 x 4 x ⅜ in)	34	80	3	tr	.1	tr	.2	17	27	73	.8	145	0	.09	.07	.6	0
	White bread, enriched[38] Soft-crumb type																	
339	Loaf, 454 g (1 lb)	36	1225	39	15	3.4	5.3	4.6	229	381	440	11.3	476	tr	1.80	1.10	15.0	tr
340	Slice (18 per loaf), 25 g	36	70	2	1	.3	.3	.3	13	21	24	.6	26	tr	.10	.06	.8	tr
341	toasted, 22 g	25	70	2	1	.2	.3	.3	13	21	24	.6	26	tr	.08	.06	.7	tr
342	Slice (22 per loaf), 20 g	36	55	2	1	.2	.2	.2	10	17	19	.5	21	tr	.08	.05	.7	tr
343	toasted, 17 g	25	55	2	1	.2	.2	.2	10	17	19	.5	21	tr	.06	.056	.7	tr
344	Loaf, 680 g (1½ lb)	36	1835	59	22	5.2	7.9	6.9	343	571	660	17.0	714	tr	2.70	1.65	22.5	tr

Item	Food, approximate measure, grams	Water (%)	Food energy (cal)	Protein (g)	Fat (g)	Saturated (g)	Oleic (g)	Linoleic (g)	Carbohydrate (g)	Calcium (mg)	Phosphorus (mg)	Iron (mg)	Potassium (mg)	Vitamin A (IU)	Thiamin (mg)	Riboflavin (mg)	Niacin (mg)	Ascorbic acid (mg)
345	Slice (24 per loaf), 28 g	36	75	2	1	.2	.2	.3	14	24	27	.7	29	tr	.11	.07	.9	tr
346	toasted, 24 g	25	75	2	1	.2	.2	.3	14	24	27	.7	29	tr	.09	.07	.9	tr
347	Slice (28 per loaf), 24 g	36	65	2	1	.2	.2	.3	12	20	23	.6	25	tr	.10	.06	.8	tr
348	toasted, 21 g	25	65	2	1	.2	.2	.3	12	20	23	.6	25	tr	.08	.06	.8	tr
349	Cubes, 30 g (1 c)	36	80	3	1	.2	.3	.3	15	25	29	.8	32	tr	.12	.07	1.0	tr
350	Crumbs, 45 g (1 c)	36	120	4	1	.3	.5	.5	23	38	44	1.1	47	tr	.18	.11	1.5	tr
	Firm-crumb type																	
351	Loaf, 454 g (1 lb)	35	1245	41	17	3.9	5.9	5.2	228	435	463	11.3	549	tr	1.80	1.10	15.0	tr
352	Slice (20 per loaf), 23 g	35	65	2	1	.2	.3	.3	12	22	23	.6	28	tr	.09	.06	.8	tr
353	toasted, 20 g	24	65	2	1	.2	.3	.3	12	22	23	.6	28	tr	.07	.06	.7	tr
354	Loaf, 907 g (2 lb)	35	2495	82	34	7.7	11.8	10.4	455	871	925	22.7	1097	tr	3.60	2.20	30.0	tr
355	Slice (34 per loaf), 27 g	35	75	2	1	.2	.3	.3	14	26	28	.7	33	tr	.11	.06	.9	tr
356	toasted, 23 g	24	75	2	1	.2	.3	.3	14	26	28	.7	33	tr	.09	.06	.9	tr
	Whole-wheat bread																	
	Soft-crumb type[38]																		
357	Loaf, 454 g (1 lb)	36	1095	41	12	2.2	2.9	4.2	224	381	1152	13.6	1161	tr	1.37	.45	12.7	tr
358	Slice (16 per loaf), 28 g	36	65	3	1	.1	.2	.2	14	24	71	.8	72	tr	.09	.03	.8	tr
359	toasted, 24 g	24	65	3	1	.1	.2	.2	14	24	71	.8	72	tr	.07	.03	.8	tr
	Firm-crumb type[38]																		
360	Loaf, 454 g (1 lb)	36	1100	48	14	2.5	3.3	4.9	216	449	1034	13.6	1238	tr	1.17	.54	12.7	tr
361	Slice (18 per loaf), 25 g	36	60	3	1	.1	.2	.3	12	25	57	.8	68	tr	.06	.03	.7	tr
362	toasted, 21 g	24	60	3	1	.1	.2	.3	12	25	57	.8	68	tr	.05	.03	.7	tr
	Breakfast cereals																		
	Hot type, cooked																		
	Corn (hominy) grits, degermed																		
363	Enriched, 245 g (1 c)	87	125	3	tr	tr	tr	.1	27	2	25	.7	27	tr[40]	.10	.07	1.0	0
364	Unenriched, 245 g (1 c)	87	125	3	tr	tr	tr	.1	27	2	25	.2	27	tr[40]	.05	.02	.5	0
365	Farina, quick-cooking, enriched 245 g (1 c)	89	105	3	tr	tr	tr	.1	22	147	113[41]	(42)	25	0	.12	.07	1.0	0
366	Oatmeal or rolled oats, 240 g (1 c)	87	130	5	2	.4	.8	.9	23	22	137	1.4	146	0	.19	.05	.2	0
367	Wheat, rolled, 240 g (1 c)	80	180	5	1	—	—	—	41	19	182	1.7	202	0	.17	.07	2.2	0
368	Wheat, whole-meal, 245 g (1 c)	88	110	4	1	—	—	—	23	17	127	1.2	118	0	.15	.05	1.5	0
	Ready-to-eat																		
369	Bran flakes (40% bran), added sugar, salt, iron, vitamins, 35 g (1 c)	3	105	4	1	—	—	—	28	19	125	12.4	137	1650	.41	.49	4.1	12
370	Bran flakes with raisins, added sugar, salt, iron, vitamins, 50 g (1 c)	7	145	4	1	—	—	—	40	28	146	17.7	154	2350	.58	.71	5.8	18
	Corn flakes																		
371	Plain, added sugar, salt, iron, vitamins, 25 g (1 c)	4	95	2	tr	—	—	—	21	(43)	9	.6	30	1180	.29	.35	2.9	9
372	Sugar-coated, added salt, iron, vitamins, 40 g (1 c)	2	155	2	tr	—	—	—	37	1	10	1.0	27	1880	.46	.56	4.6	14
373	Corn, puffed, plain, added sugar, salt, iron, vitamins, 20 g (1 c)	4	80	2	1	—	—	—	16	4	18	2.3	—	940	.23	.28	2.3	7
374	Corn, shredded, added sugar, salt, iron, thiamin, niacin, 25 g (1 c)	3	95	2	tr	—	—	—	22	1	10	.6	—	0	.11	.05	.5	0
375	Oats, puffed, added sugar, salt, minerals, vitamins, 25 g (1 c)	3	100	3	1	—	—	—	19	44	102	2.9	—	1180	.29	.35	2.9	9
	Rice, puffed																		
376	Plain, added iron, thiamin, niacin 15 g (1 c)	4	60	1	tr	—	—	—	13	3	14	.3	15	0	.07	.01	.7	0

[38]Made with vegetable shortening.
[39]Applies to product made with white cornmeal. With yellow cornmeal, value is 30 IU.
[40]Applies to white varieties. For yellow varieties, value is 150 IU.
[41]Applies to products that do not contain disodium phosphate. If disodium phosphate is an ingredient, value is 162 mg.
[42]Value may range from less than 1 mg to about 8 mg depending on the brand. Consult label.
[43]Value varies with brand. Consult label.

GRAIN PRODUCTS

NO.	FOOD AND APPROXIMATE MEASURE	Water %	Food energy cal	Protein g	Fat g	Fatty Acids Saturated g	Fatty Acids Unsaturated Oleic g	Fatty Acids Unsaturated Linoleic g	Carbohydrate g	Calcium mg	Phosphorus mg	Iron mg	Potassium mg	Vitamin A value IU	Thiamin mg	Riboflavin mg	Niacin mg	Ascorbic acid mg
377	Presweetened, added salt, iron, vitamins, 28 g (1 c)	3	115	1	0	—	—	—	26	3	14	1.1[44]	43	1250	.38	.43	5.0	15[45]
378	Wheat flakes, added sugar, salt, iron, vitamins, 30 g (1 c)	4	105	3	tr	—	—	—	24	12	83	(43)	81	1410	.35	.42	3.5	11
	Wheat, puffed																	
379	Plain, added iron, thiamin, niacin 15 g (1 c)	3	55	2	tr	—	—	—	12	4	48	.6	51	0	.08	.03	1.2	0
380	Presweetened, added salt, iron, vitamins, 38 g (1 c)	3	140	3	tr	—	—	—	33	7	52	1.6[44]	63	1680	.50	.57	6.7	20[45]
381	Wheat, shredded, plain, 1 oblong biscuit (25 g) or 25 g (½ c) spoon-size biscuits	7	90	2	1	—	—	—	20	11	97	.9	87	0	.06	.03	1.1	0
382	Wheat germ, without salt and sugar, toasted, 6 g (1 T)	4	25	2	1	—	—	—	3	3	70	.5	57	10	.11	.05	.3	1
383	Buckwheat flour, light, sifted, 98 g (1 c)	12	340	6	1	.2	.4	.4	78	11	86	1.0	314	0	.08	.04	.4	0
384	Bulgur, canned, seasoned, 135 g (1 c)	56	245	8	4	—	—	—	44	27	263	1.9	151	0	.08	.05	4.1	0
	Cake icings. See items 532–536																	
	Cakes made from cake mixes with enriched flour[46]																	
	Angelfood																	
385	Whole, 635 g (9¾-in diameter)	34	1645	36	1	—	—	—	377	603	756	2.5	381	0	.37	.95	3.6	0
386	Piece, 53 g (1/12 of cake)	34	135	3	tr	—	—	—	32	50	63	.2	32	0	.03	.08	.3	0
	Coffeecake																	
387	Whole, 430 g (7¾ x 5⅝ x 1¼ in)	30	1385	27	41	11.7	16.3	8.8	225	262	748	6.9	469	690	.82	.91	7.7	1
388	Piece, 72 g (⅙ of cake)	30	230	5	7	2.0	2.7	1.5	38	44	125	1.2	78	120	.14	.15	1.3	tr
	Cupcakes, made with egg, milk																	
389	Without icing, 25 g (2½-in diameter)	26	90	1	3	.8	1.2	.7	14	40	59	.3	21	40	.05	.05	.4	tr
390	With chocolate icing, 36 g (2½-in diameter)	22	130	2	5	2.0	1.6	.6	21	47	71	.4	42	60	.05	.06	.4	tr
	Devil's food with chocolate icing																	
391	Whole (2 layers), 1107 g (8–9-in diameter)	24	3755	49	136	50.0	44.9	17.0	645	653	1162	16.6	1439	1660	1.06	1.65	10.1	1
392	Piece, 69 g (1/16 of cake)	24	235	3	8	3.1	2.8	1.1	40	41	72	1.0	90	100	.07	.10	.6	tr
393	Cupcake, 35 g (2½-in diameter)	24	120	2	4	1.6	1.4	.5	20	21	37	.5	46	50	.03	.05	.3	tr
394	Gingerbread, whole, 570 g (8 sq in)	37	1575	18	39	9.7	16.6	10.0	291	513	570	8.6	1562	tr	.84	1.00	7.4	tr
395	Piece, 63 g (⅑ of cake)	37	175	2	4	1.1	1.8	1.1	32	57	63	.9	173	tr	.09	.11	.8	tr
	White (2 layers), with chocolate icing																	
396	Whole, 1140 g (8–9-in diameter)	21	4000	44	122	48.2	46.4	20.0	716	1129	2041	11.4	1322	680	1.50	1.77	12.5	2
397	Piece, 71 g (1/16 of cake)	21	250	3	8	3.0	2.9	1.2	45	70	127	.7	82	40	.09	.11	.8	tr
398	Yellow (2 layers), with chocolate icing Whole, 1108 g (8–9-in. diameter)	26	3735	45	125	47.8	47.8	20.3	638	1008	2017	12.2	1208	1550	1.24	1.67	10.6	2

No.	Food, approximate measure, and weight (g)	Water (%)	Food energy (cal)	Protein (g)	Fat (g)	Saturated fatty acids (g)	Oleic (g)	Linoleic (g)	Carbohydrate (g)	Calcium (mg)	Phosphorus (mg)	Iron (mg)	Potassium (mg)	Vitamin A (IU)	Thiamin (mg)	Riboflavin (mg)	Niacin (mg)	Ascorbic acid (mg)
399	Boston cream pie with custard filling — Piece, 69 g (1/16 of cake)[47]	26	235	3	8	3.0	3.0	1.3	40	63	126	.8	75	100	.08	.10	.7	tr
	Cakes made from home recipes using enriched flour[47]																	
	Fruitcake, dark																	
400	Whole, 825 g (8-in diameter)	35	2490	41	78	23.0	30.1	15.2	412	553	833	8.2	734[48]	1730	1.04	1.27	9.6	2
401	Piece, 69 g (1/12 of cake)	35	210	3	6	1.9	2.5	1.3	34	46	70	.7	61[48]	140	.09	.11	.8	tr
	Plain sheet cake																	
402	Loaf, 454 g (1 lb)	18	1720	22	69	14.4	33.5	14.8	271	327	513	11.8	2250	540	.72	.73	4.9	2
403	Slice, 15 g (1/30 of loaf)	18	55	1	2	.5	1.1	.5	9	11	17	.4	74	20	.02	.02	.2	tr
	Without icing																	
404	Whole, 777 g (9 sq in)	25	2830	35	108	29.5	44.4	23.9	434	497	793	8.5	614[48]	1320	1.21	1.40	10.2	2
405	Piece, 86 g (1/9 of cake)	25	315	4	12	3.3	4.9	2.6	48	55	88	.9	68[48]	150	.13	.15	1.1	tr
	With uncooked white icing																	
406	Whole, 1096 g (9 sq in)	21	4020	37	129	42.2	49.5	24.4	694	548	822	8.2	669[48]	2190	1.22	1.47	10.2	2
407	Piece, 121 g (1/9 of cake)	21	445	4	14	4.7	5.5	2.7	77	61	91	.8	74[48]	240	.14	.16	1.1	tr
	Poundcake[49]																	
408	Loaf, 565 g (8½ x 3½ x 3¼ in)	16	2725	31	170	42.9	73.1	39.6	273	107	418	7.9	345	1410	.90	.99	7.3	0
409	Slice, 33 g (1/17 of loaf)	16	160	2	10	2.5	4.3	2.3	16	6	24	.5	20	80	.05	.06	.4	0
	Spongecake																	
410	Whole, 790 g (9¾-in diameter)	32	2345	60	45	13.1	15.8	5.7	427	237	865	13.4	687	3560	1.10	1.64	7.4	tr
411	Piece, 66 g (1/12 of cake)	32	195	5	4	1.1	1.3	.5	36	20	74	1.1	57	300	.09	.14	.6	tr
	Cookies made with enriched flour[50,51]																	
	Brownies with nuts																	
412	Home recipe, 1, 20 g (1¾ x 1¾ x ⅞ in)	10	95	1	6	1.5	3.0	1.2	10	8	30	.4	38	40	.04	.03	.2	tr
413	Commercial recipe, 1, 20 g (1¾ x 1¾ x ⅞ in)	11	85	1	4	.9	1.4	1.3	13	9	27	.4	34	20	.03	.02	.2	tr
414	Frozen, with chocolate icing,[52] 1, 25 g (1½ x 1¾ x ⅞ in)	13	105	1	5	2.0	2.2	.7	15	10	31	.4	44	50	.03	.03	.2	tr
	Chocolate chip																	
415	Commercial, 4, 42 g (2¼ x 2¼ x ⅜ in)	3	200	2	9	2.8	2.9	2.2	29	16	48	1.0	56	50	.10	.17	.9	tr
416	Home recipe, 4, 40 g (2⅓-in diameter)	3	205	2	12	3.5	4.5	2.9	24	14	40	.8	47	40	.06	.06	.5	tr
417	Fig bars, 4, 56 g (1⅝ x 1⅝ x ⅜ in or 1½ x 1¾ x ½ in)	14	200	2	3	.8	1.2	.7	42	44	34	1.0	111	60	.04	.14	.9	tr
418	Gingersnaps, 4, 28 g (2 x 2 x ¼ in)	3	90	2	2	.7	1.0	.6	22	20	13	.7	129	20	.08	.06	.7	0
419	Macaroons, 2, 38 g (2¾ x 2¾ x ¼ in)	4	180	2	9	—	—	—	25	10	32	.3	176	0	.02	.06	.2	0
420	Oatmeal with raisins, 4, 52 g (2⅝ x 2⅝ x ¼ in)	3	235	3	8	2.0	3.3	2.0	38	11	53	1.4	192	30	.15	.10	1.0	tr
421	Plain, prepared from commercial chilled dough, 4, 48 g (2½ x 2½ x ¼ in)	5	240	2	12	3.0	5.2	2.9	31	17	35	.6	23	30	.10	.08	.9	0
422	Sandwich type (chocolate or vanilla), 4, 40 g (1¾ x 1¾ x ⅜ in)	2	200	2	9	2.2	3.9	2.2	28	10	96	.7	15	0	.06	.10	.7	0
423	Vanilla wafers, 10, 40 g (1¾ x 1¾ x ¼ in)	3	185	2	6	—	—	—	30	16	25	.6	29	50	.10	.09	.8	0
	Cornmeal																	
424	Whole-grain, unbolted, dry form, 122 g (1 c)	12	435	11	5	.5	1.0	2.5	90	24	312	2.9	346	620[53]	.46	.13	2.4	0
425	Bolted (nearly whole-grain), dry form, 122 g (1 c)	12	440	11	4	.5	.9	2.1	91	21	272	2.2	303	590[53]	.37	.10	2.3	0

44 Value varies with brand. Consult label.
45 Applies to product with added ascorbic acid. Without added ascorbic acid, value is trace.
46 Excepting angelfood cake, cakes were made from mixes containing vegetable shortening; icings with butter.
47 Excepting spongecake, vegetable shortening used for cake portion, butter for icing. If butter or margarine used for cake portion, vitamin A values would be higher.
48 Applies to product made with sodium-aluminum-sulfate-type baking powder. With low-sodium-type baking powder containing potassium, value would be about twice amount shown.
49 Equal weights of flour, sugar, eggs, and vegetable shortening.
50 Products are commercial unless otherwise specified.
51 Made with enriched flour and vegetable shortening except for macaroons, which do not contain flour or shortening.
52 Icing made with butter.
53 Applies to yellow varieties; white varieties contain only a trace.

NUTRIENTS IN INDICATED QUANTITY

NO.	FOOD AND APPROXIMATE MEASURE	Water	Food energy	Protein	Fat	Fatty Acids: Saturated	Fatty Acids: Unsaturated Oleic	Fatty Acids: Unsaturated Linoleic	Carbohydrate	Calcium	Phosphorus	Iron	Potassium	Vitamin A value	Thiamin	Riboflavin	Niacin	Ascorbic acid
		%	cal	g	g	g	g	g	g	mg	mg	mg	mg	IU	mg	mg	mg	mg
	GRAIN PRODUCTS																	
	Degermed, enriched																	
426	Dry form, 138 g (1 c)	12	500	11	2	.2	.4	.9	108	8	137	4.0	166	610[53]	.61	.36	4.8	0
427	Cooked, 240 g (1 c)	88	120	3	tr	tr	.1	.2	26	2	34	1.0	38	140[53]	.14	.10	1.2	0
	Degermed, unenriched																	
428	Dry form, 138 g (1 c)	12	500	11	2	.2	.4	.9	108	8	137	1.5	166	610[53]	.19	.07	1.4	0
429	Cooked, 240 g (1 c)	88	120	3	tr	tr	.1	.2	26	2	34	.5	38	140[53]	.05	.02	.2	0
	Crackers[38]																	
430	Graham, plain, 2, 14 g (2½ sq in)	6	55	1	1	.3	.5	.3	10	6	21	.5	55	0	.02	.08	.5	0
431	Rye wafers, whole-grain, 2, 13 g (1⅞ x 3½ in)	6	45	2	tr	—	—	—	10	7	50	.5	78	0	.04	.03	.2	0
432	Saltines, made with enriched flour, 4 11 g	4	50	1	1	.3	.5	.4	8	2	10	.5	13	0	.05	.05	.4	0
	Danish pastry (enriched flour), plain without fruit or nuts[54]																	
433	Packaged ring, 340 g (12 oz)	22	1435	25	80	24.3	31.7	16.5	155	170	371	6.1	381	1050	.97	1.01	8.6	tr
434	Round piece, 65 g (4¼ x 4¼ x 1 in)	22	275	5	15	4.7	6.1	3.2	30	33	71	1.2	73	200	.18	.19	1.7	tr
435	Piece, 28 g (1 oz)	22	120	2	7	2.0	2.7	1.4	13	14	31	.5	32	90	.08	.08	.7	tr
	Doughnuts, made with enriched flour[38]																	
436	Cake type, plain, 1, 25 g (2½ x 2½ x 1 in)	24	100	1	5	1.2	2.0	1.1	13	10	48	.4	23	20	.05	.05	.4	tr
437	Yeast-leavened, glazed, 1 50 g (3¾ x 3¾ x 1¼ in)	26	205	3	11	3.3	5.8	3.3	22	16	33	.6	34	25	.10	.10	.8	0
	Macaroni, enriched, cooked (cut lengths, elbows, shells)																	
438	Firm stage (hot), 130 g (1 c)	64	190	7	1	—	—	—	39	14	85	1.4	103	0	.23	.13	1.8	0
439	Tender stage, cold, 105 g (1 c)	73	115	4	tr	—	—	—	24	8	53	.9	64	0	.15	.08	1.2	0
440	hot, 140 g (1 c)	73	155	5	1	—	—	—	32	11	70	1.3	85	0	.20	.11	1.5	0
	With cheese																	
441	Canned,[55] 240 g (1 c)	80	230	9	10	4.2	3.1	1.4	26	199	182	1.0	139	260	.12	.24	1.0	tr
442	Home recipe (hot),[56] 200 g (1 c)	58	430	17	22	8.9	8.8	2.9	40	362	322	1.8	240	860	.20	.40	1.8	tr
	Muffins made with enriched flour[38]																	
	Home recipe																	
443	Blueberry, 1, 40 g (2⅜ x 2⅜ x 1½ in)	39	110	3	4	1.1	1.4	.7	17	34	53	.6	46	90	.09	.10	.7	tr
444	Bran, 1, 40 g	35	105	3	4	1.2	1.4	.8	17	57	162	1.5	172	90	.07	.10	1.7	tr
445	Corn (enriched degermed cornmeal and flour), 1, 40 g (2⅜ x 2⅜ x 1½ in)	33	125	3	4	1.2	1.6	.9	19	42	68	.7	54	120[57]	.10	.10	.7	tr
446	Plain, 1, 40 g (3 x 3 x 1½ in)	38	120	3	4	1.0	1.7	1.0	17	42	60	.6	50	40	.09	.12	.9	tr
	Mix, egg, milk																	
447	Corn,[58] 1, 40 g (2⅜ x 2⅜ x 1½ in)	30	130	3	4	1.2	1.7	.9	20	96	152	.6	44	100[57]	.08	.09	.7	tr
448	Noodles (egg noodles), enriched, cooked 160 g (1 c)	71	200	7	2	—	—	—	37	16	94	1.4	70	110	.22	.13	1.9	0

449	Noodles, chow mein, canned, 45 g (1 c)	1	220	6	11	—	—	—	26	—	—	—	—	—	—	—	—	—
	Pancakes[38]																	
450	Buckwheat (mix with buckwheat and enriched flours, egg and milk added), 1, 27 g (4-in diameter)	58	55	2	2	.8	.9	.4	6	59	91	.4	66	60	.04	.05	.2	tr
	Plain																	
451	Home recipe using enriched flour, 1, 27 g (4-in diameter)	50	60	2	2	.5	.8	.5	9	27	38	.4	33	30	.06	.07	.5	tr
452	Mix with enriched flour, egg and milk added, 1, 27 g (4-in diameter)	51	60	2	2	.7	.7	.3	9	58	70	.3	42	70	.04	.06	.2	tr
	Pies, piecrust made with enriched flour, vegetable shortening																	
453	Apple, whole, 945 g (9-in diameter)	48	2420	21	105	27.0	44.5	25.2	360	76	208	6.6	756	280	1.06	.79	9.3	9
454	piece, 135 g (1/7 of pie)	48	345	3	15	3.9	6.4	3.6	51	11	30	.9	108	40	.15	.11	1.3	28
455	Banana cream, whole, 910 g (9-in diameter)	54	2010	41	85	26.7	33.2	16.2	279	601	746	7.3	1847	2280	.77	1.51	7.0	9
456	piece, 130 g (1/7 of pie)	54	285	6	12	3.8	4.7	2.3	40	86	107	1.0	264	330	.11	.22	1.0	1
457	Blueberry, whole, 945 g (9-in diameter)	51	2285	23	102	24.8	43.7	25.1	330	104	217	9.5	614	280	1.03	.80	10.0	2
458	piece, 135 g (1/7 of pie)	51	325	3	15	3.5	6.2	3.6	47	15	31	1.4	88	40	.15	.11	1.4	4
459	Cherry, whole, 945 g (9-in diameter)	47	2465	25	107	28.2	45.0	25.3	363	132	236	6.6	992	4160	1.09	.84	9.8	tr
460	piece, 135 g (1/7 of pie)	47	350	4	15	4.0	6.4	3.6	52	19	34	.9	142	590	.16	.12	1.4	tr
461	Custard, whole, 910 g (9-in diameter)	58	1985	56	101	33.9	38.5	17.5	213	874	1028	8.2	1247	2090	.79	1.92	5.6	0
462	piece, 130 g (1/7 of pie)	58	285	8	14	4.8	5.5	2.5	30	125	147	1.2	178	300	.11	.27	.8	0
463	Lemon meringue, whole, 840 g (9-in diameter)	47	2140	31	86	26.1	33.8	16.4	317	118	412	6.7	420	1430	.61	.84	5.2	25
464	piece, 120 g (1/7 of pie)	47	305	4	12	3.7	4.8	2.3	45	17	59	1.0	60	200	.09	.12	.7	4
465	Mince, whole, 945 g (9-in diameter)	43	2560	24	109	28.0	45.9	25.2	389	265	359	13.3	1682	20	.96	.86	9.8	9
466	piece, 135 g (1/7 of pie)	43	365	3	16	4.0	6.6	3.6	56	38	51	1.9	240	tr	.14	.12	1.4	1
467	Peach, whole, 945 g (9-in diameter)	48	2410	24	101	24.8	43.7	25.1	361	95	274	8.5	1408	6900	1.04	.97	14.0	28
468	piece, 135 g (1/7 of pie)	48	345	3	14	3.5	6.2	3.6	52	14	39	1.2	201	990	.15	.14	2.0	4
469	Pecan, whole, 825 g (9-in diameter)	20	3450	42	189	27.8	101.0	44.2	423	388	850	25.6	1015	1320	1.80	.95	6.9	tr
470	piece, 118 g (1/7 of pie)	20	495	6	27	4.0	14.4	6.3	61	55	122	3.7	145	190	.26	.14	1.0	tr
471	Pumpkin, whole, 910 g (9-in diameter)	59	1920	36	102	37.4	37.5	16.6	223	464	628	7.3	1456	22480	.78	1.27	7.0	tr
472	piece, 130 g (1/7 of pie)	59	275	5	15	5.4	5.4	2.4	32	66	90	1.0	208	3210	.11	.18	1.0	tr
473	Piecrust (home recipe) with enriched flour and vegetable shortening, baked, 180 g (9-in diameter)	15	900	11	60	14.8	26.1	14.9	79	25	90	3.1	89	0	.47	.40	5.0	0
474	Piecrust (mix) with enriched flour and vegetable shortening, baked, 320 g (9-in diameter)	19	1485	20	93	22.7	39.7	23.4	141	131	272	6.1	179	0	1.07	.79	9.9	0
475	Pizza (cheese), baked,[19] 60 g (1/8 of 12-in diameter pie)	45	145	6	4	1.7	1.5	.6	22	86	89	1.1	67	230	.16	.18	1.6	4
	Popcorn, large kernel, popped																	
476	Plain, 6 g (1 c)	4	25	1	tr	tr	.1	.2	5	1	17	.2	—	—	—	.01	.1	0
477	With oil (coconut) and salt added 9 g (1 c)	3	40	1	2	1.5	.2	.2	5	1	19	.2	—	—	—	.01	.2	0
478	Sugar coated, 35 g (1 c)	4	135	2	1	.5	.2	.4	30	2	47	.5	—	—	—	.02	.4	0
	Pretzels, with enriched flour																	
479	Dutch, twisted, 1, 16 g (2¾ x 2⅝ in)	5	60	2	1	—	—	—	12	4	21	.2	21	0	.05	.04	.7	0
480	Thin, twisted, 10, 60 g (3¼ x 2¼ x ¼ in)	5	235	6	3	—	—	—	46	13	79	.9	78	0	.20	.15	2.5	0
481	Stick, 10, 3 g (2¼ in long)	5	10	tr	tr	—	—	—	2	1	4	tr	4	0	.01	.01	.1	0

[54]Contains vegetable shortening and butter.
[55]Made with corn oil.
[56]Made with regular margarine.
[57]Applies to product made with yellow cornmeal.
[58]Made with enriched degermed cornmeal and enriched flour.

NO.	FOOD AND APPROXIMATE MEASURE	Water %	Food energy cal	Protein g	Fat g	Fatty Acids Saturated g	Unsaturated Oleic g	Unsaturated Linoleic g	Carbohydrate g	Calcium mg	Phosphorus mg	Iron mg	Potassium mg	Vitamin A value IU	Thiamin mg	Riboflavin mg	Niacin mg	Ascorbic acid mg
	GRAIN PRODUCTS																	
	Rice, white, enriched																	
482	Instant, ready-to-serve, hot, 165 g (1 c)	73	180	4	tr	tr			40	5	31	1.3	—	0	.21	(59)	1.7	0
483	Long grain, raw, 185 g (1 c)	12	670	12	1	.2	.2	.2	149	44	174	5.4	170	0	.81	.06	6.5	0
484	cooked, hot, 205 g (1 c)	73	225	4	tr	.1	.1	.1	50	21	57	1.8	57	0	.23	.02	2.1	0
485	Parboiled, raw, 185 g (1 c)	10	685	14	1	.2	.1	.2	150	111	370	5.4	278	0	.81	.07	6.5	0
486	cooked, hot, 175 g (1 c)	73	185	4	tr	.1	.1	.1	41	33	100	1.4	75	0	.19	.02	2.1	0
	Rolls, enriched[38]																	
	Commercial																	
487	Brown-and-serve, browned, 1 26 g (1 oz)	27	85	2	2	.4	.7	.5	14	20	23	.5	25	tr	.10	.06	.9	tr
488	Cloverleaf or pan, 1 28 g (2½ x 2½ x 2 in)	31	85	2	2	.4	.6	.4	15	21	24	.5	27	tr	.11	.07	.9	tr
489	Frankfurter and hamburger, 1, 40 g	31	120	3	2	.5	.8	.6	21	30	34	.8	38	tr	.16	.10	1.3	tr
490	Hard, 1, 50 g (3¾ x 3¾ x 2 in)	25	155	5	2	.4	.6	.5	30	24	46	1.2	49	tr	.20	.12	1.7	tr
491	Hoagie or submarine, 1 135 g (11 x 3 x 2½ in)	31	390	12	4	.9	1.4	1.4	75	58	115	3.0	122	tr	.54	.32	4.5	tr
	Home recipe																	
492	Cloverleaf, 1, 35 g (2½ x 2½ x 2 in)	26	120	3	3	.8	1.1	.7	20	16	36	.7	41	30	.12	.12	1.2	tr
	Spaghetti, enriched, cooked																	
493	Firm stage, hot, 130 g (1 c)	64	190	7	1	—	—	—	39	14	85	1.4	103	0	.23	.13	1.8	0
494	Tender stage, hot, 140 g (1 c)	73	155	5	1	—	—	—	32	11	70	1.3	85	0	.20	.11	1.5	0
	Spaghetti (enriched) in tomato sauce with cheese																	
495	Home recipe, 250 g (1 c)	77	260	9	9	2.0	5.4	.7	37	80	135	2.3	408	1080	.25	.18	2.3	13
496	Canned, 250 g (1 c)	80	190	6	2	.5	.3	.4	39	40	88	2.8	303	930	.35	.28	4.5	10
	Spaghetti (enriched) with meat balls and tomato sauce																	
497	Home recipe, 248 g (1 c)	70	330	19	12	3.3	6.3	.9	39	124	236	3.7	665	1590	.25	.30	4.0	22
498	Canned, 250 g (1 c)	78	260	12	10	2.2	3.3	3.9	29	53	113	3.3	245	1000	.15	.18	2.3	5
499	Toaster pastries, 1, 50 g	12	200	3	6	—	—	—	36	54[60]	67[60]	1.9	74	500	.16	.17	2.1	(60)
	Waffles, with enriched flour[38]																	
500	Home recipe, 1, 75 g (7-in diameter)	41	210	7	7	2.3	2.8	1.4	28	85	130	1.3	109	250	.17	.23	1.4	tr
501	Mix, egg and milk added, 1 75 g (7-in diameter)	42	205	7	8	2.8	2.9	1.2	27	179	257	1.0	146	170	.14	.22	.9	tr
	Wheat flours																	
	All-purpose or family flour, enriched																	
502	Sifted, spooned, 115 g (1 c)	12	420	12	1	.2	.1	.5	88	18	100	3.3	109	0	.74	.46	6.1	0
503	Unsifted, spooned, 125 g (1 c)	12	455	13	1	.2	.1	.5	95	20	109	3.6	119	0	.80	.50	6.6	0
504	Cake or pastry flour, enriched, sifted, spooned, 96 g (1 c)	12	350	7	1	.1	.1	.3	76	16	70	2.8	91	0	.61	.38	5.1	0

No.	Food	Water (%)	Food energy (cal)	Protein (g)	Fat (g)	Saturated (total) (g)	Oleic (g)	Linoleic (g)	Carbohydrate (g)	Calcium (mg)	Phosphorus (mg)	Iron (mg)	Potassium (mg)	Vitamin A (IU)	Thiamin (mg)	Riboflavin (mg)	Niacin (mg)	Ascorbic acid (mg)
505	Self-rising flour, enriched, unsifted, spooned, 125 g (1 c)	12	440	12	1	.2	.1	.2	93	331	583	3.6	—	0	.80	.50	6.6	0
506	Whole-wheat flour, from hard wheats, stirred, 120 g (1 c)	12	400	16	2	.4	.2	.9	85	49	446	4.0	444	0	.66	.14	5.2	0
	LEGUMES (DRY), NUTS, SEEDS; RELATED PRODUCTS																	
	Almonds, shelled																	
507	Chopped (about 130 almonds), 130 g (1 c)	5	775	24	70	5.6	47.7	12.8	25	304	655	6.1	1005	0	.31	1.20	4.6	tr
508	Slivered, not pressed down (about 115 almonds), 115 g (1 c)	5	690	21	62	5.0	42.2	11.3	22	269	580	5.4	889	0	.28	1.06	4.0	tr
	Beans, dry / Cooked, drained																	
509	Great Northern, 180 g (1 c)	69	210	14	1	—	—	—	38	90	266	4.9	749	0	.25	.13	1.3	0
510	Lima, 190 g (1 c)	64	260	16	1	—	—	—	49	55	293	5.9	1163	—	.25	.11	1.3	—
511	Pea (navy), 190 g (1 c)	69	225	15	1	—	—	—	40	95	281	5.1	790	0	.27	.13	1.3	0
	Canned, solids and liquid / White with																	
512	frankfurters (sliced), 255 g (1 c)	71	365	19	18	—	—	—	32	94	303	4.8	668	330	.18	.15	3.3	tr
513	pork and tomato sauce, 255 g (1 c)	71	310	16	7	2.4	2.8	.6	48	138	235	4.6	536	330	.20	.08	1.5	5
514	pork and sweet sauce, 255 g (1 c)	66	385	16	12	4.3	5.0	1.1	54	161	291	5.9	—	—	.15	.10	1.3	—
515	Red kidney, 255 g (1 c)	76	230	15	1	—	—	—	42	74	278	4.6	673	10	.13	.10	1.5	—
516	Blackeye peas, dry, cooked (with residual cooking liquid), 250 g (1 c)	80	190	13	1	—	—	—	35	43	238	3.3	573	30	.40	.10	1.0	—
517	Brazil nuts, shelled (6–8 large kernels), 28 g (1 oz)	5	185	4	19	4.8	6.2	7.1	3	53	196	1.0	203	tr	.27	.03	.5	—
518	Cashew nuts, roasted in oil, 140 g (1 c)	5	785	24	64	12.9	36.8	10.2	41	53	522	5.3	650	140	.60	.35	2.5	—
	Coconut meat, fresh																	
519	Piece, 45 g (2 x 2 x ½ in)	51	155	2	16	14.0	.9	.3	4	6	43	.8	115	0	.02	.01	.2	1
520	Shredded or grated, not pressed down, 80 g (1 c)	51	275	3	28	24.8	1.6	.5	8	10	76	1.4	205	0	.04	.02	.4	2
521	Filberts (hazelnuts), chopped (about 80 kernels), 115 g (1 c)	6	730	14	72	5.1	55.2	7.3	19	240	388	3.9	810	—	.53	—	1.0	tr
522	Lentils, whole, cooked, 200 g (1 c)	72	210	16	tr	—	—	—	39	50	238	4.2	498	40	.14	.12	1.2	0
523	Peanuts, roasted in oil, salted, 144 g (1 c)	2	840	37	72	13.7	33.0	20.7	27	107	577	3.0	971	—	.46	.19	24.8	0
524	Peanut butter, 16 g (1 T)	2	95	4	8	1.5	3.7	2.3	3	9	61	.3	100	—	.02	.02	2.4	0
525	Peas, split, dry, cooked, 200 g (1 c)	70	230	16	1	—	—	—	42	22	178	3.4	592	80	.30	.18	1.8	—
526	Pecans, chopped or pieces (about 120 large halves), 118 g (1 c)	3	810	11	84	7.2	50.5	20.0	17	86	341	2.8	712	150	1.01	.15	1.1	2
527	Pumpkin and squash kernels, dry, hulled, 140 g (1 c)	4	775	41	65	11.8	23.5	27.5	21	71	1602	15.7	1386	100	.34	.27	3.4	—
528	Sunflower seeds, dry, hulled, 145 g (1 c)	5	810	35	69	8.2	13.7	43.2	29	174	1214	10.3	1334	70	2.84	.33	7.8	—
	Walnuts / Black																	
529	Chopped or broken kernels, 125 g (1 c)	3	785	26	74	6.3	13.3	45.7	19	tr	713	7.5	575	380	.28	.14	.9	—
530	Ground (finely), 80 g (1 c)	3	500	16	47	4.0	8.5	29.2	12	tr	456	4.8	368	240	.18	.09	.6	—
531	Persian or English, chopped (about 60 halves), 120 g (1 c)	4	780	18	77	8.4	11.8	42.2	19	119	456	3.7	540	40	.40	.16	1.1	2

[59]Product may or may not be enriched with riboflavin. Consult label.

[60]Value varies with brand. Consult label.

NO.	FOOD AND APPROXIMATE MEASURE	Water %	Food energy cal	Protein g	Fat g	Fatty Acids Saturated g	Fatty Acids Unsaturated Oleic g	Fatty Acids Unsaturated Linoleic g	Carbohydrate g	Calcium mg	Phosphorus mg	Iron mg	Potassium mg	Vitamin A value IU	Thiamin mg	Riboflavin mg	Niacin mg	Ascorbic acid mg
	SUGARS AND SWEETS																	
	Cake icings																	
532	Boiled, white plain, 94 g (1 c)	18	295	1	0	0	0	0	75	2	2	tr	17	0	tr	.03	tr	0
533	with coconut, 166 g (1 c)	15	605	3	13	11.0	.9	tr	124	10	50	.8	277	0	.02	.07	.3	0
	Uncooked																	
534	Chocolate made with milk and butter 275 g (1 c)	14	1035	9	38	23.4	11.7	1.0	185	165	305	3.3	536	580	.06	.28	.6	1
535	Creamy fudge from mix and water 245 g (1 c)	15	830	7	16	5.1	6.7	3.1	183	96	218	2.7	238	tr	.05	.20	.7	tr
536	White, 319 g (1 c)	11	1200	2	21	12.7	5.1	.5	260	48	38	tr	57	860	tr	.06	tr	tr
	Candy																	
537	Caramels, plain or chocolate, 28 g (1 oz)	8	115	1	3	1.6	1.1	.1	22	42	35	.4	54	tr	.01	.05	.1	tr
	Chocolate																	
538	Milk, plain, 28 g (1 oz)	1	145	2	9	5.5	3.0	.3	16	65	65	.3	109	80	.02	.10	.1	tr
539	Semisweet, small pieces 170 g (1 c or 6 oz)	1	860	7	61	36.2	19.8	1.7	97	51	255	4.4	553	30	.02	.14	.9	0
540	Chocolate-coated peanuts, 28 g (1 oz)	1	160	5	12	4.0	4.7	2.1	11	33	84	.4	143	tr	.10	.05	2.1	tr
541	Fondant, uncoated (mints, candy corn, other), 28 g (1 oz)	8	105	tr	1	.1	.3	.1	25	4	2	.3	1	0	tr	tr	tr	0
542	Fudge, chocolate, plain, 28 g (1 oz)	8	115	1	3	1.3	1.4	.6	21	22	24	.3	42	tr	.01	.03	.1	tr
543	Gum drops, 28 g (1 oz)	12	100	tr	tr	—	—	—	25	2	tr	.1	1	0	0	0	tr	0
544	Hard, 28 g (1 oz)	1	110	0	tr	—	—	—	28	6	2	.5	2	0	0	0	0	0
545	Marshmallows, 28 g (1 oz)	17	90	1	tr	—	—	—	23	5	2	.5	2	0	0	tr	tr	0
	Chocolate-flavored beverage powders																	
546	with nonfat dry milk, 28 g (1 oz)	2	100	5	1	.5	.3	tr	20	167	155	.5	227	10	.04	.21	.2	1
547	without milk, 28 g (1 oz)	1	100	1	1	.4	.2	tr	25	9	48	.6	142	—	.01	.03	.1	0
548	Honey, strained or extracted, 21 g (1 T)	17	65	tr	0	0	0	0	17	1	2	.1	11	0	tr	.01	.1	tr
549	Jams and preserves, 20 g (1 T)	29	55	tr	tr	—	—	—	14	4	2	.2	18	tr	tr	.01	tr	tr
550	14 g 1 packet	29	40	tr	tr	—	—	—	10	3	1	.1	12	tr	tr	tr	tr	tr
551	Jellies, 18 g (1 T)	29	50	tr	tr	—	—	—	13	4	1	.3	14	tr	tr	.01	tr	1
552	14 g 1 packet	29	40	tr	tr	—	—	—	10	3	1	.2	11	tr	tr	tr	tr	1
	Sirups																	
	Chocolate-flavored sirup or topping																	
553	Thin type, 38 g (1 fl oz or 2 T)	32	90	1	1	.5	.3	tr	24	6	35	.6	106	tr	.01	.03	.2	0
554	Fudge type, 38 g (1 fl oz or 2 T)	25	125	2	5	3.1	1.6	.1	20	48	60	.5	107	60	.02	.08	.2	tr
	Molasses, cane																	
555	Light (first extraction), 20 g (1 T)	24	50	—	—	—	—	—	13	33	9	.9	183	—	.01	.01	tr	—
556	Blackstrap (third extraction) 20 g (1 T)	24	45	—	—	—	—	—	11	137	17	3.2	585	—	.02	.04	.4	—
557	Sorghum, 21 g (1 T)	23	55	—	—	—	—	—	14	35	5	2.6	—	—	—	.02	tr	—
558	Table blends, chiefly corn, light and dark 21 g (1 T)	24	60	0	0	0	0	0	15	9	3	.8	1	0	0	0	0	0

No.	Food	Water (%)	Food energy (cal)	Protein (g)	Fat (g)	Saturated (total)	Oleic	Linoleic	Carbohydrate (g)	Calcium (mg)	Phosphorus (mg)	Iron (mg)	Potassium (mg)	Vitamin A (IU)	Thiamin (mg)	Riboflavin (mg)	Niacin (mg)	Ascorbic acid (mg)
	Sugars																	
559	Brown, pressed down, 220 g (1 c)	2	820	0	0	0	0	0	212	187	42	7.5	757	0	.02	.07	.4	0
	White																	
560	Granulated, 200 g 1 c	1	770	0	0	0	0	0	199	0	0	.2	6	0	0	0	0	0
561	12 g 1 T	1	45	0	0	0	0	0	12	0	0	tr	tr	0	0	0	0	0
562	6 g 1 packet	1	23	0	0	0	0	0	6	0	0	tr	tr	0	0	0	0	0
563	Powdered, sifted, spooned, 100 g (1 c)	1	385	0	0	0	0	0	100	0	0	.1	3	0	0	0	0	0
	VEGETABLES AND VEGETABLE PRODUCTS																	
	Asparagus, green																	
	Cuts and tips																	
564	Raw, cooked, drained, 145 g (1 c)	94	30	3	tr	—	—	—	5	30	73	.9	265	1310	.23	.26	2.0	38
565	Frozen, cooked, drained, 180 g (1 c)	93	40	6	tr	—	—	—	6	40	115	2.2	396	1530	.25	.23	1.8	41
	Spears, 4, ½-in diameter																	
566	Raw, cooked, drained, 60 g	94	10	1	tr	—	—	—	2	10	30	.4	110	540	.10	.11	.8	16
567	Frozen, cooked, drained, 60 g	92	15	2	tr	—	—	—	2	15	40	.7	143	470	.10	.08	.7	16
568	Canned, 80 g	93	15	2	tr	—	—	—	3	15	42	1.5	133	640	.05	.08	.6	12
	Beans																	
	Lima, immature seeds, frozen, cooked, drained																	
569	Thick-seeded types (Fordhook), 170 g (1 c)	74	170	10	tr	—	—	—	32	34	153	2.9	724	390	.12	.09	1.7	29
570	Thin-seeded types (baby), 180 g (1 c)	69	210	13	tr	—	—	—	40	63	227	4.7	709	400	.16	.09	2.2	22
	Snap green																	
571	Raw, cooked, drained, 125 g (1 c)	92	30	2	tr	—	—	—	7	63	46	.8	189	680	.09	.11	.6	15
	Frozen, cooked, drained																	
572	Cuts, 135 g (1 c)	92	35	2	tr	—	—	—	8	54	43	.9	205	780	.09	.12	.5	7
573	French style, 130 g (1 c)	92	35	2	tr	—	—	—	8	49	39	1.2	177	690	.08	.10	.4	9
574	Canned, drained, 135 g (1 c)	92	30	2	tr	—	—	—	7	61	34	2.0	128	630	.04	.07	.4	5
	Snap yellow or wax																	
575	Raw, cooked, drained, 125 g (1 c)	93	30	2	tr	—	—	—	6	63	46	.8	189	290	.09	.11	.6	16
576	Frozen, cooked, drained, 135 g (1 c)	92	35	2	tr	—	—	—	8	47	42	.9	221	140	.09	.11	.5	8
577	Canned, drained, 135 g (1 c)	92	30	2	tr	—	—	—	7	61	34	2.0	128	140	.04	.07	.4	7
	Beans, mature. See items 509–516.																	
	Bean sprouts (mung)																	
578	Raw, 105 g (1 c)	89	35	4	tr	—	—	—	7	20	67	1.4	234	20	.14	.14	.8	20
579	Cooked, drained, 125 g (1 c)	91	35	4	tr	—	—	—	7	21	60	1.1	195	30	.11	.13	.9	8
	Beets																	
	Cooked, drained, peeled																	
580	Whole, 2, 100 g (2-in diameter)	91	30	1	tr	—	—	—	7	14	23	.5	208	20	.03	.04	.3	6
581	Diced or sliced, 170 g (1 c)	91	55	2	tr	—	—	—	12	24	39	.9	354	30	.05	.07	.5	10
	Canned, drained																	
582	Whole, small, 160 g (1 c)	89	60	2	tr	—	—	—	14	30	29	1.1	267	30	.02	.05	.2	5
583	Diced or sliced, 170 g (1 c)	89	65	2	tr	—	—	—	15	32	31	1.2	284	30	.02	.05	.2	5
584	Beet leaves and stems, cooked, drained, 145 g (1 c)	94	25	2	tr	—	—	—	5	144	36	2.8	481	7400	.10	.22	.4	22
	Blackeye peas, immature seeds																	
585	Raw, cooked, drained, 165 g (1 c)	72	180	13	1	—	—	—	30	40	241	3.5	625	580	.50	.18	2.3	28
586	Frozen, cooked, drained, 170 g (1 c)	66	220	15	1	—	—	—	40	43	286	4.8	573	290	.68	.19	2.4	15
	Broccoli																	
	Raw, cooked, drained																	
587	Stalk, medium size, 180 g	91	45	6	1	—	—	—	8	158	112	1.4	481	4500	.16	.36	1.4	162
588	Stalk, ½-in pieces, 155 g (1 c)	91	40	5	tr	—	—	—	7	136	96	1.2	414	3880	.14	.31	1.2	140
	Frozen, cooked, drained																	
589	Stalk, 30 g (4½–5 in long)	91	10	1	tr	—	—	—	1	12	17	.2	66	570	.02	.03	.2	22
590	Chopped, 185 g (1 c)	92	50	5	1	—	—	—	9	100	104	1.3	392	4810	.11	.22	.9	105

NO.	FOOD AND APPROXIMATE MEASURE	Water %	Food energy cal	Protein g	Fat g	Fatty Acids Saturated g	Unsaturated Oleic g	Unsaturated Linoleic g	Carbohydrate g	Calcium mg	Phosphorus mg	Iron mg	Potassium mg	Vitamin A value IU	Thiamin mg	Riboflavin mg	Niacin mg	Ascorbic acid mg
	VEGETABLES AND VEGETABLE PRODUCTS																	
	Brussels sprouts																	
591	Raw, cooked, drained, 155 g (1 c)	88	55	7	1	—	—	—	10	50	112	1.7	423	810	.12	.22	1.2	135
592	Frozen, cooked, drained, 155 g (1 c)	89	50	5	tr	—	—	—	10	33	95	1.2	457	880	.12	.16	.9	126
	Cabbage																	
	Common varieties																	
593	Raw, coarsely shredded or sliced 70 g (1 c)	92	15	1	tr	—	—	—	4	34	20	.3	163	90	.04	.04	.02	33
594	finely shredded or chopped 90 g (1 c)	92	20	1	tr	—	—	—	5	44	26	.4	210	120	.05	.05	.3	42
595	Cooked, drained, 145 g (1 c)	94	30	2	tr	—	—	—	6	64	29	.4	236	190	.06	.06	.4	48
596	Red, raw, coarsely shredded or sliced 70 g (1 c)	90	20	1	tr	—	—	—	5	29	25	.6	188	30	.06	.04	.3	43
597	Savoy, raw, coarsely shredded or sliced 70 g (1 c)	92	15	2	tr	—	—	—	3	47	38	.6	188	140	.04	.06	.2	39
598	Cabbage, celery (also called pe-tsai or wongbok), raw, pieces, 75 g (1 c)	95	10	1	tr	—	—	—	2	32	30	.5	190	110	.04	.03	.5	19
599	Cabbage, white mustard (also called bokchoy or pakchoy), cooked, drained 170 g (1 c)	95	25	2	tr	—	—	—	4	252	56	1.0	364	5270	.07	.14	1.2	26
	Carrots																	
	Raw, without crowns and tips, scraped																	
600	Whole, or strips, 72 g	88	30	1	tr	—	—	—	7	27	26	.5	246	7930	.04	.04	.4	5
601	Grated, 110 g (1 c)	88	45	1	tr	—	—	—	11	41	40	.8	375	12100	.07	.06	.7	9
602	Cooked (crosswise cuts), drained 155 g (1 c)	91	50	1	tr	—	—	—	11	51	48	.9	344	16280	.08	.08	.8	9
	Canned																	
603	Sliced, drained, 155 g (1 c)	91	45	1	tr	—	—	—	10	47	34	1.1	186	23250	.03	.05	.6	3
604	Strained or junior (baby food) 28 g (1 oz)	92	10	tr	tr	—	—	—	2	7	6	.1	51	3690	.01	.01	.1	1
	Cauliflower																	
605	Raw, chopped, 115 g (1 c)	91	31	3	tr	—	—	—	6	29	64	1.3	339	70	.13	.12	.8	90
606	cooked, drained, 125 g (1 c)	93	30	3	tr	—	—	—	5	26	53	.9	258	80	.11	.10	.8	69
607	Frozen, cooked, drained 180 g (1 c)	94	30	3	tr	—	—	—	6	31	68	.9	373	50	.07	.09	.7	74
	Celery, Pascal type, raw																	
608	Stalk, large outer, 40 g (8-in long)	94	5	tr	tr	—	—	—	2	16	11	.1	136	110	.01	.01	.1	4
609	Pieces, diced, 120 g (1 c)	94	20	1	tr	—	—	—	5	47	34	.4	409	320	.04	.04	.4	11
	Collards																	
610	Raw, cooked, drained, 190 g (1 c)	90	65	7	1	—	—	—	10	357	99	1.5	498	14820	.21	.38	2.3	144
611	Frozen, cooked, drained, 170 g (1 c)	90	50	5	1	—	—	—	10	299	87	1.7	401	11560	.10	.24	1.0	56
	Corn, sweet																	
612	Raw, cooked, drained, 1 ear 140 g[61] (5 x 1¾ in)	74	70	2	1	—	—	—	16	2	69	.5	151	310[62]	.09	.08	1.1	7
613	Frozen, cooked, drained Ear, 229 g[61] (5 x 1¾ in)	73	120	4	1	—	—	—	27	4	121	1.0	291	440[62]	.18	.10	2.1	9

Item	Food, approximate measure, and weight (g)	Water (%)	Food energy (cal)	Protein (g)	Fat (g)	Saturated (g)	Oleic (g)	Linoleic (g)	Carbohydrate (g)	Calcium (mg)	Phosphorus (mg)	Iron (mg)	Potassium (mg)	Vitamin A (IU)	Thiamin (mg)	Riboflavin (mg)	Niacin (mg)	Ascorbic acid (mg)
614	Kernels, 165 g (1 c)	77	130	5	1	—	—	—	31	5	120	1.3	304	580[62]	.15	.10	2.5	8
	Canned																	
615	Cream style, 256 g (1 c)	76	210	5	2	—	—	—	51	8	143	1.5	248	840[62]	.08	.13	2.6	13
	Whole kernel																	
616	Vacuum pack, 210 g (1 c)	76	175	5	1	—	—	—	43	6	153	1.1	204	740[62]	.06	.13	2.3	11
617	Wet pack, drained, 165 g (1 c)	76	140	4	1	—	—	—	33	8	81	.8	160	580[62]	.05	.08	1.5	7
	Cowpeas. See items 585–586.																	
618	Cucumber, with peel, 6–8 slices, 28 g	95	5	tr	tr	—	—	—	1	7	8	.3	45	70	.01	.01	.1	3
619	without peel, 6½–9 slices, 28 g	96	5	tr	tr	—	—	—	1	5	5	.1	45	tr	.01	.01	.1	3
620	Dandelion greens, cooked, drained, 105 g (1 c)	90	35	2	1	—	—	—	7	147	44	1.9	244	12290	.14	.17	—	19
621	Endive, curly (including escarole), raw, small pieces, 50 g (1 c)	93	10	1	tr	—	—	—	2	41	27	.9	147	1650	.04	.07	.3	5
	Kale																	
622	Raw, cooked, drained, 110 g (1 c)	88	45	5	1	—	—	—	7	206	64	1.8	243	9130	.11	.20	1.8	102
623	Frozen, cooked, drained, 130 g (1 c)	91	40	4	1	—	—	—	7	157	62	1.3	251	10660	.08	.20	.9	49
	Lettuce, raw — Butterhead, as Boston																	
624	Head, 220 g[63] (5-in diameter)	95	25	2	tr	—	—	—	4	57	42	3.3	430	1580	.10	.10	.5	13
625	Leaves, 1 outer or 2 inner or 3 heart, 15 g	95	tr	tr	tr	—	—	—	tr	5	4	.3	40	150	.01	.01	tr	1
	Crisphead, as iceberg																	
626	Head, 567 g[64] (6-in diameter)	96	70	5	1	—	—	—	16	108	118	2.7	943	1780	.32	.32	1.6	32
627	Wedge, 135 g (¼ head)	96	20	1	tr	—	—	—	4	27	30	.7	236	450	.08	.08	.4	8
628	Pieces, chopped or shredded, 55 g (1 c)	96	5	tr	tr	—	—	—	2	11	2	.3	96	180	.03	.03	.2	3
629	Looseleaf (bunching varieties including romaine or cos), chopped or shredded pieces, 55 g (1 c)	94	10	1	tr	—	—	—	2	37	14	.8	145	1050	.03	.04	.2	10
630	Mushrooms, raw, sliced or chopped, 70 g (1 c)	90	20	2	tr	—	—	—	3	4	81	.6	290	tr	.07	.32	2.9	2
631	Mustard greens, cooked, drained, 140 g (1 c)	93	30	3	1	—	—	—	6	193	45	2.5	308	8120	.11	.20	.8	67
632	Okra pods, cooked, 10, 106 g (3 x ⅝ in)	91	30	2	tr	—	—	—	6	98	43	.5	184	520	.14	.19	1.0	21
	Onions — Mature																	
633	Raw, chopped, 170 g (1 c)	89	65	3	tr	—	—	—	15	46	61	.9	267	tr[65]	.05	.07	.3	17
634	sliced, 115 g (1 c)	89	45	2	tr	—	—	—	10	31	41	.6	181	tr[65]	.03	.05	.2	12
635	Cooked (whole or sliced), drained, 210 g (1 c)	92	60	3	tr	—	—	—	14	50	61	.8	231	tr[65]	.06	.06	.4	15
636	Young green, bulb and white portion of top, 6, 30 g (⅜-in diameter)	88	15	tr	tr	—	—	—	3	12	12	.2	69	tr	.02	.01	.1	8
637	Parsley, raw, chopped, 4 g (1 T)	85	tr	tr	tr	—	—	—	tr	7	2	.2	25	300	tr	.01	tr	6
638	Parsnips, cooked, diced, 155 g (1 c)	82	100	2	1	—	—	—	23	70	96	.9	587	50	.11	.12	.2	16
	Peas, green																	
639	Canned, whole, drained, 170 g (1 c)	77	150	8	1	—	—	—	29	44	129	3.2	163	1170	.15	.10	1.4	14
640	strained, 28 g (1 oz)	86	15	1	tr	—	—	—	3	3	18	.3	28	140	.02	.03	.3	3
641	Frozen, cooked, drained, 160 g (1 c)	82	110	8	tr	—	—	—	19	30	138	3.0	216	960	.43	.14	2.7	21
642	Peppers, hot, red, without seeds, dried (ground chili powder, added seasonings), 2 g (1 t)	9	5	tr	tr	—	—	—	1	5	4	.3	20	1300	tr	.02	.2	tr
	Peppers, sweet, whole, stem and seeds removed,																	
643	Raw, 1, 74 g	93	15	1	tr	—	—	—	4	7	16	.5	157	310	.06	.06	.4	94
644	Cooked, drained, 73 g	95	15	1	tr	—	—	—	3	7	12	.4	109	310	.05	.05	.4	70

[61] Weight includes cob. Without cob, weight is 77 g for item 612, 126 g for item 613.
[62] Based on yellow varieties. For white varieties, value is trace.
[63] Weight includes refuse of outer leaves and core. Without these parts, weight is 163 g.
[64] Weight includes core. Without core, weight is 539 g.
[65] Value based on white-fleshed varieties. For yellow-fleshed varieties, value in IU is 70 for item 633, 50 for item 634, and 80 for item 635.

NO.	FOOD AND APPROXIMATE MEASURE	Water %	Food energy cal	Protein g	Fat g	Fatty Acids Saturated g	Unsaturated Oleic g	Unsaturated Linoleic g	Carbohydrate g	Calcium mg	Phosphorus mg	Iron mg	Potassium mg	Vitamin A value IU	Thiamin mg	Riboflavin mg	Niacin mg	Ascorbic acid mg
	VEGETABLES AND VEGETABLE PRODUCTS																	
	Potatoes																	
645	Baked, peeled after baking, 1, 156 g	75	145	4	tr	—	—	—	33	14	101	1.1	782	tr	.15	.07	2.7	31
	Boiled, 1																	
646	Peeled after boiling, 137 g	80	105	3	tr	—	—	—	23	10	72	.8	556	tr	.12	.05	2.0	22
647	Peeled before boiling, 135 g	83	90	3	tr	—	—	—	20	8	57	.7	385	tr	.12	.05	1.6	22
	French-fried, 10 strips, 2½–3 in long																	
648	Raw, 50 g	45	135	2	7	1.7	1.2	3.3	18	8	56	.7	427	tr	.07	.04	1.6	11
649	Frozen, heated, 50 g	53	110	2	4	1.1	.8	2.1	17	5	43	.9	326	tr	.07	.01	1.3	11
650	Hashed brown, frozen, 155 g (1 c)	56	345	3	18	4.6	3.2	9.0	45	28	78	1.9	439	tr	.11	.03	1.6	12
	Mashed																	
651	Raw, cooked, milk added 210 g (1 c)	83	135	4	2	.7	.4	tr	27	50	103	.8	548	40	.17	.11	2.1	21
652	Raw, cooked, milk and butter added 210 g (1 c)	80	195	4	9	5.6	2.3	.2	26	50	101	.8	525	360	.17	.11	2.1	19
653	Dehydrated flakes, water, milk, butter, and salt added, 210 g (1 c)	79	195	4	7	3.6	2.1	.2	30	65	99	.6	601	270	.08	.08	1.9	11
654	Potato chips, 10, 20 g	2	115	1	8	2.1	1.4	4.0	10	8	28	.4	226	tr	.04	.01	1.0	3
655	Potato salad, with cooked salad dressing 250 g (1 c)	76	250	7	7	2.0	2.7	1.3	41	80	160	1.5	798	350	.20	.18	2.8	28
656	Pumpkin, canned, 245 g (1 c)	90	80	2	1	—	—	—	19	61	64	1.0	588	15680	.07	.12	1.5	12
657	Radishes, raw, 4, 18 g	95	5	tr	tr	—	—	—	1	5	6	.2	58	tr	.01	.01	.1	5
658	Sauerkraut, canned, solids and liquid 235 g (1 c)	93	40	2	tr	—	—	—	9	85	42	1.2	329	120	.07	.09	.5	33
	Southern peas. See items 585–586.																	
	Spinach																	
659	Raw, chopped, 55 g (1 c)	91	15	2	tr	—	—	—	2	51	28	1.7	259	4460	.06	.11	.3	28
660	cooked, drained, 180 g (1 c)	92	40	5	1	—	—	—	6	167	68	4.0	583	14580	.13	.25	.9	50
	Frozen, cooked, drained,																	
661	chopped, 205 g (1 c)	92	45	6	1	—	—	—	8	232	90	4.3	683	16200	.14	.31	.8	39
662	leaf, 190 g (1 c)	92	45	6	1	—	—	—	7	200	84	4.8	688	15390	.15	.27	1.0	53
663	Canned, drained, 205 g (1 c)	91	50	6	1	—	—	.1	7	242	53	5.3	513	16400	.04	.25	.6	29
	Squash																	
664	Summer (all varieties), diced, cooked, drained 210 g (1 c)	96	30	2	tr	—	—	—	7	53	53	.8	296	820	.11	.17	1.7	21
665	Winter (all varieties), baked, mashed, 205 g (1 c)	81	130	4	1	—	—	—	32	57	98	1.6	945	8610	.10	.27	1.4	27
	Sweet potatoes																	
666	Baked in skin, peeled, 1, 114 g (5 x 2 in)	64	160	2	1	—	—	—	37	46	66	1.0	342	9230	.10	.08	.8	25
667	Boiled in skin, peeled, 1, 151 g (5 x 2 in)	71	170	3	1	—	—	—	40	48	71	1.1	367	11940	.14	.09	.9	26
668	Candied, 1 piece, 105 g (2½ x 2 in)	60	175	1	3	2.0	.8	.1	36	39	45	.9	200	6620	.06	.04	.4	11
	Canned																	
669	Solid pack (mashed), 255 g (1 c)	72	275	5	1	—	—	—	63	64	105	2.0	510	19890	.13	.10	1.5	36
670	Vacuum pack, 1 piece, 40 g (2¾ x 1 in)	72	45	1	tr	—	—	—	10	10	16	.3	80	3120	.02	.02	.2	6

Tomatoes

Item	Food, measure, weight	Water (%)	Food energy (cal)	Protein (g)	Fat (g)	Saturated (g)	Oleic (g)	Linoleic (g)	Carbohydrate (g)	Calcium (mg)	Phosphorus (mg)	Iron (mg)	Potassium (mg)	Vitamin A (IU)	Thiamin (mg)	Riboflavin (mg)	Niacin (mg)	Ascorbic acid (mg)
671	Raw, 1, 135 g[66] (2⅗-in diameter)	94	25	1	tr	—	—	—	6	16	33	.6	300	1110	.07	.05	.9	28[67]
672	Canned, solids and liquid, 241 g (1 c)	94	50	2	tr	—	—	—	10	14[68]	46	1.2	523	2170	.12	.07	1.7	41
673	Tomato catsup, 273 g (1 c)	69	290	5	1	—	—	—	69	60	137	2.2	991	3820	.25	.19	4.4	41
674	15 g (1 T)	69	15	tr	tr	—	—	—	4	3	8	.1	54	210	.01	.01	.1	2
675	Tomato juice, canned, 243 g (1 c)	94	45	2	tr	—	—	—	10	17	44	2.2	552	1940	.12	.07	1.9	39
676	182 g (6 fl oz)	94	35	2	tr	—	—	—	8	13	33	1.6	413	1460	.09	.05	1.5	29
677	Turnips, cooked, diced, 155 g (1 c)	94	35	1	tr	—	—	—	8	54	37	.6	291	tr	.06	.08	.5	34
	Turnip greens																	
678	Raw, cooked, drained, 145 g (1 c)	94	30	3	tr	—	—	—	5	252	49	1.5	—	8270	.15	.33	.7	68
679	Frozen, cooked, drained, 165 g (1 c)	93	40	4	tr	—	—	—	6	195	64	2.6	246	11390	.08	.15	.7	31
680	Vegetables, mixed, frozen, cooked, 182 g (1 c)	83	115	6	1	—	—	—	24	46	115	2.4	348	9010	.22	.13	2.0	15

MISCELLANEOUS ITEMS

Item	Food, measure, weight	Water (%)	Food energy (cal)	Protein (g)	Fat (g)	Saturated (g)	Oleic (g)	Linoleic (g)	Carbohydrate (g)	Calcium (mg)	Phosphorus (mg)	Iron (mg)	Potassium (mg)	Vitamin A (IU)	Thiamin (mg)	Riboflavin (mg)	Niacin (mg)	Ascorbic acid (mg)
681	Baking powders for home use — Sodium aluminum sulfate with monocalcium phosphate monohydrate, 3.0 g (1 t)	2	5	tr	0	0	0	0	1	58	87	—	5	0	0	0	0	0
682	with monocalcium phosphate monohydrate, calcium sulfate, 2.9 g (1 t)	1	5	tr	0	0	0	0	1	183	45	—	—	0	0	0	0	0
683	Straight phosphate, 3.8 g (1 t)	2	5	tr	0	0	0	0	2	239	359	—	6	0	0	0	0	0
684	Low sodium, 4.3 g (1 t)	2	5	tr	0	0	0	0	2	207	314	—	471	0	0	0	0	0
685	Barbecue sauce, 250 g (1 c)	81	230	4	17	2.2	4.3	10.0	20	53	50	2.0	435	900	.03	.03	.8	13
686	Beverages, alcoholic — Beer, 360 g (12 fl oz)	92	150	1	0	0	0	0	14	18	108	tr	90	—	.01	.11	2.2	—
687	Gin, rum, vodka, whiskey 80 proof, 42 g (1½ fl oz)	67	95	—	—	—	—	—	tr	—	—	—	1	—	—	—	—	—
688	86 proof, 42 g (1½ fl oz)	64	105	—	—	—	—	—	tr	—	—	—	1	—	—	—	—	—
689	90 proof, 42 g (1½ fl oz)	62	110	—	—	—	—	—	tr	—	—	—	1	—	—	—	—	—
690	Wine — Dessert, 103 g (3½ fl oz)	77	140	tr	0	0	0	0	8	8	10	—	77	—	.01	.02	.2	—
691	Table, 102 g (3½ fl oz)	86	85	tr	0	0	0	0	4	9	10	.4	94	—	tr	.01	.1	—
692	Beverages, carbonated, sweetened, nonalcoholic — Carbonated water, 366 g (12 fl oz)	92	115	0	0	0	0	0	29	—	—	—	—	0	0	0	0	0
693	Cola type, 369 g (12 fl oz)	90	145	0	0	0	0	0	37	—	—	—	—	0	0	0	0	0
694	Fruit-flavored sodas and Tom Collins mixer, 372 g (12 fl oz)	88	170	0	0	0	0	0	45	—	—	—	—	0	0	0	0	0
695	Ginger ale, 366 g (12 fl oz)	92	115	0	0	0	0	0	29	—	—	—	0	0	0	0	0	0
696	Root beer, 370 g (12 fl oz)	90	150	0	0	0	0	0	39	—	—	—	0	0	0	0	0	0
	Chili powder. See item 642.																	
697	Chocolate — Bitter or baking, 28 g (1 oz)	2	145	3	15	8.9	4.9	.4	8	22	109	1.9	235	20	.01	.07	.4	0
	Semisweet. See item 539.																	
698	Gelatin, dry, 7 g	13	25	6	tr	0	0	0	0	—	—	—	—	—	—	—	—	—
699	Gelatin dessert prepared with gelatin dessert powder and water, 240 g (1 c)	84	140	4	0	0	0	0	34	—	—	—	—	—	—	—	—	—
700	Mustard, prepared, yellow, 5 g (1 t)	80	5	tr	tr	—	—	—	tr	4	4	.1	7	—	—	—	—	—
701	Olives, pickled, canned — Green, 4 medium or 3 extra large or 2 giant, 16 g[69]	78	15	tr	2	.2	2	.1	tr	8	2	.2	7	40	—	tr	—	—
702	Ripe, 3 small or 2 large, 10 g[69]	73	15	tr	2	.2	2	.1	tr	9	1	.1	2	10	—	tr	—	—

[66] Weight includes cores and stem ends. Without these parts weight is 123 g.

[67] Based on year-round average. For tomatoes marketed from November through May, value is about 12 mg; from June through October, 32 mg.

[68] Applies to product without calcium salts added. Value for products with calcium salts added may be as much as 63 mg for whole tomatoes, 241 mg for cut forms.

[69] Weight includes pits. Without pits, weight is 13 g for item 701, 9 g for item 702.

NUTRIENTS IN INDICATED QUANTITY

NO.	FOOD AND APPROXIMATE MEASURE	Water %	Food energy cal	Protein g	Fat g	Fatty Acids			Carbohydrate g	Calcium mg	Phosphorus mg	Iron mg	Potassium mg	Vitamin A value IU	Thiamin mg	Riboflavin mg	Niacin mg	Ascorbic acid mg
						Saturated g	Unsaturated Oleic g	Unsaturated Linoleic g										
MISCELLANEOUS ITEMS																		
703	Pickles, cucumber Dill, whole, 1, 65 g (3¾ x 1¼ in)	93	5	tr	tr	—	—	—	1	17	14	.7	130	70	tr	.01	tr	4
704	Fresh-pack, 2 slices, 15 g (1½ x ¼ in)	79	10	tr	tr	—	—	—	3	5	4	.3	—	20	tr	tr	tr	1
705	Sweet, gherkin, whole, 1, 15 g (2½ x ¾ in)	61	20	tr	tr	—	—	—	5	2	2	.2	—	10	tr	tr	tr	1
706	Relish, finely chopped, sweet, 15 g (1 t)	63	20	tr	tr	—	—	—	5	3	2	.1	—	—	—	—	—	1
707	Popsicle, 95 g (3 fl oz)	80	70	0	0	0	0	0	18	0	—	tr	—	0	0	0	0	0
	Soups, canned, condensed With equal volume of milk																	
708	Cream of chicken, 245 g (1 c)	85	180	7	10	4.2	3.6	1.3	15	172	152	.5	260	610	.05	.27	.7	2
709	Cream of mushroom, 245 g (1 c)	83	215	7	14	5.4	2.9	4.6	16	191	169	.5	279	250	.05	.34	.7	1
710	Tomato, 250 g (1 c)	84	175	7	7	3.4	1.7	1.0	23	168	155	.8	418	1200	.10	.25	1.3	15
	With equal volume of water																	
711	Bean with pork, 250 g (1 c)	84	170	8	6	1.2	1.8	2.4	22	63	128	2.3	395	650	.13	.08	1.0	3
712	Beef broth, bouillon, consomme 240 g (1 c)	96	30	5	0	0	0	0	3	tr	31	.5	130	tr	tr	.02	1.2	tr
713	Beef noodle, 240 g (1 c)	93	65	4	3	.6	.7	.8	7	7	48	1.0	77	50	.05	.07	1.0	—
714	Clam chowder, Manhattan type (with tomatoes, without milk), 245 g (1 c)	92	80	2	3	.5	.4	1.3	12	34	47	1.0	184	880	.02	.02	1.0	tr
715	Cream of chicken, 240 g (1 c)	92	95	3	6	1.6	2.3	1.1	8	24	34	.5	79	410	.02	.05	.5	tr
716	Cream of mushroom, 240 g (1 c)	90	135	2	10	2.6	1.7	4.5	10	41	50	.5	98	70	.02	.12	.7	tr
717	Minestrone, 245 g (1 c)	90	105	5	3	.7	.9	1.3	14	37	59	1.0	314	2350	.07	.05	1.0	—
718	Split pea, 245 g (1 c)	85	145	9	3	1.1	1.2	.4	21	29	149	1.5	270	440	.25	.15	1.5	1
719	Tomato, 245 g (1 c)	91	90	2	3	.5	.5	1.0	16	15	34	.7	230	1000	.05	.05	1.2	12
720	Vegetable beef, 245 g (1 c)	92	80	5	2	—	—	—	10	12	49	.7	162	2700	.05	.05	1.0	—
721	Vegetarian, 245 g (1 c)	92	80	2	2	—	—	—	13	20	39	1.0	172	2940	.05	.05	1.0	—
	Soups, dehydrated																	
722	Bouillon, 1 cube, 4 g (½ cu in)	4	5	1	tr	—	—	—	tr	—	—	—	4	—	—	—	—	—
	Mixes																	
723	Unprepared onion, 43 g (½ oz)	3	150	6	5	1.1	2.3	1.0	23	42	49	.6	238	30	.05	.03	.3	6
	Prepared with water																	
724	Chicken noodle, 240 g (1 c)	95	55	2	1	—	—	—	8	7	19	.2	19	50	.07	.05	.5	tr
725	Onion, 240 g (1 c)	96	35	1	1	—	—	—	6	10	12	.2	58	tr	tr	tr	tr	2
726	Tomato vegetable with noodles, 240 g (1 c)	93	65	1	1	0	0	0	12	7	19	.2	29	480	.05	.02	.5	5
727	Vinegar, cider, 15 g (1 T)	94	tr	tr	0	0	0	0	1	1	1	.1	15	—	—	—	—	—
728	White sauce, medium, with enriched flour 250 g (1 c)	73	405	10	31	19.3	7.8	.8	22	288	233	.5	348	1150	.12	.43	.7	2
729	Yeast, baker's dry, active, 7 g (1 pkg)	5	20	3	tr	—	—	—	3	3	90	1.1	140	tr	.16	.38	2.6	tr
730	brewer's, dry, 8 g (1 T)	5	25	3	tr	—	—	—	3	17[70]	140	1.4	152	tr	1.25	.34	3.0	tr

[70]Value may vary from 6 to 60 mg.

430

Glossary

absorption (food): the process whereby digested food moves from the small intestine into the bloodstream.

acidulate (ə-sij′-ü-lat): to make into an acid.

adrenal (ə-drēn′-əl) **glands:** two glands, each located above one of the kidneys, which produce adrenalin, a hormone essential to life.

aging: the bodily changes that gradually occur from infancy to old age.

aleurone (al′-yə-rōn): a layer in wheat beneath the bran that is rich in protein.

alkali (al′-kə-lī): a substance that has basic—rather than acidic—properties.

amino (ə-mē′-nō) **acid:** an organic acid that contains the amino (NH_2) group. The amino acids that are called ''essential'' must be supplied by food.

anabolism (ə-nab′-ə-liz′-əm): the building up of new cells. This is a type of metabolism.

anemia (ə-nĕ′-mē-ə): a physical condition characterized by a lack of hemoglobin or a shortage of red blood cells.

antibiotic: a type of drug that is administered to humans and animals to restrict the growth of harmful bacteria.

appestat: *see* hypothalamus.

arable land: land on which crops may be grown.

arteriosclerosis (är-tir̆′-ē-ō-sklə-rō′-s̆əs): a thickening and hardening of the inside walls of the arteries.

artificial sweetener: a sugar substitute that is used by diabetics or by people who want to limit their intake of calories.

ascorbic (ə-skŏr′-bik) **acid:** a water-soluble vitamin that was first extracted from lemon juice; also known as ''vitamin C.''

aseptic (ā-sep′-tik): free from bacteria.

bacterium (bak-tir′-ē-əm): a microorganism that lacks chlorophyll; helpful bacteria aid digestion and cause fermentation; harmful bacteria cause decay and disease. (*Also see* antibiotic.)

baking powder: a leavening agent used for most quick breads and cakes; contains cornstarch and soda.

balanced diet: a carefully regulated eating plan that provides the body with the variety of nutrients it needs to maintain good health.

basal (ba′-zəl) **metabolism** (mə-tab′-o-liz-əm): the minimum amount of energy required to sustain the internal life processes.

beriberi (ber′-ē-ber′-ē): a disease caused by a lack of thiamin; typical symptoms are depression, paralysis, and retention of fluid.

bile: a fluid produced by the liver and stored in the gall bladder that participates in the digestion of fats.

biotin (bĭ′-ə-tən): a B vitamin that is important to growth; found in eggs, yeast, and liver.

blanching: dipping food in boiling water or exposing it to steam, and then dipping it in cold water; stops enzyme action within food and thus prevents deterioration.

boeuf à la mode: French-style pot roast prepared with vegetables and wine.

botulism (bach′-ə-liz-əm): a type of food poisoning, often fatal, caused by a toxin that is produced by *Clostridia botulini.*

bouillabaisse (bü′-yə-bās): a French soup that contains different kinds of fish, vegetables, herbs, and seasonings.

braising (brāz′-ing): cooking meat in a small amount of water or liquid in a covered pot at a simmering temperature.

bran: the covering of whole grains like wheat and rye.

budget: an itemized forecast of expenses; should not exceed the total available income.

bulk: the end product in digestion of indigestible food materials.

café au lait (ka-fā′-ō-lā′): coffee with hot milk.

calcium (kal′-sē-əm): a mineral found in milk and many vegetables; the most abundant mineral in the body.

calorie (kal′-ə-rē): a unit of measure used to state the energy content of different foods.

candling: the placing of eggs in front of a strong light beam in order to determine their grade.

carbohydrates (kär′-bō-hī′-drāts): the name of a major class of foods that includes the sugars and starches.

cardiovascular (kärd′-ē-ō-vas′-kyə-lər) **disease:** a disease involving the heart and blood vessels.

carotene (kar′-ə-tēn): a substance that was first extracted from carrots; converted to vitamin A by the animal or human body.

cartilage (kärt′-lij): a tissue in the skeletal system.

casein (kā′-sēn): the principal protein in milk.

catabolism (kə-tab′-ə-liz′-əm): the breaking down of old useless tissues; sometimes known as "destructive metabolism."

cataract (kat′-ə-rakt): a cloudy white growth that covers the lens of the eye and obstructs vision.

crash diet: a program of eating designed to reduce weight quickly. Not recommended.

cellulose (sel′-yə-lōs): a structural plant fiber that is not broken down by the digestive process.

cerebral (sə-rē′-brəl) **hemorrhage** (hem′-rij): the discharge of blood from a ruptured blood vessel in the brain.

certified milk: milk that may or may not have been pasteurized but has been inspected and found to have a low bacterial count. If it has not been pasteurized, it deteriorates quickly.

choice grade: The second-best grade of beef; the grade used most often in the home. It has less fat and less marbling than prime grade.

cholesterol (kə-les′-tə-rōl′): a fatlike waxy substance derived from fat that is found in all animal tissue.

clabber (klab′-er): a thick curd or gel formed when lactic acid unites with a protein in milk called "casein."

Clostridia (klä-strid′-ē-ə) *botulini* (bät′-u-lini-ī): the bacteria that produce the toxin that causes botulism.

Clostridia (klä-strid′-ē-ə) ***perfringens*** (pər-frin′-jenz): a bacteria widespread in soils, feces, and sewage that causes food-poisoning.

coenzyme (kō-en′-zim): a substance such as a vitamin that joins with a protein molecule to form an enzyme.

collagen (käl′-ə-jen): a protein substance that holds body cells together.

colostrum (kə-läs′-trəm): a yellowish fluid secreted from a mother's breast for about ten days after the infant is born.

complementary proteins: a combination of proteins in which the strong amino acids of one protein counterbalance the weak amino acids of another protein.

complete protein: a protein that contains enough of all the essential amino acids needed to maintain life and support natural growth. ,

complex carbohydrate (kär′-bō-hī′-drāt): a carbohydrate containing starch and substances such as cellulose (fiber) and pectin, which cannot be digested by human beings.

connective tissue: threadlike strands that tie the cells of an organ together; bind the muscle fibers in little bundles; also bind the muscles to the bones.

constipation (kän-stə-pā-shən): a prolonged inability to eliminate feces. As a result of constipation, feces become dry and hardened.

convenience food: a food that has been processed and packaged to minimize preparation time and effort.

converted rice: rice treated by a process that forces nutrients in the hull into the grain. When the hull is removed, these nutrients are retained in the rice.

coronary atherosclerosis (ath′-ə-rō′-sklə-rō-sis): thickening of the walls of the heart arteries caused by the buildup of fatty materials in the arteries.

coronary occlusion (ə-klū′-zhən): an obstruction of a blood vessel that blocks the passage of blood to or from the heart and causes a heart attack.

coronary thrombosis (thräm-bō′-səs): a heart attack caused by a blood clot occurring within a blood vessel.

creaming: softening and blending fat and sugar until smooth and light with a spoon or electric mixer.

crock pot: a thick earthenware pot used for all-day cooking and for tenderizing tough meats.

crystalline (kris′-tə-lən) **candy:** a candy, such as fudge, in which sugar retains its crystalline form. (*Also see* noncrystalline candy.)

cubing: cutting into small equal-sided pieces.

curd: the solid part of milk used after processing as cheese.

cured meat: meat that is preserved through a chemical process, for example the action of salt or brine over a period of time.

cutting in: mixing a solid, such as fat, with a dry mixture, such as flour, with knives, a pastry blender, fingertips, electric mixer or blender.

DDT: a pesticide banned by the U. S. government because of its harmful effects on animals and people.

deep-frying: cooking in fat in a deep pan; the steam formed by the water in the food cooks the food.

dental caries (kar′-ēz): tooth decay.

descriptive label: a label on packages of processed foods that identifies the product and lists ingredients and nutrients in the food.

diabetes (dī-ə-bēt′-ēz): a disease in which the body has a deficiency of insulin, resulting in an excess of unburned sugar in the blood.

dietician: a person who is skilled in applying the science of nutrition to feeding people.

digestion: the process of breaking down food into nutrients that can be absorbed and used by the body.

d

disaccharide (dī-sak′-ə-rīd): a sugar that contains two simple sugars per molecule, e.g. sucrose, maltose, lactose. Disaccharides are also known as "double sugars."

eating pattern: the combined eating habits of an individual or a society, including kinds of foods eaten, methods of preparation, and meal times.

edema: retention of water in the tissues.

electrocardiogram (ē-lek′-trō-kärd′-e-ə-gram): the printout of a device that monitors the activity of the heart.

electronic heating (high—frequency): a method of canning that is currently being investigated.

empty calories (kal′-ə-rēs): calories that provide the body with energy but no nutrients.

emulsify (i-məl′-sə-fī): to hold together two or more ingredients that would otherwise be separate.

endocrine (en′-də-drən) **glands:** glands that control the metabolic processes by producing secretions that are distributed in the bloodstream.

endosperm (en′-də-spərm): the part of the grain that remains after the milling process. The endosperm is rich in starch.

enriched: a term that indicates that riboflavin, thiamin, niacin, and iron have been added to a food after that food has been refined.

epidermis (ep-ə-dər′-məs): the outermost layer of the skin.

epithelial (ep′-ə-thĕ′-lē-əl) **cells:** cells that form the protective layer of skin, known as the "epidermis."

erythrocyte (i-rith′-rə-sīt): a flexible disc in the blood, commonly called the "red blood cell" or the "red corpuscle," that enables the body to use nourishment and oxygen.

extrinsic factor: vitamin B_{12}; must combine with the intrinsic factor before it can be absorbed by the digestive tract.

fad diet: an eating plan that is popular for a limited period of time, although it lacks a nutritionally sound foundation.

fallacy: an erroneous idea; a concept that is contradicted by facts.

family service: a type of table service in which each food is brought to the table in a serving dish. Dishes are passed around the table, and persons serve themselves from each dish.

fast-food chains: chains of restaurants specializing in quickly prepared, quickly served meals.

fasting: not eating for a meal, a day, or a longer period of time.

fatty acids: acids provided by fat containing chains of oxygen, hydrogen, and carbon atoms.

fermented milk: milk that has been curdled by bacteria—for example, yogurt and buttermilk.

fiber (fi′-bər): an elongated plant cell that resembles a thread; helps in the absorption of nutrients into the bloodstream.

filled milk: a milk substitute that contains nonfat milk solids that may or may not be the same as those solids found in natural milk.

fixed expense: a regular, recurring expense that does not fluctuate—for example, food or housing.

flash canning: a method of food processing in which the food is brought to a high temperature for a short period of time.

flexible expense: a household or personal expense that may vary according to budget needs.

folding in: combining two mixtures by gently cutting down through the ingredients and turning them over, repeating until the contents are thoroughly blended.

434

folacin (fō´-lə-sin), or **folic** (fō´-lik) **acid:** a B vitamin essential for growth, tissue repair, formation of red blood cells, reproduction, and lactation.

food: material that is consumed by animals, including human beings, to help support the vital body functions.

food chain: energy cycle in which lower organisms are food for higher organisms. For example, plants are eaten by animals; animals are eaten by humans.

food fallacy: erroneous opinion about food.

food grade: a standard of food quality that has been established by the U. S. Department of Agriculture.

food quack: a person, who knowingly presents incorrect information about nutrition.

food supplement: something that is ingested in addition to the regular diet—for example, pills containing vitamins and minerals.

formula diet: a reducing diet in which the foods consumed are prepared as liquids.

fortified: a term that indicates food to which nutrients, which may or may not have been in the unprocessed food, have been added.

fortified milk: milk that has an increased nutritional value due to the addition of nutrients—for example, vitamin D, vitamin A, or milk solids.

freeze-drying: a combination of two methods of preserving food that reduces weight and bulk.

fructose (frək´-tōs): a type of sugar found in fruit and honey.

full-term baby: a baby that has been carried by its mother for the full nine-month gestation period.

galactose (gə-lak´-tōs): a monosaccharide sugar that is produced by the body through the digestion of lactose.

garnish: a food added to a dish for the main purpose of improving the appearance of the dish.

germ: part of a grain kernel that is lost in the milling process.

glucose (glü´-kōs): a simple sugar; used by body cells for energy.

gluten (glüt´-ən): a protein that gives dough its elastic quality.

glycerol (glis´-ə-rōl): a syrupy alcohol obtained from fat.

glycogen (glī´-kə-jən): a form of starch made by the body from glucose and stored in the liver or muscle tissues.

goiter (gȯit´-ər): an enlargement of the thyroid gland caused by a lack of iodine.

good grade: the third-best grade of beef.

gourmet (gùr´-mā): a person who enjoys foods that are prepared with imagination; one who considers food preparation an art rather than a means of satisfying hunger.

gristle (gris´-əl): a smooth, shiny type of connective tissue on the ends of bones; also known as ''cartilage.''

hemoglobin (hē-mə-glō´-bən): the thick part of the blood; carries oxygen from the lungs to the tissues.

hemorrhagic (hem-ər-raj´-ik) **anemia** (ə-ne´-me-ə): a deficiency of hemoglobin caused by severe bleeding.

homogenized (hō-mäj´-ə-nizd) **milk:** milk that has been processed so that the fat is evenly distributed throughout.

hormone (hȯr´-mōn): a substance produced by an endocrine gland that regulates body processes; there are different hormones for different processes.

hors d'oeuvre (ȯr-derv´): a French-style appetizer or first course.

humus (hyü-məs): the portion of the soil that has developed from the decaying of plant or animal matter.

hydrogenation (hī-dräj-e-nā´-shən): the addition of hydrogen to an unsaturated fat (oil) to harden it; margarine is made from oil in this way.

g

h

hypervitaminosis (hī'-pər-vī'-tə-min-ō'-sis): a condition that results from excessive intake of certain vitamins, especially A or D vitamins.

hypothalamus (hī-pō-thəl'-ə-məs): the portion of the brain that is related to appetite control.

imitation milk: a milk substitute that contains water, vegetable oil, and either a milk protein or a soybean protein.

incomplete protein: a protein that is missing some of the essential amino acids.

insecticide (in-sek'-tə-sīd): an agent that destroys insects. *See also* pesticide.

insulin (in'-sə-lən): a hormone secreted by the pancreas that enables cells to oxidize glucose and release energy from food.

intrinsic factor: a substance in gastric juice that helps the body absorb vitamin B_{12}.

iron-deficiency anemia (ə-nē'-mē-ə): a shortage of hemoglobin caused by an unblanced diet or by loss of blood; also known as "nutritional anemia."

kwashiorkor (kwäsh-ē-ȯr'-kȯr): a disease that is related to a lack of protein in the diet; characterized by retention of fluids, change in skin color, and lack of growth.

lactase (lak'-tās): an enzyme that is present in the intestines of young mammals.

lactation (lak-tā'-shən): the secretion of milk.

lactose (lak'-tōs): a type of sugar contained in milk.

legume (leg'-yüm): a plant that takes nitrogen from the air and soil to form protein; Examples are dried beans, peas, lentils, and peanuts.

life expectancy: The number of years a person may expect to live, depending on health.

linoleic (lin-ə-lē'-ic) **acid:** a polyunsaturated fatty acid that is generally found in vegetable oil.

lipase (līp'-ās): an enzyme in the small intestine that participates in the digestion of fat.

lipid (lip'-īd): a chemist's term for fat.

macrocytic (mak'-rō-sit-ik) **anemia** (ə-nē'-mē-ə): a condition characterized by a shortage of red blood cells containing too little hemoglobin.

magnesium (mag-nē'-zē-əm): a mineral that is essential to life.

malnutrition: a deficient state of the body caused by a lack of nourishment.

marbling: thin streaks of fat through the lean muscle of meat.

marinate (mar'-ə-nāt): to soak meat or fish in liquid to make it more tender and flavorful.

meat extender: a product usually made from grains or legumes used in meat dishes—particularly with ground meat—to make them stretch to serve more people.

megablastic (meg'-ə-blas-tik) **anemia** (ə-nē'-mē-ə): see macrocytic anemia.

metabolism (mə-tab'-ə-liz-əm): the chemical changes that take place within the body—especially the building up and breaking down of the body cells.

milk solids: the total dry nutrients in milk.

mineral: type of nutrient necessary to bodily functions. Mineral elements in the body include calcium, phosphorus, sulfur, magnesium, iron, iodine, and zinc.

monocalcium phosphate: an ingredient in some baking powders.

monosaccharide: a sugar containing one simple sugar per molecule, e.g. glucose, fructose, galactose.

monosodium phosphate: an ingredient in some baking powders.

mono-unsaturated fats: fats, such as oleic acid in egg yolks, in which molecules have one double-bonded carbon.

myocardial (mi-ə-kärd'-ē-əl) **infarction** (in-fark'-shən): the death of tissues in the muscular layer of the heart due to an obstruction in a local blood vessel.

436

natural food: a food supposed to have been packaged or processed without additives.

noncrystalline (non'-kris-tə-len) **candy:** candy such as caramel or toffee in which the sugar has been prevented from forming crystals.

nucleus (nu'-klē-əs): a thick round structure in the center of a cell.

nutrients (nü'-trē-ənts): the chemical substances in food that are used by the body for growth, repair of tissues, and energy. They include carbohydrates, proteins, fats, minerals, and vitamins.

nutrition (nü-trish'-ən): the study of the process by which the body makes use of food.

nutritional needs: the requirements of the body for the chemical substances foods supply.

obesity (ō-bē'-sət-ē): a condition in which a person weighs at least 15 to 20 percent more than the recommended weight for her or his height and frame.

organic food: health food term for food grown using only animal or vegetable fertilizers, not commercial fertilizers or pesticides.

osteoporosis (äs'-tē-ō-pō-rō'-sis): a bone disease believed to result from loss of calcium: bones shrink and become porous, which frequently causes them to fracture.

overweight: a term describing people who weigh at least 10 percent more than the recommended weight for their height.

ovum (o'-vəm): the mammalian egg; if fertilized, it develops into an embryo in the uterus.

oxalic (äk-sal'-ik) **acid:** an acid contained in some leafy vegetables such as spinach, Swiss chard, beet tops, and rhubarb.

oxidation (äk'-sə-dā'-shən): a chemical process that is accompanied by the release of energy and heat.

pan broiling: cooking on top of the stove in a heavy skillet or on a griddle with little or no fat.

papillae (pə-pil-ē): small protuberances on the tongue in which are located the taste buds.

parathyroid (par-ə-thir'-ôid) **glands:** glands located in the neck that secrete a hormone that controls the level of calcium in the bloodstream.

pasteurization (pas'-chə-rə-zā'-shən): a means of destroying harmful bacterial by heating liquid for a specific time at a certain temperature.

pectin (pek-tən): A carbohydrate found especially in cooked fruits; used for jelly making; it combines with cholesterol, which is then eliminated with the pectin.

pellagra (pəl-lag'-rə): a disease caused by a deficiency of niacin; attacks the skin, the gastrointestinal tract, and the nervous system.

peristalsis (per-ə-stäl'-səs): wavelike contractions of the small intestines that move food bulk along the digestive tract, for purposes of digestion, absorption, and elimination.

pernicious (per-nish'-əs) **anemia** (ə-nē'-mē-ə): a disease in which the red blood cells increase in size, but become fewer in number.

pesticide: a chemical or ''natural'' agent used to kill small animals or insects that are harmful to plants or animals. *See also* insecticide.

phlebitis (flə-bīt'-əs): the inflammation of a vein—especially, of a vein in a limb—due to the presence of a blood clot.

phosphorus (fäs'-fə-rəs): an essential mineral contained in many foods; combines with calcium to build and repair bones and teeth.

photosynthesis (fōt'-ə-sin'-thə-səs): a process that occurs within green plants, in which the chlorophyll in the plant uses solar energy to create carbohydrates from carbon dioxide and water.

placenta (plə-sent′-ə): an organ consisting of spongy tissue and a network of blood vessels attached to the wall of the mother's uterus and connected to the baby by the umbilical cord; allows nutrients to pass from the mother to the unborn baby.

plaque (plak): a deposit of cholesterol and other fatty material in the connective tissue of blood vessel walls.

plasma (plaz′-mə): the fluid portion of the blood; contains antibodies, hormones, and digested foods.

polysaccharide: a sugar containing more than two simple sugars per molecule, e.g. starches and cellulose.

polyunsaturated fats: fats which have two or more double-carbon bonds in each molecule, such as linoleic acid, found in vegetable oil.

pot-au-feu (pät′-ō-fə): a thick French soup that traditionally contains many types of foods.

predator: an organism that kills other organisms for food.

premature baby: a baby that is born before the completion of the nine-month gestation period; the bodies of premature babies are usually underdeveloped in one or more ways.

pressure canning: a method of processing nonacid vegetables and meat products.

prime grade: the highest grade of beef; most often available only in restaurants.

processed meat: meat that is preserved by canning, freezing, freeze-drying, drying, or pickling.

progesterone: hormone that prepares the reproductive organs for gestation.

protein (prō′-tēn): the largest and most complex molecule found in food; consists of a group of amino acids.

protopectin (prō′-tə-pek-tən): a substance found in fruits that tends to cement the structure of the fruit cells; can interfere with the body's absorption of the nutrients in a fruit.

ptyalin (tī′-ə-lən): an enzyme in the salivary juice that splits up simple sugars and breaks starch into smaller molecules.

puréeing: putting cooked food through a blender, food mill, or sieve to form a smooth product.

putrefaction (pü-trə-fak′-shən): the decay of organic material especially the decay caused by putrefactive bacteria.

pyridoxine (pir-ə-däk′-sēn): one of the B vitamins; known as vitamin B_6.

pyruvic (pi-rū′-vik) **acid:** an acid that accumulates in the blood and tissues when the body has a shortage of thiamin.

quick bread: any bread product leavened with a quick-acting leavening agent.

raw milk: milk that has not been pasteurized.

restored: a term that indicates that nutrients lost in processing are restored to the refined, ready-to-eat grain product.

retina (ret′-nə): the part of the eye that receives the image formed by the lens.

riboflavin (rī′-bə-flā′-vən): a B vitamin, first discovered in milk, that is necessary for normal growth and for healthy skin and hair.

rickets (rik′-əts): a disease caused by a deficiency of vitamin D in which the bones grow soft and may possibly be deformed.

ripened meat: meat that has hung in a refrigerated warehouse long enough for the enzymes to act on the lean and connective tissues, making the meat more tender, more juicy, and more delicate in flavor.

saccharin: an artificial sugar substitute.

salmonella (sal-mə-nel′-ə): a group of bacteria responsible for a common type of food poisoning.

salt-rising bread: a form of leavened bread in which salt is added to the yeast to prevent the formation of bacteria.

SAS: *see* sodium aluminum sulfate.

saturated fats: fats in which within each molecule every carbon atom is linked to an atom of hydrogen; found in beef fat and butter for example.

sautéeing: cooking food in a skillet or saucepan with a small amount of fat until just tender.

scalding: heating a liquid to just under the boiling point.

scalloping: baking food in layers with a sauce.

scurvy: a disease caused by lack of vitamin C, or ascorbic acid; characterized by anemia, joint pain, swollen and bleeding gums.

self-rising flour: soft-wheat or all-purpose flour with salt and leavening ingredients (such as baking powder or baking soda) added to it.

shortening: the fat used to make a flour mixture tender.

sieving: pressing food through a strainer.

simmering: cooking a liquid or food in a liquid at a temperature just below the boiling point.

sodium aluminum sulfate (SAS): an ingredient in some baking powders that leavens by forming carbon dioxide in the presence of heat.

sodium cyclamate (sī′-klə-māt): a sugar substitute removed from the market after tests indicated that it might cause cancer.

soil depletion: the removal of nutrients from farmland.

sourdough: fermented yeast dough used as leavening.

stamina (stam-ə-nə): endurance; ability to remain active over extended time periods.

standard grade: the lowest grade of beef; usually sold to processors and used for purposes other than human consumption.

standard of identity: a term indicating that the ingredients of a food meet FDA standard; products covered by standards of identity do not have to list their ingredients.

staphylococcus (staf′-ə-lō-käk′-əs): a group of spherical bacteria that form a toxin that causes food poisoning.

stroke: the rupture or obstruction of an artery in the brain; a blood clot that occurs in the brain.

strontium (strän′-chəm) **90:** a radioactive byproduct of atomic explosions that may cause bone cancer or leukemia in the human body.

sulfuring (səl′-fər-ing): a method of retaining color and protecting vitamin C in light-colored fruits.

tartrate (tär′-trāt): a substance that contains the leavening agent tartaric acid.

tenderizing: making meat more tender by soaking in brine, by injecting enzymes or other curing agents into the meat, by breaking the fibers, or by cooking.

thiamin (thī′-ə-mən): a B vitamin that helps the body burn glucose and is necessary for the utilization of protein.

thyroid (thīr′-ôid): a gland in the throat that secretes a hormone that affects growth, physical development, and the rate of metabolism.

thyroxin (thī-räk′-sən): a hormone secreted by the thyroid gland that regulates the cells' use of energy.

toxemia: condition that may develop during pregnancy; results from kidney malfunction; symptoms include high blood pressure and weight gain from fluid retention.

traditional food: a food served over many years for a particular religious, ethnic, or geographical reason.

tryptophane (trip′-tə-fān): an essential amino acid; it also can be used by the body to manufacture the B vitamin, niacin.

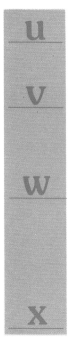

umbilical (əm·bil′·i·kəl) **cord:** the tissue that connects the unborn baby to the placenta. The umbilical cord is cut at the time of birth.

unit price: the cost of a product in relation to a unit of measure—for example, the cost per kilogram or pound.

unleavened bread: bread made without the leavening agents to make it rise.

vegetarians: people whose diets consist primarily of plant foods (vegetables, fruits, grains, nuts): they eat no meat, and sometimes, no animal products (milk, eggs).

villi (vil′ī): tiny folds of fingerlike tissue that line the intestine wall.

vitamin (vī′·tə·minz): nutrients essential for many body processes.

volatile acid: an acid present in canned foods. While a volatile acid affects the color of some foods, it does not affect their taste or nutritive value.

weaning: helping a child to become accustomed to solid foods and taking liquids from a cup, instead of mother's milk or a bottle.

whey (hwā): the watery portion of milk that is separated from the curd in the making of cheese.

whole milk: milk that contains all the nutrients of natural milk.

womb (wüm): the uterus; the organ in which the human embryo is carried and nourished.

work centers: places in the kitchen that can be used efficiently in the preparation of a meal.

xerophthalmia (zer·of·thal′·mē·ə): a disease characterized by lack of moisture in the eye; caused by a deficiency of vitamin A.

Index

Department of Agriculture **56:** U.S. Department of Agriculture **59:** J. Gerard Smith **60-61:** J. Gerard Smith **62:** Owen Franken, Stock/Boston **65:** William Hubbell, Woodfin Camp & Associates **71** *top left:* Kellogg Co. **71** *top right:* American Dairy Association **71** *bottom left:* Photo Media **71** *bottom right:* General Foods **76-77:** Dudley-Anderson-Yutzy **78:** Sheila R. Turner, Monkmeyer Press **79:** DPI **80** *both:* Paul Conklin, Monkmeyer Press **82:** Elinor S. Beckwith **84** *top:* Al Rubin, Stock/Boston **84** *bottom:* J. Albertson, Stock/Boston **85:** Upjohn Co. **86:** Paul Conklin, Monkmeyer Press **89:** United Fresh Fruit and Vegetable Association **91:** DPI **94-95:** Lewis & Neale **96:** DPI **97:** Owen Franken, Stock/Boston **99:** Dole **102:** Mimi Forsyth, Monkmeyer Press **103:** Paul Conklin, Monkmeyer Press **104:** United Dairy Industry Association **105:** Shostal Associates **106** *left:* Green Giant Company **106** *right:* Paul Conklin, Monkmeyer Press **108:** Elinor S. Beckwith **110:** Green Giant Company **111** *top:* Maria B. Wooden Associates **111** *bottom:* Shostal Associates **116-117:** J. Gerard Smith **118:** Cary Wolinsky, Stock/Boston **119:** Paul Conklin, Monkmeyer Press **124:** Monkmeyer Press **130-131:** Lewis & Neale **132-133** *all:* U.S. Department of Agriculture **134:** Elinor S. Beckwith **135:** Elinor S. Beckwith **136:** Paul Conklin, Monkmeyer Press **138** *both:* United Dairy Industry Association **139:** United Dairy Industry Association **141** *top left:* American Dairy Association **141** *top right:* Thomas J. Lipton Co. **141** *bottom:* United Dairy Industry Association **144-145:** J. Gerard Smith **146:** National Live Stock and Meat Board **147** *top:* Thomas J. Lipton Co. **147** *bottom:* Cary Wolinsky, Stock/Boston **148:** Oscar Mayer & Co. **149:** National Medical Audiovisual Center **152:** National Live Stock and Meat Board **153** *top:* Alfred Owezarzak, Taurus **153** *bottom:* Rotker **154:** J. Alex Langley, DPI, **156:** National Live Stock and Meat Board **157:** National Medical Audiovisual Center **160-161:** Lewis & Neale **164** *left:* National Live Stock and Meat Board **164** *right:* U.S. Department of Agriculture **169** *top left:* Hugh Rogers, Monkmeyer Press **169** *center left:* Pet Incorporated **169** *bottom left:* Thomas J. Lipton Co. **169** *top and bottom right:* National Oceanic and Atmospheric Administration **170:** U.S. Department of Agriculture **171** *left:* DPI **171** *right:* National Oceanic and Atmospheric Administration **175** *top:* Thomas J. Lipton Co. **175** *bottom:* National Live Stock and Meat Board **177:** Lewis & Neale, American Spice Trade Association **180:** Ivor Parry, DPI **181** *top:* Owen Franken, Stock/Boston **181** *bottom:* Paul Conklin, Monkmeyer Press **183:** Tony Howarth, Woodfin Camp & Associates **186-187:** Shostal Associates **188** *left:* Jay Lyons, DPI **188** *top and bot-*

tom right: Bill Gillette, Stock/Boston **189** *all:* Shostal Associates **190** *left:* Shostal Associates **190** *top right:* Bill Bridge, DPI **190** *bottom right:* John Running, Stock/Boston **191:** Photo Media **192:** John Running, Stock/Boston **193:** Paul Conklin, Monkmeyer Press **194** *top:* Seafood Marketing Authority **195:** J. Gerard Smith **199:** Elinor S. Beckwith **202-203:** Lewis & Neale **204:** Paul Conklin, Monkmeyer Press **205:** Durum Wheat Institute **206** *left:* Armour Food Co. **206:** *right:* Photo Media **207** *both:* Paul Conklin, Monkmeyer Press **208:** Elinor S. Beckwith **210:** American Dairy Association **211:** DPI **212** *top:* Durum Wheat Institute **212** *bottom:* Paul Conklin, Monkmeyer Press **213** *top:* Oscar Mayer & Co. **213** *bottom:* Pepperidge Farm **216-217:** J. Gerard Smith **218:** Owen Franken, Stock/Boston **219** *top:* Owen Franken, Stock/Boston **219** *bottom:* Photo Media **220** *top left:* U.S. Department of Agriculture **220** *top right:* Mike Mazzaschi, Stock/Boston **220** *bottom:* O. Christian Irgens **221:** Paul Conklin, Monkmeyer Press **222:** United Fresh Fruit & Vegetable Association (Dudley-Anderson-Yutzy) **225** *top:* Shostal Associates **225** *bottom left and right:* Elinor S. Beckwith **228-229:** J. Gerard Smith **231** *both:* Elinor S. Beckwith **232:** Creamer Dickson Basford **235:** Raoul Hackel, Stock/Boston **237:** Lewis & Neale, Lea & Perrins **239:** Ellis Herwig, Stock/Boston **240** *top:* National Marine Fisheries Service **240** *bottom:* John Hardy, DPI **245:** J. Gerard Smith **246-247:** J. Gerard Smith **248:** DPI **249** *top:* Chris Reeberg, DPI **249** *bottom:* American Heart Association **251** *both:* Paul Conklin, Monkmeyer Press **252** *top:* DPI **252** *bottom:* Cary Wolinsky, Stock/Boston **253** *both:* National Live Stock and Meat Board **255** *top:* U.S. Department of Agriculture **255** *bottom:* Wheat Flour Institute **257:** National Live Stock and Meat Board **260** Photo Media **261** *all:* Mirro Aluminum Company **264-265:** American Dairy Association **266:** Rhoda Sidney, Monkmeyer Press **267** *left:* Paniska, DPI **267** *right:* Paul Conklin, Monkmeyer Press **269** *top:* J. Paul Kirouac, Monkmeyer Press **269** *bottom:* Shostal Associates **272:** Maria B. Wooden Associates **275:** Shostal Associates **276:** Wayne Miller, Magnum Photos **280-281:** J. Gerard Smith **282:** Leonard Freed, Magnum Photos **282** *all:* American Heart Association **284** *top:* Raoul Hackel, Stock/Boston **284** *bottom:* Rhoda Sidney, Monkmeyer Press **286** *top:* Sam Falk, Monkmeyer Press **286** *bottom:* Hugh Rogers, Monkmeyer Press **288:** DPI **289** *top:* Hal McCusick, DPI **289** *bottom:* Elinor S. Beckwith, DPI **290** *top:* John Marmaras, Woodfin Camp & Associates **290** *bottom:* U.S. Department of Agriculture **291:** Mimi Forsyth, Monkmeyer Press **294-295:** Lewis & Neale **296:**

Elinor S. Beckwith, DPI **297:** DPI **298** *top:* Lou Niznik, DPI **298** *bottom:* Irene Bayer, Monkmeyer Press **299** *top:* Rick Smolan, Leo de Wys **299** *bottom left:* Elinor S. Beckwith, DPI **299** *bottom right:* Marvin Newman, Woodfin Camp & Associates **300:** Lewis & Neale, Lea & Perrins **301** *left:* Photo Media **301** *right:* Monkmeyer Press **304-305:** Lewis & Neale **306** *left:* DPI **306** *right:* Anthony Howarth, Woodfin Camp & Associates **307:** Doug Schild Studio, DPI **308:** DPI **309:** Photo Media **310:** Newman Saylor & Gregory **311** *both:* DPI **312** *top:* Bannett, DPI **312** *bottom:* American Dairy Association **313:** Rhoda Sidney, Monkmeyer Press **314** *top left:* Bernard Wolf, DPI **314** *bottom left:* Murray Greenberg, Monkmeyer Press **314** *right:* Werner Stoy, DPI **317:** J. Gerard Smith **318-319:** J. Gerard Smith **320** *both:* Paul Conklin, Monkmeyer Press **322:** Paul Conklin, Monkmeyer Press **323:** Eric Simmons, Stock/Boston **324** *top:* Paul Conklin, Monkmeyer Press **324** *bottom:* Elinor S. Beckwith **327:** Paul Conklin, Monkmeyer Press **329:** Tana Hoban, DPI **332-333:** J. Gerard Smith **334:** S. Faludi, DPI **335:** Wil Blanch, DPI **336** *left:* Leo de Wys **336** *right:* Photo Media **338** *top:* DPI **338** *bottom:* Paul Conklin, Monkmeyer Press **339:** Paul Conklin, Monkmeyer Press **340** *top:* Bob Witt, DPI **341** *top:* William Hubbell, Woodfin Camp & Associates **341** *bottom:* U.S. Department of Agriculture **342:** U.S. Department of Agriculture **350:** DPI **351** *top left:* American Spice Trade Association **351** *top right:* Reynolds Metals **351** *bottom:* McIlhenny Co. **352** *left:* California Strawberry Advisory Board **352** *top right:* Florida Citrus Commission **352** *bottom right:* United Fresh Fruit & Vegetable Association **355:** Elinor S. Beckwith **356** *top:* Knox Gelatine **356** *bottom:* Rice Council **359:** Elinor S. Beckwith **360** *top:* American Dairy Association **360** *bottom:* Processed Apples Institute **363:** Land O' Lakes **367** *top:* National Macaroni Institute **367** *bottom right:* United Fresh Fruit and Vegetable Association **370** *top left:* Reynolds Metals **370** *top right:* Processed Apples Institute **370** *bottom:* American Spice Trade Association **371:** Thomas J. Lipton Co. **373:** Reynolds Metals **375:** U.S. Department of Agriculture **376:** Reynolds Metals **378:** Elinor S. Beckwith **379:** Universal Oil Products Co. **383:** Elinor S. Beckwith **385:** Pepperidge Farm **386** *top:* Diamond Walnuts **386** *bottom:* National Macaroni Institute **388-389:** Elinor S. Beckwith **392-393** *top left:* Kohn & Hass Co. **392-393** *top center:* Del Monte **392-393** *top right:* Anderson Clayton Co. **392-393** *bottom left:* Reynolds Metals **392-393** *bottom right:* CPC International **397:** Elinor S. Beckwith **398:** Elinor S. Beckwith **399:** Elinor S. Beckwith **Back cover:** J. Gerard Smith